POSITIVE MENTAL HEALTH, FIGHTING STIGMA AND PROMOTING RESILIENCY FOR CHILDREN AND ADOLESCENTS

POSITIVE MENTAL HEALTH, FIGHTING STIGMA AND PROMOTING RESILIENCY FOR CHILDREN AND ADOLESCENTS

Edited by

MATTHEW HODES

SUSAN GAU

AMSTERDAM • BOSTON • HEIDELBERG • LONDON
NEW YORK • OXFORD • PARIS • SAN DIEGO
SAN FRANCISCO • SINGAPORE • SYDNEY • TOKYO

Academic Press is an imprint of Elsevier

Academic Press is an imprint of Elsevier
125 London Wall, London EC2Y 5AS, UK
525 B Street, Suite 1800, San Diego, CA 92101-4495, USA
50 Hampshire Street, 5th Floor, Cambridge, MA 02139, USA
The Boulevard, Langford Lane, Kidlington, Oxford OX5 1GB, UK

British Library Cataloguing-in-Publication Data
A catalogue record for this book is available from the British Library

Library of Congress Cataloging-in-Publication Data
A catalog record for this book is available from the Library of Congress

ISBN: 978-0-12-804394-3

For information on all Academic Press publications
visit our website at https://www.elsevier.com/

Working together
to grow libraries in
developing countries

www.elsevier.com • www.bookaid.org

Publisher: Nikki Levy
Acquisition Editor: Emily Ekle
Editorial Project Manager: Timothy Bennett
Production Project Manager: Nicky Carter
Designer: Matthew Limbert

Typeset by TNQ Books and Journals

Contents

I

CONCEPTUAL APPROACHES

1. Positive Mental Health—What Is It, How Is It Recognized, and Can It Be Achieved?

B. FALISSARD

2. ICD-11—Comparison With DSM-5 and Implications for Child & Adolescent Psychiatric Disorders

M.E. GARRALDA

II

RISK AND RESILIENCE

3. Disorders of Brain Development: Understanding Childhood Psychopathology

F.P. MACMASTER, M. SEMBO, L.M. LANGEVIN, K. MA AND P. CROARKIN

4. Genetic Process in Resilience and Vulnerability and the Consequence of Abuse

M. PESKIN AND G. ZALSMAN

5. Resilience and Developmental Health in Autism Spectrum Disorder

P. SZATMARI, L. ZWAIGENBAUM, S. GEORGIADES, M. ELSABBAGH, C. WADDELL,
T. BENNETT, S. BRYSON, E. DUKU, E. FOMBONNE, P. MIRENDA, W. ROBERTS, I. SMITH,
T. VAILLANCOURT AND J. VOLDEN

6. Mental Health Promotion for Indigenous Youth

L.J. KIRMAYER, E. SHEINER AND D. GEOFFROY

7. Psychological Consequences of Parental Migration for Left-Behind Children

Y. ZHENG

III

INTERVENTIONS AND TREATMENTS

8. Mental Health Literacy for Students and Teachers: A "School Friendly" Approach

S. KUTCHER, Y. WEI AND M. HASHISH

9. Transforming Cultures for the Mental Health Care of Young People: The Service Reform Imperative

P. MCGORRY AND S. GOLDSTONE

10. Evidence-Based Parenting Interventions: Current Perspectives and Clinical Strategies

D.J. HAWES AND J. ALLEN

11. Psychopharmacological Treatment for Depression in Children and Adolescents: Promoting Recovery and Resilience

M.R. CHAPMAN, J.L. HUGHES, B.D. KENNARD, T.L. MAYES AND G.J. EMSLIE

12. Treatment of Eating Disorders in Children and Adolescents

J. DERENNE AND J. LOCK

13. Seclusion in the Management of Highly Disturbed Children and Adolescents

M. YURTBASI, G.A. MELVIN AND M.S. GORDON

Contributors

J. Allen   University College London, London, United Kingdom

T. Bennett   McMaster University, Hamilton, ON, Canada

S. Bryson   Dalhousie University, Halifax, NS, Canada

M.R. Chapman   UT Southwestern Medical Center, Dallas, TX, United States

P. Croarkin   Mayo Clinic College of Medicine, Rochester, MN, United States

J. Derenne   Stanford University School of Medicine, Stanford, CA, United States

E. Duku   McMaster University, Hamilton, ON, Canada

M. Elsabbagh   McGill University, Montreal, QC, Canada

G.J. Emslie   UT Southwestern Medical Center, Dallas, TX, United States

B. Falissard   University of Paris-Sud, Paris, France

E. Fombonne   Oregon Health & Science University (OHSU), Portland, OR, United States

M.E. Garralda   Imperial College London, London, United Kingdom

D. Geoffroy   Jewish General Hospital, Montreal, QC, Canada

S. Georgiades   McMaster University, Hamilton, ON, Canada

S. Goldstone   Orygen, The National Centre of Excellence in Youth Mental Health, Parkville, VIC, Australia

M.S. Gordon   Monash University, Notting Hill, VIC, Australia; Monash Health, Monash Medical Centre, Clayton, VIC, Australia

M. Hashish   Dalhousie University and IWK Health Centre, Halifax, NS, Canada

D.J. Hawes   The University of Sydney, NSW, Australia

J.L. Hughes   UT Southwestern Medical Center, Dallas, TX, United States

B.D. Kennard   UT Southwestern Medical Center, Dallas, TX, United States

L.J. Kirmayer   McGill University, Montreal, QC, Canada; Jewish General Hospital, Montreal, QC, Canada

S. Kutcher   Dalhousie University and IWK Health Centre, Halifax, NS, Canada

L.M. Langevin   University of Calgary, Calgary, AB, Canada

J. Lock   Stanford University School of Medicine, Stanford, CA, United States

F.P. MacMaster   University of Calgary, Calgary, AB, Canada

K. Ma   University of Calgary, Calgary, AB, Canada

T.L. Mayes   UT Southwestern Medical Center, Dallas, TX, United States

P. McGorry   Orygen, The National Centre of Excellence in Youth Mental Health, Parkville, VIC, Australia

G.A. Melvin   Monash University, Notting Hill, VIC, Australia

P. Mirenda   University of British Columbia, Vancouver, BC, Canada

M. Peskin   Tel Aviv University, Tel Aviv, Israel

W. Roberts   University of Toronto, Toronto, ON, Canada

M. Sembo   University of Calgary, Calgary, AB, Canada

E. Sheiner   Jewish General Hospital, Montreal, QC, Canada

I. Smith   Dalhousie University, Halifax, NS, Canada

P. Szatmari   University of Toronto, Toronto, ON, Canada

T. Vaillancourt   University of Ottawa, Ottawa, ON, Canada

J. Volden   University of Alberta, Edmonton, AB, Canada

C. Waddell   Simon Fraser University, Vancouver, BC, Canada

Y. Wei   Dalhousie University and IWK Health Centre, Halifax, NS, Canada

M. Yurtbasi   Monash University, Notting Hill, VIC, Australia

G. Zalsman   Tel Aviv University, Tel Aviv, Israel; Columbia University, New York, NY, United States

Y. Zheng   Beijing Anding Hospital, Capital Medical University, Beijing, P.R. China; The Chinese Society of Child and Adolescent Psychiatry; The International Association for Child and Adolescent Psychiatry and Allied Professions (IACAPAP)

L. Zwaigenbaum   University of Alberta, Edmonton, AB, Canada

Introduction

M. Hodes[1,2], S. Shur-Fen Gau[3,4]

[1]Imperial College London, London, United Kingdom; [2]Central and North West London NHS Foundation Trust, London, United Kingdom; [3]National Taiwan University Hospital (NTUH) and College of Medicine, Taipei, Taiwan; [4]National Taiwan University, Taipei, Taiwan

INTRODUCTION

The International Association for Child and Adolescent Psychiatry and Allied Professions (IACAPAP) aims to promote the mental health and development of children and adolescents worldwide. It seeks to achieve this by contributing to the training and professional development of the child and adolescent mental health professionals by disseminating up-to-date and high-quality information through its publications, organization of biennial international congresses, and study groups. IACAPAP has a long tradition of publishing monographs released to coincide with the congresses, with the first one published in 1970. We are pleased to introduce this monograph prepared for the IACAPAP congress to be held in Calgary, Alberta, Canada in September 2016.

Innovations in IACAPAP's dissemination strategy, most dramatically a move to greater access of materials through the organization's website (http://iacapap.org/) including the freely available ebook, the IACAPAP Textbook of Child and Adolescent Mental Health has prompted a rethink regarding the place of the monographs. Traditionally the monographs had followed the themes of the numerous congresses, and their contents provided summaries of disorders and treatments in the child and adolescent mental health field. With the growth of the website and textbook, the monograph has been focused to address congress themes, regional or social issues, new topics, and selective reviews in child and adolescent mental health treatments and other innovations. By way of illustration, the 2014 monograph was released to coincide with the first IACAPAP congress to take place in Africa (in Durban) and so provided significant coverage of child and adolescent mental health in low- and middle-income countries (Raynaud, Hodes, & Gau, 2014). This monograph addresses the themes of the 2016 Calgary Congress entitled "Fighting Stigma, Promoting Resiliency and Positive Mental Health," as well as including evidence-based reviews of selective treatment areas.

A further change for the monograph, in keeping with IACAPAP's move to more Internet-based open access to materials, is that for the first time it will become available online, one year after the congress, accessed via the IACAPAP website. We are delighted that Elsevier, the new publisher of the monographs, supports this free access, and so will contribute to IACAPAP's mission to disseminate high-quality information as widely as possible.

CONCEPTUAL ISSUES

The book begins with some conceptual issues. Falissard provides a nuanced historical and cultural perspective on positive mental health and in so doing problematizes the concept itself. For him, doctors including psychiatrists have become so fascinated by diseases and disorders that they have lost the "person," and so this gap has been filled by notions of happiness and well-being. However these ideas themselves are problematic as there is no accepted definition of happiness and positive health, and Falissard aptly reminds us of the WHO statement that "From a cross-cultural perspective, it is nearly impossible to define mental health comprehensively. It is, however, generally agreed that mental health is broader than a lack of mental disorders" (WHO, 2001).

The situation is also complicated by the continually changing classificatory systems for psychiatric disorders, which does not help the conceptual confusion. When the major classificatory systems, the World Health Organization's International Classification of Diseases (ICD) and the USA's Diagnostic and Statistical Manual (DSM) of psychiatric disorders are revised, there is a great increase in preparatory work and publications addressing the conceptual and empirical basis for the changes. We are at such a juncture now, as DSM-5 was published in 2013 (American Psychiatric Association, 2013), and we are expecting the next revision of the WHO system (ICD-11) to be released in 2016 or 2017. Garralda writes lucidly about the classificatory systems for child and adolescent psychiatric disorders, beginning by summarizing the history and principles of psychiatric classification. She then describes the main changes that have taken place in relation to some of the most important disorders with childhood onset in DSM-5 and the expected changes in ICD-11. The focus is on autism spectrum disorders, dissocial and conduct disorders, and the new DSM-5 category disruptive mood dysregulation disorder. The chapter considers some issues for the future of psychiatric classification, most importantly whether it will be replaced by systems that are based on the neurobiological basis of psychopathology. The concluding section describes a number of clinically relevant issues such as the lack of knowledge about child and adolescent psychiatric disorders among the general population and in primary care, use of categorical and continuous systems of classification, and stigma and labeling.

RISK AND RESILIENCE

The second section begins with a comprehensive summary of the brain mechanisms as revealed by neuroimaging that underlies most of the child and adolescent psychiatric disorders associated with high impairment and distress seen in clinical services. McMaster and colleagues describe the salient features of brain imaging, and then for each of the disorders describe the associated anatomical basis and neurochemical abnormalities. It is illuminating to consider the way the functional imaging studies illustrate the mechanisms of action of psychopharmacological treatments, and it is hoped that such understanding will facilitate the discovery and refinement of new treatments in the future. The chapter is relevant to the theme of stigma as it is hoped that understanding the biological basis of the disorders will help challenge blame and negative attributions often associated with them.

Genetic influences on risk vulnerability and resilience, in the context of child maltreatment, are addressed by Zalsman and Peskin. While abuse will adversely affect all exposed children, only some will develop psychopathology and it is now becoming clearer what are some of the genetic increasing this vulnerability. The authors explain the potential role of polymorphisms in the promoter region of the monoamine oxidase A gene, corticotropin-releasing hormone type 1 receptor gene that influences the hypothalamic-pituitary-adrenal axis, and the serotonin transporter promoter gene, and others. The authors describe how genes may involve different mechanisms including those affecting brain structural integrity.

The concept of resilience has been applied to autism spectrum disorder (ASD) in a very original chapter by Szatmari and colleagues. While there is emerging and strengthening evidence for the neurobiological abnormalities associated with ASD, as outlined by McMaster et al., for Szatmari and colleagues this is an adversity against which the concept of resilience can be considered.

Their well-informed chapter outlines the meanings of good outcomes for young people with ASD and demonstrates considerable heterogeneity of outcomes, and the various reasons for this.

Adversities of very different kinds have been experienced by indigenous people in many countries. Kirmayer and colleagues summarize the appalling histories of coercion, forced community displacement, and often separation of children from families in many indigenous communities including those in Canada. The resulting socioeconomic hardships, intergenerational trauma, and disrupted parent child–relationships has been associated with high levels of psychopathology and suicide. To try to reverse these processes, programs are described that promote resilience, and require a holistic perspective and the re-embedding of individuals in their social and natural environments. In this way, the indigenous people can experience a more integrated sense of self. For these authors the notion of positive health is useful as it refers to this more sociocentric, rather than individualistic notion of well-being.

The impact of rather different socioeconomic processes are explored in the chapter by Zheng describing the plight of "left-behind" children. These are young people who have one or both parents who migrate for work opportunities and financial reasons. Globally, millions of children are cared for by single parents or grandparents, with variable but sometimes only occasional contact over years with the parent(s) who has departed. This is a phenomenon that has occurred in China among other countries, in the context of rapid industrialization and urbanization. Often there are adverse psychological consequences for the children, and Zheng describes the range of difficulties, such as problems with lower mood and greater anxiety and antisocial behavior, social isolation, and lower scholastic attainment. The studies reviewed suggest that there are a number of risk factors, and that resilience may be increased by maintaining parent–child communication.

INTERVENTIONS AND TREATMENTS

In thinking about mental health service provision, a perennial issue is how are child and adolescent disorders, distress, and impairment recognized, and then what are the optimal referral pathways for timely service access. Kutcher and colleagues propose that a school-based perspective can achieve the important task of improving the mental health literacy of pupils and teachers, and this will be crucial in promoting mental health including facilitating service access. They have developed and evaluated a program embedded in the school system that seeks to improve knowledge of mental health problems, reduce stigma, and facilitate appropriate access to specialist mental health services. They provide data that suggests their program is effective.

McGorry and Goldstone agree with Kutcher and colleagues that young people's knowledge and awareness of mental health problems are important, but in addition they argue traditional mental health services create barriers to appropriate access and engagement. They go on to make the case for youth-focused mental health services embedded in a primary care model with links to other community service settings that offer a biopsychosocial approach. The services offer easy access in non-stigmatizing settings. The services they describe following this model demonstrate young people with undifferentiated symptoms and distress who may not have clearly diagnosable or severe psychiatric disorders, but the services are supported by links to more specialist services for those who need them. Their data suggests high uptake of the services, and benefit associated with contact, usually after only a small number of sessions.

The first of four chapters that address treatments is by Hawes & Allen who provide a summary of the mechanisms and evidence for the efficacy of the best established parenting programs. The authors skillfully summarize the steps required for engagement and treatment planning, then go on to describe the evidence for the efficacy of some of the main parenting programs focusing especially on conduct problems in younger children. Interestingly parenting programs have not been shown to be effective for childhood internalizing problems in addition to cognitive behavioral therapy (CBT), and reasons for this are discussed.

Many child and adolescent psychiatric disorders require knowledge of the role of psychological treatment as well as psychopharmacological treatments for effective management. Chapman and colleagues provide a very informative chapter in the fast moving field of the treatment of depression, focusing on drug treatments, addressing their benefits, and providing practical information about their use. They also address themes of prevention and promotion of resilience in maintaining good health. A further example of the need to think broadly is provided in the comprehensive overview of the treatment of child and adolescent eating disorders by Derenne and Lock. They describe the need to consider eating and weight stabilization, a range of psychological treatments, and sometimes intensive treatments in residential settings or day programs.

The most distressed, impaired, and uncontained children and adolescents need management in secure settings. This is a subject that has been sensitively discussed by Yurtbasi and colleagues. They discuss psychiatric ward and contextual factors associated with seclusion, and suggest appropriate practice. They also consider seclusion in non-clinical settings, in schools. The authors are at pains to point out that there is limited evidence on this topic and the problems in carrying out good studies. While seclusion is best avoided, and has ethical implications, the practice is still needed in many settings to promote recovery and improved mental health and functioning.

We would like to thank all the authors for contributing such rich and well-researched chapters for this volume. We hope that it will be a fitting complement to the 2016 IACAPAP congress as well as a book that stands alone as a coherent volume.

References

American Psychiatric Association. (2013). *Diagnostic and statistical manual of mental disorders* (5th ed.). Washington, DC: American Psychiatric Association.

Raynaud, J.-P., Hodes, M., & Gau, S. S.-F. (2014). *From research to practice in child and adolescent mental health*. Lanham, MD: Rowman & Littlefield.

WHO. (2001). *The world health report 2001 – Mental health: New understanding, new hope*. Geneva: World Health Organisation.

PART I

CONCEPTUAL APPROACHES

Positive Mental Health—What Is It, How Is It Recognized, and Can It Be Achieved?

B. Falissard

University of Paris-Sud, Paris, France

INTRODUCTION

Since its birth, psychiatry has struggled against a conceptual blur that has, with time, contributed to forming its inmost identity. What are mental disorders? Do they "really" exist? Is there any kind of normality in the functioning of the mind? What is mental health? Is it different from psychiatry? And so forth. All of these questions are regularly debated in the media, from specialized literature to the mainstream press.

Recently, a new concept has emerged, that of positive mental health. It is perhaps more than just an item added to a long list. Indeed, from its very beginnings, psychiatry has dealt with mental distress. The notion of positive mental health seems to have upset the paradigm: the implicit objective is now to make people happy, rather than solely dealing with their distress. This difference is more than symbolic, and this is what we are going to discuss in the present chapter.

WE ALL WANT OUR YOUNG PEOPLE TO BE HAPPY

At first sight, positive mental health and its implicit positioning toward a search for happiness seems to sum up the very nature of the aims of mental health professionals: we want children and teenagers to be well and happy with their lives. And because young people are so important in society, because they are the future, and because they are cherished, it is natural for everybody to want the best for children and adolescents.

Positive Mental Health, Fighting Stigma and Promoting Resiliency for Children and Adolescents
http://dx.doi.org/10.1016/B978-0-12-804394-3.00001-2

In fact, things are not so simple, and this is one important aspect of clinical practice. The feelings we have for our patients and the feelings parents and caregivers have about their young people is extraordinarily complex and ambivalent. In the depths of our emotional lives, it is not always easy to disentangle positive and negative emotions and intentions. It can be recalled that this was discussed in the excellent paper by Daniel Winnicott, "Hate in the Counter-Transference" (Winnicott, 1994). Even mothers have many reasons to hate their babies:

> "The baby is an interference with her private life, a challenge to preoccupation. […] He is ruthless, treats her as scum, an unpaid servant, a slave. She has to love him, excretions and all, […] His excited love is cupboard love, so that having got what he wants he throws her away like orange peel. […] At first he does not know at all what she does or what she sacrifices for him. Especially he cannot allow for her hate. […] He is suspicious, refuses her good food, and makes her doubt herself, but eats well with his aunt. After an awful morning with him she goes out, and he smiles at a stranger who says: "Isn't he sweet!" […] He excites her but frustrates - she mustn't eat him or trade in sex with him."

There are even sociological reasons to hate babies and children. One day they will become adults with power, and when that time comes, we will be old—and at their mercy.

But let us temporarily forget these unwelcome preliminaries and concentrate on the general consensus: we all want happiness for our youngsters.

THE QUESTION OF HAPPINESS

But what does "happiness" mean, after all? Surprisingly, this common and fascinating word raises numerous problems. Philosophy has tried to address most of them over two millennia, and some answers have been proposed (Haybron, 2011). They consist less in definitive solutions than in a number of interesting views, among which are a certain number of theories of happiness. Three appear to be most influential.

The first is hedonism. According to hedonism, happiness comes from the predominance of pleasant experiences over unpleasant ones.

The second theory is subtly but importantly different. It is the emotional state perspective. According to this theory, happiness is related to our emotional state, and there can be a gap between feeling pleasure and being in a positive mood. For instance, an anxious person who eats a tasty cake to deal with his/her anxiety will obviously experience some pleasure. But it is possible that this person, at the same time, will not experience happiness because of his/her ever-present anxiety and, perhaps, because of added guilt. Negative emotions can emerge from pleasure.

The third theory relates to life satisfaction, and here we clearly have another perspective. Life satisfaction is a personal, introspective, and global judgment about what a human being considers he/she is and has done with his/her life. And this may or may not be related to pleasure or experiencing positive emotions. A classic example is the emblematic figure of the ill-fated and unrecognized artist. Hopeless, misunderstood, and melancholic all of his/her life, he/she obtains recognition for his/her genius only at the end of his/her life, if not posthumously.

It is therefore difficult to be clear about happiness. And because of the considerable theoretical diversity, some authors have proposed very extreme opinions. For instance, the opinion that happiness simply does not exist. This is A. Schopenhauer's message: do not try to achieve happiness, just avoid unnecessary suffering (Schopenhauer, 2009).

WHAT PSYCHOMETRICS TELL US ABOUT HAPPINESS AND WELL-BEING

Even if they are obviously very normative, some authors have devised instruments devoted to the measurement of happiness or well-being. With these instruments it is possible to carry out statistical analyses of happiness. In particular, it is possible to determine whether or not happiness is a unidimensional concept, or whether it is merely the opposite of distress. Of course, considering the complexity of the concept, any results should be considered very cautiously.

Regarding the dimensional structure of happiness, some studies are in favor of an approximate unidimensionality. More precisely, as has been seen above, there are indeed several dimensions in the concept of happiness (such as autonomy, control of the environment, personal growth, positive relationships with others, purpose in life, self-acceptance, etc.), but these dimensions are positively correlated, so that a model with a single second-order super-factor has an acceptable fit (Ryff & Keyes, 1995; Stones & Kozma, 1985). In other words, from a statistical point of view, happiness is not a pure concept, but it is made up of several facets that have a common core, and this common core can be measured.

To the question: "is happiness simply the opposite of distress?" the answer is clearly "No." Although measurements of happiness are negatively correlated with measurements of distress in most studies, the correlation is moderate at best. Moreover, the patterns of correlations between positive and negative sub-dimensions of happiness and distress can be complex. For instance, a person is unlikely to be both satisfied with life and depressed, but may be satisfied and anxious (Headey, Kelley, & Wearing, 1993). On the other hand, some covariates can have specific effects on positive or negative measurements: socioeconomic status (SES) seems to have, in absolute value, a greater influence on "ill-being" than on well-being. The reverse is true for having a well-developed social network, while health tends to be more markedly associated with ill-being (Headey, Holmstrom, & Wearing, 1985).

Recently, UNESCO (Child Well-being in Rich Countries, n.d.) has used psychometric measurements of this kind to provide a comparative overview of child well-being in wealthy countries.

WHAT POPULATION-BASED STUDIES TELL US ABOUT CHILD WELL-BEING

The UNESCO study is interesting, because in the same document it provides objective socioeconomic indicators alongside more subjective measurements of children's life satisfaction obtained from a self-administered questionnaire (children aged 11 to 15).

The socioeconomic indicators were distributed across five dimensions: material well-being, health and safety, education, behaviors and risks, and housing and environment. A series of 29 countries—the United States, Canada, and 27 European nations—were ranked according to these dimensions.

The main results are summarized as follows:

- The Netherlands and most Scandinavian countries are the top-ranking countries.
- The Baltic countries, Greece, Romania, and the United States are the lowest-ranking countries.
- The relationship between per capita Gross Domestic Product and overall child well-being is not clear. Indeed, the Czech Republic is ranked higher than Austria, Slovenia higher than Canada, and Portugal higher than the United States.
- The consequences of child development in the early years are likely to have substantial and sustained effects on the well-being of children.

The concept of well-being appears to be potentially useful, especially to help in public policy decision-making as suggested by the last bullet point. This is one of a number of possible explanations for the rise of "positive psychology" at the start of the 21st century.

POSITIVE PSYCHOLOGY

According to some of its figureheads, positive psychology is defined as "the scientific study of positive human functioning and flourishing on multiple levels that include the biological, personal, relational, institutional, cultural, and global dimensions of life." (Seligman & Csikszentmihalyi, 2000).

From this definition, positive psychology is clearly not a philosophical movement, but a scientific discipline. It is a de facto branch of psychology: the notions of "functioning" and "flourishing" are related to behavior and to the mind, respectively. From a more institutional point of view, it can be noted that Martin Seligman, a leader in the domain, was the president of the American Psychological Association in 1998.

There are postulates that structure positive psychology. In particular, certain emotions and traits that can be considered "positive" and others that are considered "negative". For instance, joy, relief, and pride are positive emotions, while optimism and kindness are positive traits. On the other hand, sadness and anger are negative emotions, while impulsiveness is a negative trait. Positive psychology thus uses methods from fields as different as neuroscience, cognitive science, genetics, or epidemiology to study "positivity." The number of papers that have been published in the international literature on the subject during the last two decades has been particularly impressive.

Alongside these scientific studies, therapeutic interventions have been developed to promote positive feelings, positive behaviors, or positive cognitions. Some encouraging results have been published concerning the evaluation of these interventions (Sin & Lyubomirsky, 2009).

Positive psychology appears ultimately as the crystallization of ancient traditions of promoting happiness and well-being. This crystallization has been made possible in the last few decades by the catalytic effect of modern and high-tech sciences, such as neuroscience, genetics, and other quantitative approaches. The advent of "positive psychology" can also be considered the movement of emancipation of psychology from psychopathology and psychiatry. This is explicit in many texts, such as this passage by Seligman (2004): "for the last half century psychology has been consumed with a single topic only - mental illness."

This is not the first occurrence in which medicine, in its most narrow sense, has been extended to a broader concept. The emergence of the notions of health and mental health, as promoted by WHO, has followed similar logic.

WHO AND THE DEFINITION OF HEALTH

For a long time, health was considered the opposite of being in a pathological state. This was brilliantly described in a famous sentence attributed to the surgeon René Leriche in 1936: "Health is life, lived in the silence of the organs."

In 1946, WHO proposed a radically different perspective: "Health is a state of complete physical, mental, and social well-being and not merely the absence of disease or infirmity" (Constitution of the World Health Organization 1946, 2002). This position is much more ambitious: health no longer derives from the absence of problems (silence of the organs) but from a positive state (complete physical, mental, and social well-being). Many have criticized such a complete change. The most provocative denunciation that I have heard of the historic WHO definition of health was during a PhD viva, some years ago, when a colleague said that "complete physical, mental, and social well-being" could only occur after an orgasm or a shot of heroin.

Perhaps because of these problems of interpretation, in 1986 WHO proposed some elements of clarification on its definition of health: "To reach a state of complete physical, mental, and social well-being, an individual or group must be able to identify and to realize aspirations, to satisfy needs, and to change or cope with the environment." (WHO: The Ottawa Charter for Health Promotion, 2015).

Here WHO comes up against the problems we pointed out in the previous section on the philosophy of happiness. There are several distinct theories of happiness, and WHO has tried to combine at least two of them, which is not an easy task. The original definition in 1946 was oriented toward the search for some kind of ultimate pleasant experience, while the 1986 definition emphasized the new notion of satisfaction. But satisfaction is an emotion related to the fulfillment of a need, and it is not clear why an emotion of this sort should be included in the definition of health. It is even more surprising to note that the 1946 definition corresponds to a very exhilarating feeling, while satisfaction, at the core of the 1986 definition, is more closely associated with a peaceful state. Exhilaration and peacefulness are opposite feelings, and they appear here in definitions of the same notion. This raises questions, at the very least.

When considering the definition that WHO gives of mental health, things do not get any simpler. In 2001, in the World Health Report (WHO. The World Health Report 2001 – Mental Health, 2015) it was proposed that:

"Concepts of mental health include subjective well-being, perceived self-efficacy, autonomy, competence, intergenerational dependence, and self-actualization of one's intellectual and emotional potential, among others. From a cross-cultural perspective, it is nearly impossible to define mental health comprehensively. It is, however, generally agreed that mental health is broader than a lack of mental disorders.

An understanding of mental health and, more generally, mental functioning is important because it provides the basis on which to form a more complete understanding of the development of mental and behavioural disorders.

In recent years, new information from the fields of neuroscience and behavioural medicine has dramatically advanced our understanding of mental functioning. Increasingly, it is becoming clear that mental functioning has a physiological underpinning, and is fundamentally interconnected with physical and social functioning and health outcomes."

The first part of this text is particularly opaque, but concludes on the need to develop a new area extending beyond the limits of psychiatry. The second part calls on science, in particular neuroscience, for legitimation of the project. And this is surprising. It can even appear somewhat paradoxical that the notion of "mental health" should become valid and relevant because it can be linked to the physiology of the brain. Of course it is against the most basic dualistic position, but this is not necessarily a problem. What is really surprising is that the notion of "health" does not require the same kind of backup at all. It is even the opposite: health is defined without any mention of the body, the organs, or the biology of human beings. To define the notion of mental health, it is the brain that is considered, which is clearly not the case for the notion of health per se.

There are obviously relationships between health, medicine, mental health, and psychiatry that are unclear, and that needs to be considered.

HEALTH VERSUS MEDICINE; MENTAL HEALTH VERSUS PSYCHIATRY

In the previous section we looked at the definitions of health and mental health, and this is not straightforward. Concerning the definition of medicine, it has only the appearance of simplicity. Simplicity is seen in the consensus that exists across dictionaries. If you look in the Oxford or Collins dictionary (for English), or the dictionary of the French Academy of Medicine, "medicine/médecine" is in all cases the science/discipline/practice of preventing, diagnosing, and curing disease.

Because the object of medicine is disease, it is dealing with negativity and not with positivity, and this provides a *raison d'être* for positive psychology or positive mental health. As discussed above, there is room left for people who wish to develop the notion of well-being instead of simply dealing with "ill-being."

In fact these definitions of medicine can and *should* be challenged. Obviously, medicine should deal primarily with patients and not diseases. Indeed, a patient is not defined as a person with a disease.

Georges Canguilhem has admirably explained what a patient is (Canguilhem & Foucault, 1991):

"The doctor is called by the patient. It is the echo of this pathetic call which qualifies as pathological all the sciences which medical technology uses to aid life. Thus it is that there is a pathological anatomy, a pathological physiology, a pathological histology, a pathological embryology. But their pathological quality is an import of technical and thereby subjective origin. There is no objective pathology. Structures or behaviors can be objectively described but they cannot be called "pathological" on the strength of some purely objective criterion. Objectively, only varieties or differences can be defined with positive or negative vital values."

By this definition, a patient is a person who calls for a doctor and this call is "pathetic" (ie, linked to suffering). A doctor therefore has to respond to this call. This is specifically his/her job, and all the rest (pathology, diagnosis, treatment) should be organized and determined by this goal. In psychiatry, a psychiatric patient is likewise not defined as a person with a mental disorder. Rather, psychiatry is the discipline that has answers to offer to people who call for help because they are suffering in their mind or as a result of their behavior.

This definition has immediate and important consequences. First, medicine (and psychiatry in particular) is not devoted to ensuring happiness. Of course, happiness can be a significant side effect, but it will always be merely a consequence of a call that has been answered. Second, the notion of satisfaction is particularly delicate in medicine. If, as discussed earlier, satisfaction derives from the fulfilling of a need, it is difficult to obtain satisfaction from a doctor. A patient may lack information, an attentive ear, solutions to his/her problems, etc. and can thus be satisfied if responses are provided for these needs. But the actual state of being a patient does not correspond to a need or a lack, and cannot therefore be satisfied. Most often, a patient is not merely a person who has something wrong (ie, a disease) which needs to be corrected, leading to some kind of satisfaction. The call from the patient is in general more complex, in particular in chronic diseases, which are frequent in psychiatry. Sometimes there is a slight ambiguity in patient status and in the way patients experience their symptoms. This is one reason why the notion of cure raises so many problems and why alternative concepts, such as recovery, are currently proposed.

The definition of medicine as an answer to a distress call prevents psychiatry from repeating tragic errors that have been made in the past as a result of straightforward, blind applications of unreasonable theories of happiness. Making people happy despite themselves (ie, without any call on their part) has led to disasters. The way psychiatry has dealt with political opponents in the USSR or with homosexuals in many countries should encourage extreme caution when considering any normative perspective on happiness (King & Bartlett, 1999; Luty, 2014).

Medicine as an answer to a call, however, is also likely to have drawbacks. The call of a patient may be ambiguous or distorted by his/her environment, and the response may be limited. In schizophrenia, for instance, positive symptoms have been stressed, because they are so apparent, while psychiatrists have long neglected the treatment of negative symptoms, which are now considered a major issue in the patient's existence. Likewise, in attention deficit hyperactivity disorder (ADHD), hyperactive and impulsive symptoms have been the focus of clinicians, while inattention, because it may be less problematic in daily life, has been somewhat neglected. Yet it is now acknowledged that their role in patient prognosis is crucial (Pingault et al., 2013).

THE PARTICULAR NATURE OF CHILD AND ADOLESCENT PSYCHIATRY

In his definition of what a patient is, G. Canguilhem added a footnote: "It is understood that we are not dealing here with mental illnesses where the patients' ignorance of their state often constitutes an essential aspect of the disease." Hence, for this author, a psychiatric patient should perhaps not be defined in the same way as a patient with a somatic disorder. However, this opinion of psychiatric patients as often being "ignorant of their state" is a rather preconceived idea. Of course we need to remember that *The Normal and The Pathological* was published in 1966, and that the representations and realities of psychiatry were very different at that time. It is now well-known that even if there is a deficit in self-awareness in some psychiatric disorders, most patients are able to reliably self-report on how they assess their existence. This is even true for schizophrenic patients with significant executive impairment (Baumstarck et al., 2013). Conversely, it is a well-known fact today that denial is not rare in somatic diseases, especially among people with cancer (Vos & de Haes, 2007). Thus, the definition proposed by Canghuilhem could and should also apply to psychiatric patients, except perhaps when the patient is experiencing the most intense levels of psychotic episode.

This solves the question for adult psychiatry, but unfortunately not for child and adolescent psychiatry. Indeed, many young patients with autism or ADHD who see a child and adolescent psychiatrist are there because of their parents or because of the school, but not because of a personal appeal resulting from suffering in their minds or because of their behavior.

This is a real ethical issue that has so far not drawn enough discussion, and for which we have no definite solution. One proposal would be to consider that the "patient" in child and adolescent psychiatry is a community and not a person. The call leading to the consultation emerges from a group, and even if it is a child or an adolescent who actually presents, it is the group as a whole who is suffering and will even sometimes participate in, and benefit from, the treatment.

SYNTHESIS

From a philosophical point of view, happiness is a complex topic. Hedonism, the emotional state perspective, and life satisfaction are leading theories of happiness. These three theories are only partly compatible.

For a long time, many have found happiness in the development of positive emotions, traits, or behaviors. This was already the case in ancient Greece. In the 16th century, Spinoza stressed the need to favor joyful passions and shun sad ones (Spinoza, The Ethics IV, proposition 41). Positive psychology is a scientific update of these traditions.

Positive mental health has been developed to escape limitations inherent in psychiatry, but the concept suffers from inconsistencies. By construction, psychiatry addresses ill-being. Mental health is an attempt to bring together the traditional psychiatric approach and the more recent perspective of positive psychology. From an epistemological point of view, this fusion is frail for the following reasons:

> *Medicine is not an art or a science that treats diseases, but the discipline that produces doctors who respond to their patients' call.* Medicine is not designed to make patients happy. Medicine addresses the existential shift that comes from being a patient, and this is not reducible to pain, suffering, or ill-being (even if in practice, it is essential to treat pain, suffering, ill-being, and disease).
>
> *Psychiatry is the medical discipline that proposes answers to people who call for help because they are suffering in their mind or as a result of their behavior.* Because of the nature of mental disorders, patients can sometimes find it difficult to ask for help. This definition of psychiatry should therefore be considered as a principle and not a rule.

CONCLUSION

The object of medicine and psychiatry is distress in human beings. Distress in body or mind can be so intense that there is a need to call for help.

Across the centuries, physicians and scientists have progressively identified diseases and disorders from regular patterns of symptoms and biological abnormalities. Physicians are so fascinated by diseases that, with time, medicine has become the discipline that diagnoses and treats diseases instead of the discipline that treats patients.

Because of this shift, and because physicians are more inclined to prefer the great pleasure and glory that comes with successful treatment to the silent efficacy of a good prevention intervention, today there is a gap between the expectations of society concerning medicine, and what is offered by physicians in general and psychiatrists in particular. Because of this gap, new concepts have been introduced to challenge the powerful and well-established field of medicine. Health, mental health, and positive mental health are among these concepts. Unfortunately, their definitions raise many issues. Today, there is a risk that a good initiative might fail, particularly because there is no single definition of happiness, and because happiness is not the mere opposite of distress. Solid societal legitimacy is required to be able to determine what is "good" for people, and health care providers do not have this legitimacy. This is particularly true in the field of psychiatry.

Health care providers, whether they are physicians or not, should thus restrict themselves to the treatment of distress. But that is not to say that medicine and psychiatry do not need to evolve. Caring for the patient instead of being obsessed with disorders, and investing more in prevention are two urgent needs.

References

Baumstarck, K., Boyer, L., Boucekine, M., Aghababian, V., Parola, N., Lançon, C., & Auquier, P. (2013). Self-reported quality of life measure is reliable and valid in adult patients suffering from schizophrenia with executive impairment. *Schizophrenia Research, 147*(1), 58–67. http://dx.doi.org/10.1016/j.schres.2013.03.008.

Canguilhem, G., & Foucault, M. (1991). *The normal and the pathological* (C.R. Fawcett, Trans.). New York: Zone Books.

Child Well-being in Rich Countries: A Comparative Overview. (n.d.). Retrieved from: http://www.unicef-irc.org/publications/683.

Constitution of the World Health Organization 1946. (2002). *Bulletin of the World Health Organization, 80*(12), 983–984.

Haybron, D. (2011). Happiness. In E. N. Zalta (Ed.), *The Stanford encyclopedia of philosophy (fall 2011)*. Retrieved from: http://plato.stanford.edu/archives/fall2011/entries/happiness/.

Headey, B., Holmstrom, E., & Wearing, A. (1985). Models of well-being and ill-being. *Social Indicators Research, 17*(3), 211–234. http://doi.org/10.1007/BF00319311.

Headey, B., Kelley, J., & Wearing, A. (1993). Dimensions of mental health: life satisfaction, positive affect, anxiety and depression. *Social Indicators Research, 29*(1), 63–82. http://dx.doi.org/10.1007/BF01136197.

King, M., & Bartlett, A. (1999). British psychiatry and homosexuality. *The British Journal of Psychiatry, 175*(2), 106–113. http://doi.org/10.1192/bjp.175.2.106.

Luty, J. (2014). Psychiatry and the dark side: eugenics, Nazi and Soviet psychiatry. *Advances in Psychiatric Treatment, 20*(1), 52–60. http://doi.org/10.1192/apt.bp.112.010330.

Pingault, J.-B., Côté, S. M., Galéra, C., Genolini, C., Falissard, B., Vitaro, F., & Tremblay, R. E. (2013). Childhood trajectories of inattention, hyperactivity and oppositional behaviors and prediction of substance abuse/dependence: a 15-year longitudinal population-based study. *Molecular Psychiatry, 18*(7), 806–812. http://dx.doi.org/10.1038/mp.2012.87.

Ryff, C. D., & Keyes, C. L. M. (1995). The structure of psychological well-being revisited. *Journal of Personality and Social Psychology, 69*(4), 719–727. http://dx.doi.org/10.1037/0022-3514.69.4.719.

Schopenhauer, A. (2009). *Die Kunst, glücklich zu sein (4., unveränderte Auflage. edition)*. München: Beck C. H.

Seligman, M. E. P. (2004). *Authentic happiness: Using the new positive psychology to realize your potential for lasting fulfillment* (reprint). New York: Atria Books.

Seligman, M. E. P., & Csikszentmihalyi, M. (2000). Positive psychology: an introduction. *American Psychologist, 55*(1), 5–14. http://dx.doi.org/10.1037/0003-066X.55.1.5.

Sin, N. L., & Lyubomirsky, S. (2009). Enhancing well-being and alleviating depressive symptoms with positive psychology interventions: a practice-friendly meta-analysis. *Journal of Clinical Psychology, 65*(5), 467–487. http://dx.doi.org/10.1002/jclp.20593.

Spinoza, B. (2013). *Ethics*. Heraklion Press.

Stones, M. J., & Kozma, A. (1985). Structural relationships among happiness scales: a second order factorial study. *Social Indicators Research, 17*(1), 19–28. http://dx.doi.org/10.1007/BF00354110.

Vos, M. S., & de Haes, J. C. J. M. (2007). Denial in cancer patients, an explorative review. *Psycho-Oncology, 16*(1), 12–25. http://doi.org/10.1002/pon.1051.

WHO. The Ottawa Charter for Health Promotion. (July 20, 2015). Retrieved July 20, 2015, from: http://www.who.int/healthpromotion/conferences/previous/ottawa/en/.

WHO. The World Health Report 2001-Mental Health: New Understanding, New Hope. (July 21, 2015). Retrieved July 21, 2015, from: http://www.who.int/whr/2001/en/.

Winnicott, D. W. (1994). Hate in the counter-transference. *The Journal of Psychotherapy Practice and Research, 3*(4), 348–356.

ICD-11—Comparison With DSM-5 and Implications for Child & Adolescent Psychiatric Disorders

M.E. Garralda

Imperial College London, London, United Kingdom

INTRODUCTION

Since the mental disorder sections of the International Statistical Classification of Diseases, 10th revision (ICD-10) (WHO, 1992) and the *Diagnostic and Statistical Manual of Mental Disorders*, fourth edition (DSM-IV) (American Psychiatric Association, 1994) were updated in 1992 and 1994 there has been a steady growth of research and knowledge about the nature and treatment of mental disorders. Mental health services have also been expanding worldwide. The classification of disorders remains crucial to communication between all those involved with the services, and diagnoses are increasingly made as a requirement for service function and development. The two most widely used classification systems are the World Health Organization's ICD which has a worldwide perspective, and the USA's American Psychiatric Association's DSM. Their most recent revisions aim to reflect changes in our understanding of mental health disorders, clinical consensus, and utility.

This chapter addresses the classification of child and adolescent mental health disorders in the recently published DSM-5, and the changes proposed for ICD-11. It describes the rationale and historical context for classification in mental health, and more specifically recent changes to neurodevelopmental and disruptive/dissocial disorders. It considers proposals for alternative classifications and discusses challenges for child mental health clinics in implementing diagnostic procedures.

Positive Mental Health, Fighting Stigma and Promoting Resiliency for Children and Adolescents
http://dx.doi.org/10.1016/B978-0-12-804394-3.00002-4

HISTORICAL CONTEXT FOR ICD CLASSIFICATIONS

The historical and conceptual backgrounds of current classifications of mental health disorders have been comprehensively discussed by Cooper and Sartorius (2013), and this section will draw on their observations. Cooper and Sartorius highlight the fact that in the absence of an agreed-upon way of describing problems in diagnostic terms, early medical publications had to rely on detailed case histories of patients. The lack of a standard usage of diagnostic terms meant that the results of treatments could not be carried over into settings other than the unit where they were used. This became a particular problem with the development of psychotropic medications in the first part of the 20th century, but the absence of an internationally agreed-upon classification also meant that the emerging epidemiological studies had limited translation value across countries.

It was only in 1949 that ICD-6 for the first time included a section on mental disorders, but even the following seventh revision of the ICD in the 1950s was still little more than a list of approved names attached to a list of code numbers. By then different classifications had proliferated (28 different systems were identified at one point), and this led to what was described as "the chaotic state of the classifications in current use in psychiatry." The modern era and major breakthrough in psychiatric classification was signaled by the development by British psychiatrists of a Glossary of Mental Disorders and Guide to the Classification in 1974 in Chapter V of ICD-8. This was aided by the development and publication in the international literature of symptomatic rating scales, and of standardized research psychiatric interviews such as the Present State Examination developed at the Institute of Psychiatry in London, which became widely used in international studies, and by the Mental Status Schedule in the United States.

In the United States, the American Psychiatric Association (APA) published the predecessor of DSM in 1844 (DSM-5, 2013). This was a statistical classification of institutionalized mental patients designed to aid communication about the types of patients cared for in these hospitals. Later, the Office of the Surgeon General produced a psychiatric classification to help assess the mental health of military personal in World War II, which was updated and extended by the APA, and became DSM-I, published in 1952. This in addition to the eighth revision of ICD published by the WHO in 1968 led to DSM-II. However, both classifications reflected the then prevalent psychodynamic approach in the United States, and there was little description of symptoms. DSM-III was published in 1980, and represented a major shift, as it contained a narrative description of the clinical features of different disorders. It was said to be welcome by editors of major psychiatric journals, though it may not have been so popular with clinicians. The existence of increasingly sound classification systems and research methods allowed a number of epidemiological studies from many countries, demonstrated the feasibility of universal recognition of disorders, and compared prevalence rates across communities and internationally.

In the 1980s there was a concerted effort to harmonize DSM and ICD classifications, and their 4th and 10th versions, respectively, were remarkably similar conceptually, in diagnostic terms and descriptions. The recent development of DSM-5 and ICD-11 has been guided by consideration that they should be useful in both primary care and specialist psychiatry, for billing for services, for the production of national statistics about mental disorders or public health purposes, and to serve as internationally useful common language for researchers. They also have to reflect opinions of psychiatrists and other mental health personnel and practices in different settings and cultures.

RECOMMENDED PROPERTIES OF AN INTERNATIONAL CLASSIFICATION

It is recommended that the properties of an international classification include the following features (Cooper & Sartorius, 2013), and clearly both classificatory revisions have striven to meet them, namely to be:

- based upon points of agreement between mental health professionals
- sufficiently simple and understandable to allow easy use with common disorders
- sufficiently well-liked as a tool of information exchange
- conservative and theoretically familiar to be attractive and acceptable to a wide variety of users with different levels of knowledge and backgrounds
- stable and subject to change only when sufficient scientific knowledge becomes available to openly justify any innovations
- able to take into account languages into which it will be translated
- in a position to offer continuity between successive revisions for stability, economic, and scientific reasons

CLASSIFICATION AND TAXONOMY: RATIONALE

In essence, classification is a tool for communication, so when researchers, clinicians, or policy-makers refer to a feature, they mean the same thing (Taylor & Rutter, 2008).

To classify is to arrange things in groups that have some characteristic in common (Cooper & Sartorius, 2013). Scientifically, classification is part of the discipline of taxonomy, supported by extensive and reliable data, whereby a set of names or nomenclature is agreed-upon and descriptions or glossaries are worked out. These are then refined into definitions, containing a list of properties unique to the object defined. Definitions should be mutually exclusive and jointly exhaustive. A group of objects with similar characteristics constitutes a "taxon," and while recognizing some imprecision in the boundaries, most psychiatric disorders are taxons. However, because they can only be identified by subjective descriptions, their taxonomic qualities are not as high as conditions based on more objective measurements. Hence, the detailed description of diagnostic criteria and the development of reliable measurements that are correlated with clinical symptoms and syndromes, alongside the recognition that psychiatric diagnoses are guide points or hypotheses for understanding, communication, and treatment setting, rather than immutable statements of objective phenomena.

In practice, however, classification is also meant to reflect the presence of diseases requiring particular treatments. This is complicated by the way in which individual disorders can manifest in different subjects and circumstances, making them at times appear fluid and arbitrary in contrast with fixed and stable diagnostic entities. Moreover, there is not often a clear separation between early clinical changes and treatable disorders, and this lays at the root of the debate about the advantages and disadvantages of the dimensional versus the dichotomous approach to health problems. When is elevated blood pressure a disease requiring treatment? When are high levels of inattention in a child an expression of an attention deficit disorder, and when is apparent adolescent turmoil a depressive disorder? What constitutes a disease requiring a medical or mental health label is not always straightforward, and there can be disagreements between doctors, nurses, and patients. Classificatory systems nevertheless follow the taxonomical, dichotomous tradition, and aim to describe the crucial symptoms that cluster together into clinically recognizable entities opening the way to potentially efficacious treatments.

CLASSIFICATION IN PSYCHIATRY

Psychiatry diverges from general medicine, where the main purpose is to identify and treat physical diseases established by clinical syndromes supported by abnormal physical signs or laboratory findings. Psychiatry, rather, puts emphasis on the concept of disorder supported by patient distress and suffering, and causing impairment and interference with activities.

Both ICD-10 and DSM-IV defined disorders in similar ways, implying the existence of a clinically recognizable set of symptoms or behaviors associated in most cases with distress and interference with personal functions. Clinically recognizable sets of symptoms or behaviors were crucial, so that social deviance or conflict alone, without personal dysfunction, would not be a mental disorder. However, there was a difference between the two classificatory systems: in DSM-IV, clinically significant distress and impairment in social, occupational, or other important areas of functioning were regarded as intrinsic aspects of disorders, whereas in ICD-10, disorders would cause distress and impairment in most, but not all, cases. While it seems conceptually best not to include the consequences of disorders in their definition, it is still the case that there are a number of disorders, such as simple schizophrenia, which are defined by impairment in functionality. Pragmatically, psychiatric syndromes that do not cause distress and impairment seem unlikely to lead to seeking help from health services. The debate on whether to include impairment in the definition of disorders has veered to the side of inclusion, so that both DSM-5 and ICD-11 specify in the description of different disorders that the symptoms or deficits limit or are sufficiently severe to cause impairment in everyday functioning such as personal, family, social, educational, or occupational domains, or in other important areas of functioning.

The two classificatory systems use contrasting approaches to psychiatric diagnosis: the narrative approach—also called prototype matching—follows the convention of psychiatric textbooks in providing a narrative of the presentation: it gives prominence to the main features and mentions other features which may be or not be regarded as diagnostic. This is the approach followed by the Clinical Descriptions and Diagnostic Guidelines version of ICD and is the one more popular with clinicians (Reed, Mendonca Correia, Esparza, Saxena, & Maj, 2011). The second approach, adopted by DSM-5, provides a list of diagnostic or "operational" criteria, with instructions about how many and what combinations are required for a given diagnosis, and is more popular with researchers.

ICD-11 AND DSM-5: COMPATIBILITY AND DIVERGENCE

DSM-5 was developed on the back of several meetings planned to review basic issues related to classification. These were followed by a series of scientific review meetings involving leading experts from the United States and other countries, and led to a task force, which created working groups in order to develop proposals for groups of disorders to be used in field tests and inform the final version.

WHO similarly created an advisory group for ICD-11 to set up working groups in order to prepare proposals on individual disorders. In addition, WHO carried out a survey of opinions of psychiatrists and set up parallel groups to work on the classification of mental health disorders to be used in primary care. To harmonize proposals with DSM-5, officials of WHO and APA met on a number of occasions and they agreed on a "meta-structure of the classification" which divides disorders into clusters:

- neurocognitive (identified by neural substrate abnormalities)
- neurodevelopmental (with early and continuing cognitive deficits)
- psychoses (identified by clinical features and biomarkers for information processing defects)
- emotional disorders (with temperamental antecedents of negative emotionality)
- externalizing (with temperamental antecedents of disinhibition)

Clinical Significance

DSM-5 has developed a generic diagnostic criterion to establish disorder thresholds based on distress or disability, usually worded as "the disturbance causes clinically significant distress or impairment in social, occupation or other important areas of functioning." Similar wording is likely to be applied to qualify clinical significance in ICD-11. In addition and where applicable, DSM-5 applies specific criteria for defining disorder severity (mild, moderate, severe, extreme), descriptive features, and course (such as partial remission or recurrent).

The overall philosophy of both DSM-5 and ICD-11 has been one of reducing the number of diagnosable psychiatric disorders, leaving the best validated and clinically relevant. The general convention is to allow multiple diagnoses when present.

Both systems provide *subtypes*, and *specifiers* or *qualifiers* (both terms will be used interchangeably in this chapter) for increased specificity. Subtypes define mutually exclusive and jointly exhaustive phenomenological subgroups within a diagnosis, while specifiers are not jointly exhaustive and more than one type may be given for each disorder. Specifiers provide an opportunity to define a homogeneous subgrouping of individuals, sharing certain features that may be relevant for management. The specifier "provisional" can be used when there is a strong presumption that a diagnosis will be met. As discussed later in the chapter, the multiaxial system is not retained in either scheme.

CLASSIFICATION IN CHILD AND ADOLESCENT PSYCHIATRY

As in other fields, classification in child and adolescent psychiatry is a tool for communication among clinicians and researchers, for application of research to clinical problems, guidance on practice, explanations to patients, and clinical reimbursement. For all these purposes, a good scientific classification system should have the virtues of clarity, comprehensiveness, acceptability to users and fidelity to nature. A scheme should also be flexible and change as understanding alters (Taylor & Rutter, 2008).

The differences in emphasis between ICD and DSM outlined above are unlikely to have a major effect on classification as used in clinical child psychiatric practice. They are, however, more of a problem for research and will need to be taken into account in case definitions, as even minor differences can influence findings. Examples include whether pervasiveness is central to an attention deficit hyperactivity disorder (ADHD) diagnosis or not; whether age of onset is of relevance for the diagnosis of separation anxiety disorder; and whether individual items such as numbing of general responsiveness are included in the definition of post-traumatic stress disorder (Taylor & Rutter, 2008).

Earlier ICD classifications supported a multidimensional and multiaxial framework for child psychiatric diagnoses, as did DSM-IV for disorders across the age range. The multiaxial system is particularly well suited to child psychiatry, since clinically alongside psychiatric disorders, the presence of developmental delays and learning disability, medical problems, and psychosocial risks are all taken into account in the psychiatric formulation of individual children and young people. The multiaxial system avoided having to choose between two disorders in what was in effect a hierarchical classification.

Nevertheless DSM-5 working parties concluded that the previous multiaxial system was no longer advisable, because of its complexity and the fact that clinicians were not commonly using multidimensions. The global assessment of functioning was moreover thought to lack conceptual clarity and have questionable psychometrics in clinical practice (DSM-5, 2013). The enhanced convergence of child and adult psychiatric disorders within the revised classificatory systems has in effect meant a loss of the child psychiatric multiaxial approach. This is nevertheless partly compensated by the use of psychiatric comorbidity and by the introduction of clinically relevant diagnostic specifiers or qualifiers, for example, to note the presence of intellectual disability in autism.

The previous hierarchical approach whereby one disorder would take precedence and encompass any accompanying symptoms from others is now complemented by the ability to diagnose different disorders, provided that the symptoms of each are sufficiently extensive and impairing to justify more than one diagnosis, and are not better explained by one psychiatric disorder. The development of specifiers also counteracts possible disadvantages of the general philosophy of both DSM-5 and ICD-11 of reducing the number of diagnosable psychiatric disorders, as they identify additional homogeneous subgroupings, which may represent a clinical summary of social, psychological, and biological factors with management implications.

THE PROPOSED CHILD AND ADOLESCENT PSYCHIATRIC DISORDERS IN ICD-11 AND THEIR CONVERGENCE WITH DSM-5

WHO's priorities for the development of ICD-11 include increasing its clinical utility in global worldwide mental health settings and improving the identification and diagnosis of mental disorders among children and adolescents.

A decision was made early in the process of ICD-11 preparatory work to modify the placement of child psychiatric disorders, to spread and merge them across ICD-11 categories. For this to work, it was essential for all diagnoses to provide a lifetime perspective and an explicit set of instructions for the ways in which manifestations vary with age (Rutter, 2011), and this has been adopted by both DSM and ICD. Likewise, the way in which gender and cultural factors may affect clinical presentations is explained and integrated as applicable. DSM-5 is actually organized around developmental and life considerations (DSM-5, 2013). It begins with diagnoses thought to reflect developmental processes that manifest early in life, namely, neurodevelopmental, schizophrenia spectrum, and other psychotic disorders, followed by diagnoses that are more commonly manifested in adolescence and young adulthood such as bipolar, depressive, and anxiety disorders, and it ends with diagnoses relevant to adulthood and later life such as neurocognitive disorders.

Within this overall framework, the diagnostic categories—most characteristic of childhood—are those with onset in the first few years of life, the neurodevelopmental and disruptive-dissocial disorders, and these will be addressed here in some detail. For reference purposes the ICD-10 classification of children's psychiatric disorders is summarized in Table 2.1.

TABLE 2.1   Child Psychiatric Disorders in ICD-10

---

1. Disorders of psychological development, involving early developmental tasks addressing intellectual, learning and communication tasks
   a. Specific developmental disorders of speech and language/communication; of scholastic skills/learning; of motor function
   b. Pervasive developmental disorders, involving social development, communication and behavior.

2. Behavioral and emotional disorders with onset usually occurring in childhood and adolescence, including those affected by emotional/behavioral immaturities of childhood
   a. Hyperkinetic disorders
   b. Conduct disorders
   c. Emotional disorders with onset specific to childhood
   d. Disorders of social functioning with onset specific to childhood and adolescence
   e. Tic disorders and others including enuresis, encopresis; feeding disorders, pica, stereotyped movement disorder, stuttering, cluttering.

3. Disorders that apply across the age and developmental age, including mental retardation.

THE NEURODEVELOPMENTAL CLUSTER OF DISORDERS IN DSM-5 AND ICD-11

The DSM-5 study group charged with the task of reviewing the early developmental disorders considered it in the light of two newly proposed DSM-5 categories of brain dysfunction: neurodevelopmental disorders and major cognitive disorders of later life. Disorders would be appropriately placed within a neurodevelopmental cluster if they exhibited similar and overlapping risks and clinical manifestations, and a shared course or developmental profile. They would need to meet the cluster criteria of affected neurodevelopmental function and evolve through processes that alter trajectories in normal brain development. They would have in common an onset in early life during the early developmental period, have the potential to induce lifelong impairments, and symptoms would be characterized by either delays, excess, or deviance in achieving milestones (Andrews, Pine, Hobbs, Anderson, & Sunderland, 2009).

The resulting DSM-5 definition outlines persistent behavioral and cognitive disorders that affect brain-based functions, including intellectual function and learning, communication and social function, and attention and motor control; the onset is during the developmental period; the disorders cause impairment in activities and performance; and can persist into adulthood (Andrews et al., 2009). ADHDs are regarded as meeting these requirements and are therefore included under neurodevelopmental disorders.

The proposed ICD-11 neurodevelopmental disorders are generally congruent with those included in DSM-5, although there may be slight differences as outlined in Table 2.2, partly due to the need to take into account

TABLE 2.2   Neurodevelopmental Disorders Proposed for ICD-11 and in DSM-5

ICD-11	DSM-5
Disorders of intellectual development	Intellectual disabilities

• developmental speech/language disorders
   includes language, speech sound, fluency
	• communication disorders
	   includes language, speech sound, fluency, and social (pragmatic)

• autism spectrum disorder	• autistic spectrum disorder
• attention deficit disorders	• attention deficit hyperactivity disorder
• specific developmental learning disorders	• specific learning disorder
• specific coordination disorder	• motor disorders includes coordination, stereotypic, tics
• stereotyped movement disorder/tic disorder	

other disorders and overall ICD-11 terminology. Notably intellectual disability replaces mental retardation and is a newcomer to the neurodevelopmental disorders cluster, as are attention deficit disorders.

AUTISM SPECTRUM DISORDERS (ASD): SYNDROME CONSOLIDATION AND THE NEW DYAD OF IMPAIRMENTS

In line with DSM-5, ICD-11 introduces important differences to the definition of autism, including a consolidation under this umbrella term of a number of related disorders (ie, autism, Asperger's syndrome, disintegrative and pervasive developmental disorders). The previously defining triad of impairment becomes a dyad with anomalies in two key dimensions: social communication and restricted repetitive behaviors. The diversity of the syndrome is represented through subtypes or qualifiers to acknowledge the presence of intellectual disability or language disorder, and in ICD-11, possibly also the loss of previously acquired developmental skills. It is now made explicit that autistic spectrum disorders are seen across the life span.

These changes reflect research findings and differences in the conceptualization of autistic spectrum disorders, and are congruent with its increasing recognition in individuals with average intellectual levels and language development. In restricting impairments to a dyad—in social communication and restricted repetitive behaviors—the diagnosis of autism has lost language delay as an intrinsic autistic dimension. Lord and Jones (2012) argued that this was a response to the fact that not all children with ASD have language delays and by later school years many are fluent speakers. Conversely language delay is not specific to autism and the majority of young children referred because of language delay do not have autistic spectrum disorder nor severe developmental delays.

Nevertheless current language level and use by the child still play a significant role in the diagnosis, course, and treatment of ASD. All behaviors that contributed to the former dimension of communication with the exception of overall language delay have been retained, within the rubric of social-communication or of fixated interests and repetitive behaviors. Abnormalities in social nonverbal language such as in the use of gaze and gestures in verbal conversation and social aspects of imaginative play are included under social communication; repetitive aspects of language, such as stereotyped speech, delayed echolalia, repeated questions and vocalizations, neologisms and restricted aspects of play under autistic restricted repetitive behaviors. The validity of the revised dyad was examined by Mandy et al. (2012) in a study of 708 verbal children and young people with mild-to-severe autistic difficulties. Factor analysis of clinical features confirmed the superiority of the dyadic over the triadic diagnostic approach; it assigned the autistic sensory abnormalities to the repetitive and restricted behaviors symptom cluster.

There has been debate and discrepant estimates on whether these changes in diagnostic features will bring about alterations in the number of individuals receiving an ASD diagnosis (Swedo et al., 2012; Kent et al., 2013; Huerta, Bishop, Duncan, Hus, & Lord, 2012). It must be acknowledged that although classificatory system revisions take care to change criteria as little as possible, it seems regrettable but inevitable that changes will have an effect on the frequency and nature of disorders, and potentially affect the extent to which research findings before and after revisions apply to the same group of patients.

Autism Spectrum Disorders: The Role of Intellectual and Language Function Levels

Not uncommonly, children with ASD also have intellectual disability and/or developmental language delays or deficits, and this is crucial to the level of support required and general management. To help acknowledge this in the diagnostic process, DSM-5 has three severity level specifiers, which rely to a considerable extent on the presence of associated deficits in these areas. For example, a child with few words of intelligible speech and little in the way of social interactions will be regarded as requiring very substantial support under severity specifier level 3. Other specifiers address the presence of accompanying intellectual or language impairment more directly and also of known medical/genetic conditions or environmental factors. ICD-11 is similarly likely to acknowledge that individuals with autism spectrum disorder frequently exhibit co-occurring limitations in intellectual and functional language abilities, and that these and possibly also loss of previously acquired skills in the absence of a causative neurological disorder are factors to consider for appropriate individualization of supports, treatment planning, and selection of effective interventions.

SPECIFIC LANGUAGE DISORDERS

The specific language disorders in ICD-11 include developmental language disorder, speech sound disorder, and speech fluency disorder.

Developmental language disorder is characterized by persistent difficulties arising during early childhood in the acquisition, understanding, production, or use of language which causes significant limitations in the ability to communicate. To record uneven deficits in language development, clinicians will be able to use qualifiers to state whether the problem affects both receptive and expressive language or whether it affects primarily expressive or pragmatic language. The pragmatic language qualifier characterizes persistent and substantial difficulties in the understanding and use of language in social contexts, for example, making inferences, understanding verbal humor, and resolving ambiguous meanings.

Instead of a pragmatic language qualifier, DSM-5 has a separate social (pragmatic) communication disorder, though its validity has been challenged in part because of the paucity of research evidence and the high levels of concomitant disorders of language structure and cognition (Norbury, 2014). Nevertheless, descriptively there is a great deal of congruence between DSM-5's social (pragmatic) communication disorder and ICD-11's pragmatic language qualifier, making it likely that either will identify the same children and problems. Both classifications highlight the lack of repetitive and restricted interests in the differential diagnosis with ASD.

THE CLASSIFICATION OF DISRUPTIVE, DISSOCIAL, AND CONDUCT DISORDERS

DSM-5's disruptive disorders are diagnosed under a "disruptive, impulse-control and conduct disorders" heading and include:

- oppositional defiant disorder (ODD), with specifiers for severity (mild, moderate, or severe)
- intermittent explosive disorder
- conduct disorder with three subtypes: childhood onset, adolescent onset, unspecified onset; and two specifiers: a) with limited prosocial emotions, and b) severity (mild, moderate, severe)
- antisocial personality disorder (with dual coverage with cluster B personality disorders)
- pyromania
- kleptomania
- other specified disruptive, impulse control, and conduct disorders
- unspecified disruptive, impulse control, and conduct disorders

The introduction of the limited pro-social emotions specifier accords with the growing literature on "callous and emotional traits" in children being identifiable, relatively stable, and linked to the more severe, aggressive, and stable pattern of antisocial behavior (Frick & White, 2008). However, more validating research and clinical experience on treatment implications is needed before its usefulness is fully established.

The same proviso applies to conduct disorder subtyping by age of onset and demonstration that these subcategories are both comprehensive and mutually exclusive. The age of onset subtypes includes *childhood onset* which is distinguished from the adolescent onset subtype by being especially common in males, and involving physical aggression, disturbed peer relationships, comorbid neurodevelopmental anomalies, and possibly an earlier oppositional defiant disorder; by full criteria being met before puberty, and a tendency to persist. Although there is empirical support for this early childhood onset subgroup, it is also the case that many children with childhood onset anti-social behavior do not fit this pattern, and that this pattern is also found in young people with conduct disorder starting in adolescence (Fairchild, van Goozen, Calder, & Goodyer, 2013). The childhood onset nomenclature runs the risk that clinicians will a priori and erroneously judge prepubertal children with conduct disorder as universally having a poor prognosis. An added difficulty with persistence and poor outcome being part of the definition is that this only becomes clear retrospectively, making diagnosis somewhat paradoxically more appropriate for adolescents and young adults than for prepubertal children.

Given the limited clinical experience in their use and the particularly negative connotations of some qualifiers/subtypes, it would seem advisable for them to be regarded in practice as tentative, and for field clinical trials to be carried out to assess their clinical validity and usefulness.

In ICD-11 it is proposed that the disruptive diagnoses cluster will be named "disruptive behavior and dissocial disorders" and include:

- oppositional defiant disorder, with qualifier/subtype: with and without chronic irritability-anger
- conduct-dissocial disorder, with qualifier/subtypes: childhood and adolescent onset
- both disorders have a qualifier with limited pro-social emotions

Intermittent explosive disorder, kleptomania, and pyromania may be classified in this section or under the separate cluster of impulsive disorders.

The most important difference between the two classificatory systems is the approach taken to the diagnosis of children presenting with both oppositional behavior and marked irritability. Whereas in ICD-11 they would be regarded as having oppositional defiant disorders qualified with marked irritability, DSM-5 has created the separate category disruptive mood dysregulation disorder or DMDD.

IS DMDD A VALID DIAGNOSIS?

The assessment, diagnosis, and treatment of children with severe irritability and anger has become a hotly debated topic in childhood psychopathology.

Clearly some children display consistently high levels of reactivity and irritability in a way that is distressing and impairing to them, and is regarded as a form of emotional dysregulation. In recent years, severe and impairing irritability in children came to be understood by some clinicians and researchers, especially in the United States, as a manifestation of mania and bipolar disorder, and treated accordingly (Lochman et al., 2015). Many of these children also meet diagnostic requirements for oppositional defiant disorder, and it is now established that a number of children with ODD have marked emotional dysregulation and that in these children ODD shows continuity with mood and anxiety disorders.

In an effort to clarify links between irritability and bipolar disorder, researchers at the US National Institute of Mental Health outlined a syndrome called severe mood dysregulation, or SMD, characterized by chronic abnormal levels of anger or sadness, and hyperarousal, evidenced by insomnia or agitation and heightened verbal or physical reactivity. SMD and severe irritability/anger in childhood were found to predict anxiety and depressive disorders in adolescence and adulthood, rather than bipolar disorders. DSM-5 chose to diagnose children with SMD with frequent and severe temper outburst and persistent irritably with a new disorder named disruptive mood dysregulation disorder, or DMDD, located with the depressive disorders group.

The addition of this new category met with negative reactions among many professionals because it was regarded as not sufficiently distinct from ODD and because it could lead to overuse of mood-regulating medications in children. Field studies appeared to indicate limited reliability, and very high rates of overlap with other disorders (Lochman et al., 2015). ICD-11 has therefore chosen a different and more conservative approach in adding a specifier/qualifier to oppositional defiant disorder to indicate the presence of chronic irritability and anger, rather than adopting this new disorder.

The different subtypes and qualifiers of the disruptive and conduct or dissocial disorder cluster are a result of new research findings. They have generated a great deal of interest but also controversy, and may best be regarded as work in progress. Further validating work is likely to be required before we can be confident that they will be retained in their present form in ICD-12 and DSM-6.

FUTURE APPROACHES TO CLASSIFICATION: THE RESEARCH DOMAIN CRITERIA (RDoC)

A challenge to the development of future versions of both DSM-5 and ICD-11 may come from research into brain function underlying mental health problems. The US National Institute for Mental Health is advocating an alternative approach to classification, with the development of Research Domain Criteria, or RDoC, as the basis for a new classification framework for research on mental disorders (Insel et al., 2010). The basic argument is that while current diagnostic categories are largely based on clinical consensus, they fail to align with findings emerging from clinical neuroscience and genetics or genomics, their boundaries have not been predictive of treatment response, and they may not capture fundamental underlying pathophysiological mechanisms of dysfunction. The RDoC project aims to create a framework for research on pathophysiology, especially genomics and neuroscience, which ultimately would inform future classification schemes.

The RDoC classification rests on three assumptions: first, a conceptualization of mental illnesses as dysfunction or disorders of brain circuits; second, this can be identified with the tools of clinical neuroscience, such as electrophysiology, functional neuroimaging, and new methods for quantifying connections in vivo; and third, data from genetics and clinical neuroscience will yield bio-signatures to complement clinical symptoms and signs for clinical management. RDoC will address broad domains of function that affect both the biology and psychology of mental illness such as negative emotionality and cognition through different levels of analysis (genetic, molecular, and cellular), progressing on the one hand to the brain circuit level and to the other to the level of individual, family environment, and social context.

Possible fundamental changes in future medical classificatory systems in the light of new scientific and therapeutic discoveries are unlikely to be confined to mental disorders. Fast-moving developments in genetic and molecular biology and the "precision revolution" in medicine may mean for example that tumors will be classified according to their genetic mutant features rather than to site and pathology as at present, and treatment targeted at individual patients' genetic cancer mutations.

Whether RDoC or other initiatives have an impact on the classification of mental health disorders may depend on its ability to lead to major breakthroughs in our understanding of their nature and management.

CLASSIFICATION SYSTEMS AND THE PRACTICE OF CHILD AND ADOLESCENT PSYCHIATRY AND CAMHS

The use of psychiatric diagnosis and international classificatory systems is not always popular with some clinicians and multidisciplinary Child and Adolescent Psychiatric or Mental Health Services (CAMHS). A broad diagnostic-*less* approach or locally developed idiosyncratic classifications have been in use and claimed to be better suited to individuals' or services' interests, philosophies, theories and ways of working. However, in an increasingly globalized world, and given the growth in knowledge of child mental health problems, there is now a strong drive to follow a common terminology that is global in its reach and increasingly empirically-based. The ICD and DSM revisions provide the best available means of facilitating well-informed communications about mental health problems in children and young people between professionals, with children and families and for administrative purposes, across different countries. WHO has also developed a Global Clinical Practice Network for mental health with worldwide clinician representation, to support its goal of reducing global disease burden of mental disorders by developing a more clinically useful and globally applicable diagnostic manual: this practice network might prove to be a useful tool for international research into promotion and prevention in mental health (Reed et al., 2015).

Possible challenges for CAMHS in adopting the diagnostic classificatory approach are outlined in the next section.

Limited Knowledge in the General Population and Among Referring Primary Care Workers About Child and Adolescent Mental Health Problems

This limited knowledge is understandable in view of the comparatively recent development of a body of knowledge and expertise in the field. Unlike pediatric disorders such as asthma or diabetes, there is a lack of a common language with families and referring primary care workers to describe children's problems. As general public awareness of selected disorders such as autism and ADHD increases, there is a tendency for families and referrers to adhere to these in preference to others, such as general intellectual disability or oppositional defiant disorder. In addition, the lack of expertise in primary care—whether health, educational or social—in the management of comparatively mild child mental health problems has meant that CAMHS and therapists in effect have been expected to deliver both a primary care type service—where treatment tends to be generic and the use of diagnoses is less central—and disorder-related specialist work.

Better general knowledge about different types of child psychiatric disorders and new expertise by primary care workers in the management of milder problems may result from recent electronic teaching packages—such as the Mind-Ed program in the United Kingdom—and by continuing efforts to close the gap between primary care and specialist CAMHS (www.mind. org.uk; Kramer & Garralda, 2015). In primary care, for example, the use of targeted inquiry can successfully assist general practitioners in the differentiation between adolescent emotional turmoil and depressive disorder, and in putting into place well-informed management strategies. It may be expected this will lead to the more severe and complex problems being referred to specialist CAMHS and to the growth of disorder-specific services.

The Importance of Generic Psychosocial Influences for Child and Adolescent Mental Health

The undeniable role of dysfunctional psychosocial, family, and school environments for the development and/or maintenance of child psychiatric disorders has strongly influenced how problems have been viewed and managed in CAMHS and the use of generic over disorder-specific treatments. Some children, for example, are presented with difficulties involving stress in parent–child relationships without necessarily being linked to mental health problems in the child (Carrey & Gregson, 2008). Expertise in CAMHS has often focused on techniques to reduce stress, convey therapeutic empathy and understanding to the child, and improve parenting techniques and family relationships. These techniques in expert hands can be beneficial for children with any type and level of difficulty, in the same way that antipyretics are helpful for many types of febrile illness, or advice and expert help to engage in a healthy lifestyle for many different types of physical disorders. Some of these trans-diagnostic techniques will remain important and helpful.

Nevertheless, diagnosis of individual disorders as described in ICD and DSM has been central to empirical evaluations of both psychotherapeutic and medical treatments for child and adolescent mental health problems. Specific disorder-based treatments include certain kinds of family therapy for anorexia nervosa, parenting work for conduct disorders, cognitive behavioral therapies for mood disorders, specific medications for ADHD, schizophrenia, or other psychotic states, and for anxiety and depressive disorders. Increasingly specialist diagnostic and treatment CAMHS are being developed for disorders such as autism, ADHD, mood disorders, and obsessive compulsive disorder, and pediatric liaison services for children with joint medical and psychiatric problems. Bodies such as NICE (National Institute for Health and Care Excellence) in the United Kingdom—which aims to help practitioners deliver the best possible care for physical and mental disorders, to provide the most effective treatments based on the most up-to-date evidence, and provide value for money—have published guidelines on a number of diagnosis-based child psychiatric disorders (https://www.nice.org.uk).

Even so, it is well-established that in child psychiatric practice, specific techniques will often need to be complemented by trans-diagnostic interventions as mentioned above.

The Usefulness of a Combined Categorical/Dimensional Approach

Within multidisciplinary CAMHS, different staff members will have varying levels of expertise in the diagnosis of CAMH problems. Although a key aspect of diagnosis is the integration of individual features into clinically useful categories, in practice diagnosis is helpfully complemented by dimensional approaches (Taylor & Rutter, 2008), with the use of rating scales—generic or specific—to reliably document symptom severity and clinical change. A combined categorical/dimensional approach is also helpful to identify children and young people with subsyndromal but impairing symptoms. An example of a particularly user-friendly generic measure for CAMHS is HoNOSCA (Health of the Nation Outcome Scales for Children and Adolescents), a clinician-rated scale with good international interrater reliability, which has been validated as an appropriate proxy for diagnosis and is fit for use by diagnosticians and therapists alike, for clinical and administrative purposes, and for research (Garralda, 2009).

"Children Do Not Read Textbooks": Problem Complexity

There is a notion that children's problems do not easily fit into diagnostic categories, exemplified by the phrase "children do not read textbooks." This may be related to limitations in disorder specificity of existing classifications, or to insufficiently focused clinical inquiry. It may, however, also reflect the fact that many children with the more severe problems seen in specialist CAMHS display challenging psychiatric and neurodevelopmental comorbidities, all of which need to be identified and inform their management. For a number of cases this will call for a broad, carefully monitored management plan, one that takes into account individual psychopathological manifestations and uses different therapeutic tools at different time points.

In some cases comorbid disorders will be early manifestations of an emerging personality disorder. Personality disorders are conceptualized in ICD-11 as "a relatively enduring and pervasive disturbance in how individuals experience and interpret themselves, others and the world" resulting in maladaptive patterns of cognition, emotional experience and behavior, and significant problems in psychosocial functioning and interpersonal relationships. Personality disorders will be diagnosed by the severity of the interpersonal difficulties and qualified not in terms of traditional categories but of predominant features (negative affective, dissocial, disinhibition, anankastic, detachment) (Tyrer, Reed, & Crawford, 2015). These difficulties may well be adult manifestations of childhood psychiatric, neuro-developmental, dissocial, and mood disorders. Future research should help clarify the extent of their developmental congruence and shared underlying risks.

Diagnoses, Labels, Stigmatization

Does making a diagnosis label and stigmatize children? Is a particular diagnosis more or less stigmatizing than having general "mental health issues"? Does a diagnosis of conduct disorder stigmatize children over and above the negative consequences of dissocial or antisocial behavior per se, or does it on the contrary help others understand it with a kinder, well-informed perspective? Do the adverse consequences of pigeon-holing children through diagnosis outweigh the advantages of being offered efficacious treatments? These topics have been and will continue to be discussed and are addressed elsewhere in this book. In balancing the advantages and disadvantages of child psychiatric diagnoses, it is important to acknowledge the innate wish to understand problems by giving them a meaningful name and by accessing professional expertise to help with management and coping. Nevertheless it is also obviously important to be sensitive to children's and families' views on these issues and to act accordingly.

Diagnosis and Formulation

Because of their multilayered etiology and management, it is well-recognized that child psychiatric diagnoses need to be supplemented by a formulation of the children's problems that reflects the individuality of their predicament (Carrey & Gregson, 2008). A popular way of reflecting this in practice is through grids outlining underlying risk and protective predisposing, precipitant and maintaining factors in the child, family or circumstance/environment, the identification of maintaining factors being especially relevant for management.

FINAL CONSIDERATIONS

It is of course important to recognize that psychiatric disorders are human constructs and works in progress. As attributed to Jaspers, "the idea of a disease entity is not an objective to be reached, but our most fruitful point of orientation." Diagnoses need to adapt and change in the light of new knowledge and expertise. The ultimate goal is to integrate knowledge, aid communication between all those involved, and open the way for new and better understanding of mental health problems.

It is increasingly accepted that the "child is the father of the man" (and the mother of the woman!) and that child and adolescent mental health problems should be "everybody's business." The continuing improvement in our understanding of child psychiatric disorders, their assessment and management should help achieve a better recognition by society and medicine of their importance for children, families and adults alike, and contribute to a better adjusted population.

Declaration of Interests

The author chairs WHO's ICD-11 Working Groups on Neurodevelopmental Disorders and Disruptive Dissocial Disorders, but the views expressed in this chapter are the author's and not representative of WHO or of its Working Groups. The descriptions of ICD disorders in this chapter reflect work in progress.

References

American Psychiatric Association. (1994). *Diagnostic and statistical manual of mental disorders* (4th ed.). Washington DC: American Psychiatric Association.

American Psychiatric Association. (2013). *Diagnostic and statistical manual of mental disorders* (5th ed.). Washington DC: American Psychiatric Association.

Andrews, G., Pine, D. S., Hobbs, M. J., Anderson, T. M., & Sunderland, M. (2009). Neurodevelopmental disorders: cluster 2 of the proposed meta-structure for DSMV and ICD11. *Psychological Medicine, 39*, 2013–2023.

Carrey, N., & Gregson, J. (2008). A context for classification in child psychiatry. *Journal of the Canadian Academy of Child and Adolescent Psychiatry, 17*, 50–57.

Cooper, J. E., & Sartorius, N. (2013). *A companion to the classification of mental disorders.* Oxford: Oxford University Press.

Fairchild, G., van Goozen, S. H. M., Calder, A. J., & Goodyer, I. M. (2013). Review: evaluating and reformulating the developmental taxonomic theory of antisocial behaviour. *Journal of Child Psychology and Psychiatry, 54*, 924–940.

Frick, J. P., & White, S. F. (2008). Research Review: the importance of callous unemotional traits for developmental models of aggressive and antisocial behaviour. *Journal of Child Psychology and Psychiatry, 49*, 359–375.

Garralda, M. E. (2009). Accountability of specialist child and adolescent mental health services. *British Journal of Psychiatry, 194*, 389–391.

Huerta, M., Bishop, S. L., Duncan, A., Hus, V., & Lord, C. (2012). Application of DSM-5 criteria for autism spectrum disorder to three samples of children with DSM-IV diagnoses of pervasive developmental disorders. *American Journal of Psychiatry, 169*, 1056–1064.

Insel, T., Cuthbert, B., Riegarvey, M., Heinssen, R., Pine, D. S., Quinn, K., ... Wang, P. (2010). Research domain criteria (RDoC): toward a new classification framework for research on mental disorders. *American Journal of Psychiatry, 167*, 748–751.

Kent, R. G., Carrington, S. J., Le Couteur, A., Gould, J., Wing, L., Maljaars, J., ... Leekam, S. R. (2013). Diagnosing autism spectrum disorder: who will get a DSM-5 diagnosis? *Journal of Child Psychology and Psychiatry, 54*, 1242–1250.

Kramer, T., & Garralda, M. E. (2015). Assessment and treatment in non-specialist community health care settings. In A. Thapar, D. S. Pine, J. F. Leckman, S. Scott, M. J. Snowling, & E. A. Taylor (Eds.), *Rutter's child and adolescent psychiatry* (6th ed.) (pp. 623–635). Oxford: Wiley-Blackwell. ISBN: 978-1-118-38196-0. Chapter 49.

Lochman, J. E., Evans, S. C., Burke, J. D., Roberts, M. C., Fite, P. J., Reed, G. M., ... Garralda, M. E. (2015). An empirically based alternative to DSM-5's disruptive mood dysregulation disorder for ICD-11. *World Psychiatry, 14*, 30–33.

Lord, C., & Jones, R. M. (2012). Re-thinking the classification of autism spectrum disorders. *Journal of Child Psychology and Psychiatry, 53*, 490–509.

Mandy, P. L., Charman, T., & Skuse, D. H. (2012). Testing the construct validity of proposed criteria for *DSM-5* autism spectrum disorder. *Journal of the American Academy of Child and Adolescent Psychiatry, 51*, 41–50.

Norbury, C. F. (2014). Practitioner review: social (pragmatic) communication disorder conceptualization, evidence and clinical implications. *Journal of Child Psychology and Psychiatry, 55*, 204–216.

Reed, G. M., Mendonca Correia, J., Esparza, P., Saxena, S., & Maj, M. (2011). The WPA-WHO global survey of psychiatrists' attitudes towards mental disorders classifications. *World Psychiatry, 10,* 118–131.

Reed, G. M., Rebello, T. J., Pike, K. M., Medina-Mora, M. E., Gureje, O., Zhao, M., … Saxena, S. (May 2015). *WHO's global clinical practice network for mental health* (Vol 2). www.thelancet.com/psychiatry.

Rutter, M. (2011). Research review: child psychiatric diagnosis and classification: concepts, findings, challenges and potential. *Journal of Child Psychology and Psychiatry, 52,* 647–660.

Swedo, S. E., Baird, G., Cook, E. H., Happe, F. G., Harris, J. C., Kaufmann, W. E., … Wright, H. H. (2012). Commentary from the DSM-5 workgroup on neurodevelopmental disorders. *Journal of the American Academy of Child and Adolescent Psychiatry, 51,* 347–349.

Taylor, E., & Rutter, M. (2008). Classification. In M. Rutter, D. Bishop, D. Pine, S. Scott, J. S. Stevenson, E. A. Taylor, & A. Thapar (Eds.), *Rutter's child and adolescent psychiatry* (5th ed.). Oxford: Blackwell. Chapter 2.

Tyrer, P., Reed, G. M., & Crawford, M. J. (2015). Personality disorder 1- classification, assessment, prevalence, and effect of personality disorder. *Lancet, 385,* 727–734.

WHO. (1992). *The ICD-10 classification of mental and behavioural disorders: Clinical descriptions and diagnostic guidelines.* Geneva: World Health Organization.

PART II

RISK AND RESILIENCE

Disorders of Brain Development: Understanding Childhood Psychopathology

F.P. MacMaster[1], M. Sembo[1], L.M. Langevin[1], K. Ma[1], P. Croarkin[2]

[1]University of Calgary, Calgary, AB, Canada; [2]Mayo Clinic College of Medicine, Rochester, MN, United States

INTRODUCTION

For many decades, understanding the underlying biological underpinnings of neuropsychiatric diseases in children and adolescents has been elusive. However, with the advent of new methods to evaluate brain structure, chemistry, and function, investigators are beginning to understand the role brain development plays in neuropsychiatric disorders. The application of these new neuroscientific techniques to describe the biology of mental disorders can lead to improved diagnosis and innovative treatments. Moreover, studies of brain development may find the critical timeperiods during which brain abnormalities could lead to mental illness. Indeed, most mental disorders begin during childhood and adolescence. This would indicate a role of brain development. In this chapter, we first discuss core brain imaging techniques. Second, we address normal brain development. Third, we summarize relevant findings from brain imaging studies of mental illness in childhood and adolescence.

NEUROSCIENTIFIC METHODS TO STUDY OF BRAIN DEVELOPMENT IN VIVO

Until recently, our understanding of the biology of brain development was limited to post-mortem work. This was insufficient to develop an

Positive Mental Health, Fighting Stigma and Promoting Resiliency for Children and Adolescents
http://dx.doi.org/10.1016/B978-0-12-804394-3.00003-6

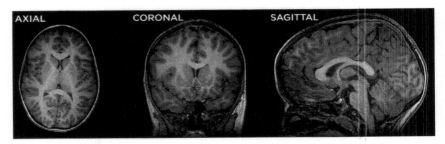

FIGURE 3.1   Sample magnetic resonance imaging scan showing the axial, coronal, and sagittal views.

understanding of mental illness that occurs in childhood and adolescence. The introduction of brain imaging techniques overcame this obstacle. As magnetic resonance imaging (MRI) does not use ionizing radiation as computed tomography (CT) does, the safety profile allows for repeated measures over time safely. Further, MRI has supplanted quantitative CT in brain research due to its better resolution and tissue contrast.

Brain Structure

Studies of human brain morphology include the examination of specific structures, volume, and shape. Data for morphological analysis is typically obtained by two methods: (1) MRI (see Figs. 3.1 and 3.2) and (2) CT, both of which are performed on living human brains and have been non-invasively applied to children and adolescents. Initial studies focused on determining the presence of visible lesions, based on traditional radiological methods. Initially this appeared to have meager utility, as mental illness does not always involve a visible lesion but is often associated with distributed changes across a number of brain regions. As the field evolved, more quantitative approaches were employed, including discriminative examinations of related conditions, including bipolar disorder (BD) and major depressive disorder (MDD). Using brain volume analysis, researchers determined that the anterior cingulate cortex was smaller in individuals with MDD than BD (MacMaster, Carrey, Langevin, Jaworska, & Crawford, 2014). Since BD and MDD initially present very similarly, the ability to distinguish these disorders through quick and non-invasive means has many implications for faster treatments and beneficial outcomes. MRI-based analyses also help to forge new pathways for earlier diagnosis of pathological conditions as related to a typical cohort. In one study aimed at investigating attention-deficit/hyperactivity disorder (ADHD), researchers discovered thickness reductions in the prefrontal cortex, a region involved in response

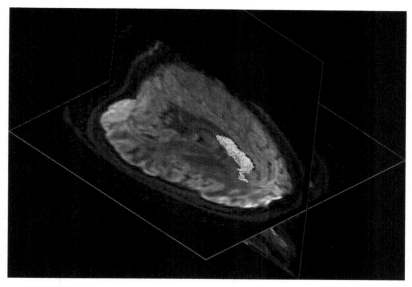

FIGURE 3.2   Sample diffusion tensor image showing white matter tracts.

inhibition and attention when compared to healthy controls (Yang, Carrey, Bernier, & MacMaster, 2012). Current conceptualizations of cortical thickness and other basic morphological studies using MRI are validated and enhanced using diffusion tensor imaging, which permits the study of the integrity and organization of white matter tracts (see Fig. 3.2). Combinatorial approaches such as these are currently being used to help understand the overlapping neurobiology of ADHD and motor disorders, as these conditions are frequently comorbid (Langevin, MacMaster, Crawford, Lebel, & Dewey, 2014). Multimodal studies have also advanced the understanding of white matter changes in children through adulthood (Lebel, Walker, Leemans, Phillips, & Beaulieu, 2008). Structural studies therefore offer insight into the foundations of normal development, as well as critical information on disease course, and the effects of intervention, if any.

Brain Chemistry

The physiological functioning of the brain in childhood psychopathology is not well understood. However, examination of different bioactive compounds in the brain can yield many clues as to disease onset and progression, and also informs potential targets for intervention. Major advances in the field of molecular central nervous system (CNS) imaging have allowed the development of three commonly used tools for understanding brain chemistry in the context of mental health disorders. Single photon emission computed tomography (SPECT), positron emission tomography (PET), and magnetic resonance spectroscopy (MRS) provide specific advantages and disadvantages inherent in their approach at both the diagnostic and pharmaceutical level.

SPECT and PET have limited use in children and adolescents due to the requirement for injection of radioactive isotopes. However, the utility of both methods has been exemplified in studies aimed at improving the understanding of mental illness in children and adolescents (Ernst, 1999). In autism spectrum disorders (ASD), PET has been used to evaluate the role of serotonin in brain development and its connection to ASD, demonstrating that asymmetry in the synthesis of serotonin was associated with specific behavioral sequelae (Chandana et al., 2005). PET additionally allows for the study of regional cerebral blood flow, glucose metabolism, and neurochemistry—including certain neurotransmitters, transporters, and receptors. Despite these advantages, the application of radioisotopes in young people has not been studied longitudinally, and benefits must be weighed heavily against the potential for harm. Controlled studies are also challenging to conduct due to inherent ethical concerns.

MRS methods are akin to MRI in that no ionizing radiation is used, effectively bypassing the safety limitations of PET and SPECT. However, the capacity to probe various biological compounds is more limited. Spectra that are quantifiable using MRS include phosphorus (^{31}P), carbon (^{13}C), fluorine (^{19}F), sodium (^{23}Na), and proton (^{1}H) compounds. Phosphorous and proton MRS are the two most commonly used in studies involving children and adolescents (see Stanley et al., 2008; MacMaster et al., 2008). Proton MRS permits the study of a wide variety of neurotransmitters, hormone, and metabolic compounds, which may play a role in both the onset and severity of disease. ^{1}H-MRS provides measures of N-acetyl-aspartate, a neuronal marker; creatine/phosphocreatine, involved in energy metabolism; choline compounds, membrane components; myoinositol, a secondary messenger involved in signal transduction; and glutamate, glutamine, and γ-aminobutyric acid (GABA)—all of which occur in relatively high concentrations in brain (see Fig. 3.3). ^{31}P-MRS allows for the analysis of membrane synthesis (phosphomonoesters (PMEs) like phosphoethanolamine and phosphocholine) and breakdown (phosphodiesters (PDEs) like glycerophosphoethanolamine and glycerophosphocholine), along with substrates of energy metabolism. Coupled with existing diagnostic paradigms, using magnetic resonance imaging to predict and describe psychopathological conditions allows for more precise, accurate, and standardized predictions, and may lead to improved response and interventions.

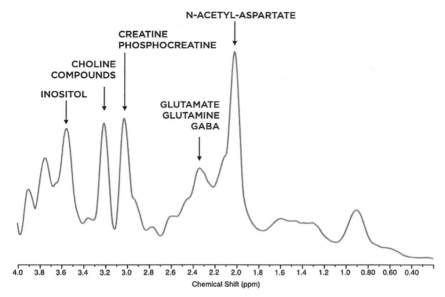

FIGURE 3.3   Sample spectra using proton (¹H) magnetic resonance spectroscopy.

Brain Function

Functional MRI, or fMRI, has become a prominent tool in the study of development and mental illness in children and adolescents. Fundamentally, fMRI detects changes in blood flow, thus requiring the use of carefully designed neurobehavioral paradigms to generate activation signals, and perturb the resting neuronal circuitry (see Fig. 3.4). fMRI task-based studies have been used to examine inhibitory control in youth with obsessive-compulsive disorder (OCD) compared to healthy controls (Woolley et al., 2008), uncovering reduced activation in frontal brain centers—a region involved in response inhibition and attentional processes. New methical techniques being developed for fMRI allow for the examination of "baseline" or "resting-state" activity. The study of the default mode network, regions of the brain displaying synchronous activity while not engaged in higher-order tasks, offers an innovative method for determining differences in brain function between groups and conditions, including age-related changes in connectivity within specific networks (Vinette & Bray, 2015).

Considerations

There are two practical considerations regarding the execution of MRI based studies in pediatric and adolescent participants. First, the

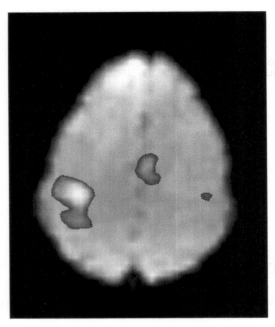

FIGURE 3.4 Sample functional magnetic resonance imaging data showing brain activity during a simple finger-tapping task.

requirement for remaining still can be challenging even for healthy children. Further, movement artifact is common in children with mental illness and other neurodevelopmental conditions, including ADHD and motor disorders. Second, anxiety induced by being in a confined space can limit comfort and the capacity to acquire accurate images. Although this reaction occurs in a minority of patients, the effect of motion artifacts is a major technological impediment to the utility of imaging data. Sedation is an option for more emergent, clinical scan procedures, but due to its inherent risks it is not typically applied in research studies involving children and adolescents. Training subjects with a "mock scanner" (see Fig. 3.5) prior to the actual scan reduces subjective distress and heart rate, facilitating the successful completion of most research studies. Other technical considerations in structural brain imaging include the tremendous variation in brain structure, function, and chemistry over the course of childhood into adolescence. Cognitive task-based imaging data may be influenced by performance on tasks and functions under scrutiny. Children may participate poorly on a task in the scanner should they consider it too difficult or too boring. Tailoring task difficulty to individual abilities and age helps ensure consistent performance across subjects at different developmental stages.

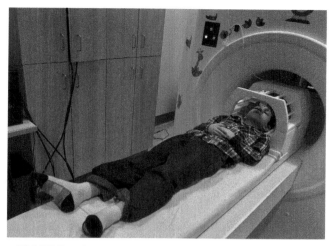

FIGURE 3.5 Picture showing a mock scanner environment.

TYPICAL DEVELOPMENT

Complete understanding of typical brain development is the key requirement for examining abnormal changes that accompany mental illness. Overall brain size increases significantly from in utero through to 2 years of age. It is during this time that synaptogenesis, the formation of synapses between brain cells (neurons), is most active. In the time frame leading up to early adolescence, two major dynamic processes are ongoing in the maturing brain. These are (1) synaptic pruning and (2) myelination. Synaptic pruning is the process of synapse elimination, associated with both regulation of required synaptic connections, and terminal pruning associated with learning and memory. Myelination is formation of the myelin sheath around a nerve to allow for improved conduction. It is thought that increased myelination, connectivity, and changing functional activation patterns indicate that increasingly efficient connections between brain regions are being made from childhood into adulthood.

Gray matter volume (consisting of neuronal bodies, neuropil, glia synapses, and capillaries) peaks in mid-childhood into early adolescence, briefly plateaus then decreases following puberty (Courchesne et al., 2000). Gray matter volume maturation roughly parallels changes in local cerebral metabolic rates for glucose as a function of age (Chugani, 1998) (see Fig. 3.6 for schematic). These changes represent the consequence of synaptic pruning—an increase in the efficiency of neural processing. It is essential to note that brain development is heterochronous; meaning the timing, degree, and rate of cortical and subcortical gray

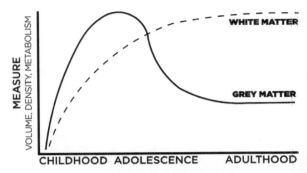

FIGURE 3.6   Simple schematic showing the general developmental trend for the brain from childhood through adulthood.

matter change are regionally specific. White matter volume increases more linearly through childhood into adolescence (Courchesne et al., 2000), with connections being formed during maturation. The corpus callosum, which connects the right and left hemispheres of the brain and topographically maps onto the cortex, with both sex-specific synaptogenesis in associated cortical regions, appears to parallel the increase in associative reasoning skills (Thompson et al., 2000). Interestingly, the dorsolateral prefrontal cortex (DLPFC), a brain region critical in executive function, shows the most dramatic increase in white matter during the infant and early childhood period, when individual inhibitory and attentional processes develop.

Biological sex also plays an important role in the development of the brain. Parietal and frontal gray matter volume was found to peak earlier in females and then decline after puberty, while temporal lobe gray matter volume reached its peak in both sexes at approximately the same time (Giedd et al., 1999). Subcortically, basal ganglia, hippocampus, and amygdala also appear to be influenced by sex (Durston et al., 2001). Gray matter loss in the basal ganglia is dramatic in boys between the ages of 6 to 12 years. In girls, the hippocampus increases more than in boys with age, while the reverse is true for the amygdala. These maturational alterations coincide with sex-specific differences in the timing of puberty and suggest a role for gonadal hormones on brain development. Differential sex trajectories of specific brain regions may be reflected in preponderance of specific disorders within each sex that are associated with those regions (ie, basal ganglia—OCD and ADHD in males, and MDD in females). Finally, the pituitary gland demonstrates a striking gender difference (MacMaster et al., 2007), with females developing a larger pituitary gland than males, particularly during adolescence. Again, this may be associated with the differential timing of puberty in males and females.

FINDINGS IN MENTAL ILLNESS

ADHD

Attention-deficit/hyperactivity disorder begins in childhood and occurs in approximately 5% of children. Diagnostic criteria include a pattern of persistent inattention or hyperactivity-impulsivity that must be present in multiple settings (home, school, work), and negatively influence academic and social functioning. This pattern of behavior interferes severely with activities of daily living and/or development. Inattentive symptoms include difficulty focusing on a task and a lack of persistence, and are not due to a lack of comprehension, hostility, or defiance. Hyperactivity refers to inappropriate and excessive motor activity, fidgeting, or talkativeness. Impulsive symptoms are actions that are taken without forethought and that have a high potential of harm to the child. In order to be diagnosed with ADHD, a child must display several developmentally inappropriate symptoms of inattention or hyperactivity-impulsivity in at least two different settings for a minimum of six months before the age of 12 years. Children with ADHD are often rejected by their peers, and in turn are at higher risk for academic problems, school dropout, delinquency, substance abuse, and higher rates of psychopathology.

ADHD is reasonably consistent in expression throughout the lifespan. Consequently, studies of the disorder in children, close to the onset of the illness, are relevant to understanding ADHD into adulthood. Fundamental deficits in attention, arousal, and impulse control distinguish children with ADHD, while symptoms of inattention predominate in later life. The core brain region implicated in these functions is the prefrontal cortex—the seat of "executive" control. Given the pivotal role in attention and inhibition, the prefrontal cortex is a key target in the investigation of the pathophysiology of ADHD. Smaller prefrontal cortical volumes and thickness have been reliably noted in MRI studies of children with ADHD (Almeida et al., 2010; Yang et al., 2012). A landmark study of children with ADHD demonstrated that the structural maturation of the prefrontal cortex lags behind typically developing children by 2–3 years (Shaw et al., 2007). The behavioral ramifications of frontal executive development delays can represent significant deficits in age-appropriate behaviors and failure to achieve academic success at their grade level. Phosphorus magnetic resonance spectroscopy (^{31}P-MRS) has demonstrated lower concentrations of membrane phospholipid precursors in older ADHD children as compared to healthy children (Stanley et al., 2008, 2006), suggesting a possible disruption of the neuronal processes and synaptogenesis in children with ADHD.

Developmental studies of ADHD have highlighted the importance of regional brain connections, and have described a bottom-up trajectory to developmental dysfunction—beginning in the basal ganglia and progressing to the prefrontal cortex. Abnormalities in the basal ganglia have been consistently observed in children with ADHD prior to the onset of alterations in frontal brain regions (Carrey et al., 2012; Castellanos et al., 1994; Soliva et al., 2010). Converging evidence from independent samples using different measures (volumetric and spectroscopic methods) have found early deficits in the basal ganglia (Carrey et al., 2012; Stanley et al., 2008, 2006), which may in turn affect prefrontal cortex development (Stanley et al., 2008, 2006; Yang et al., 2012). ^{1}H-MRS studies of children with ADHD found greater concentrations of frontal-striatal glutamatergic levels in medication-free pediatric patients as compared to age- and sex-matched controls (Carrey et al., 2012, 2003; Carrey, MacMaster, Sparkes, Khan, & Kusumakar, 2002; MacMaster, Carrey, Sparkes, & Kusumakar, 2003). This bottom-up change in developmental trajectory may be at the heart of ADHD and warrants further longitudinal studies.

The basal ganglia and its substructures—caudate, putamen, and globus pallidus—have been implicated in the pathophysiology of several other disorders, including Tourette's syndrome, motor disorders, and OCD. This may account for the high degree of comorbidity among these conditions in children. Developmental coordination disorder (DCD) is commonly comorbid with ADHD in children. Recently, it was found that children with comorbid DCD and ADHD had more widespread decreases in cortical thickness when compared to children with a diagnosis of DCD or ADHD alone (Langevin, MacMaster, & Dewey, 2014). This cortical thinning was found to be concentrated in the frontal, parietal, and temporal lobes, and was associated with poorer motor and attentional functioning. Structural studies of white matter in comorbid DCD and ADHD also found reductions in fractional anisotropy (FA) (ie, white matter integrity) in both frontal and parietal regions (Langevin et al., 2014). In children with ADHD alone, abnormalities were concentrated in frontal regions of the corpus callosum. In children with DCD, regions of the corpus callosum that connect parietal brain regions and the left superior longitudinal fasciculus were implicated. These studies suggest that comorbidity of DCD and ADHD may be reflected in a combined neurobiology that is distinct from the individual disorders.

Stimulants including methylphenidate are the first-line treatment for ADHD. A meta-analysis of fMRI studies that examined the effect of stimulants on brain function in ADHD found that stimulants consistently enhanced right inferior frontal cortex and insula activation, with a smaller effect on putamen activation (Rubia et al., 2014). The inferior frontal cortex and insula play critical roles in cognitive control and are commonly implicated in ADHD. In children with ADHD who respond to methylphenidate, greater caudate gray matter is observed compared to non-responders in the caudate (Moreno et al., 2014). This finding is consistent with previous studies that show that a larger posterior hippocampus predicts a better response to antidepressants in adults with major depressive disorder (MacQueen & Frodl, 2011; MacQueen, Yucel, Taylor, Macdonald, & Joffe, 2008). The feasibility of imaging to predict treatment response has yet to be fully investigated in child and adolescent psychiatry, and relies on furthering neuroimaging research into pediatric and adolescent mental illness.

Anxiety Disorders

Anxiety disorders include multiple conditions associated with fear, anxiety, and related behavioral disturbances. Although anxiety disorders differ from one another in the types of objects or situations that induce avoidant behavior, they share the common symptom of excessive or persistent fear or anxiety that is not developmentally appropriate. Generalized anxiety disorder (GAD) involves excessive worry that the individual finds hard to control and that causes significant distress in social, occupational, or other areas of functioning. Children with GAD worry excessively about their competence and performance, or about catastrophic events, with the focus of the worry shifting from one concern to another. This excessive worry impairs the individual's ability to do things quickly and efficiently, and can cause fatigue, difficulty concentrating, and sleep disturbances. GAD therefore has negative social, academic, and occupational implications. Anxiety disorders such as GAD differ from stress-induced fear or typical anxiety by their persistence, and overestimation of situational danger. Diagnosing clinicians must ascertain whether fear is excessive or out of proportion based on the available contextual information. Many anxiety disorders develop in childhood and will persist if untreated.

The amygdala represents a major component of cortical-limbic circuitry, and plays an important role in the processing of anxiety or fear. Indeed, fMRI studies have found exaggerated amygdala activation in response to fearful faces in children with GAD (McClure et al., 2007). Functional connectivity between the amygdala and medial prefrontal cortex, insula, and cerebellum is disturbed (Hamm et al., 2014), and volumetric studies have also demonstrated greater cortical thickness in brain regions involved in fear learning and extinction, and mentalization (Strawn et al., 2014). In response to a continuous performance task with emotional distractors, greater activation in the left medial prefrontal cortex and right ventrolateral prefrontal cortex was observed in adolescents with GAD (Strawn et al., 2012). Functional alterations in GAD may also reflect hypoactivity, indicating function-dependent deficits. When treated with either medication or cognitive behavior therapy, right ventrolateral prefrontal cortex activation related to emotional faces increased in children with GAD (Maslowsky et al., 2010). Subcortical regions are also affected in GAD.

The right putamen is larger compared to controls, with mistreated children also showing larger left thalamic volumes (Liao et al., 2014). Combinatorial deficits underscore the emerging consensus that brain structure and circuitry is heavily influenced by previous experiences. GAD is therefore characterized by the aberrant activation of the amygdala. Further research is required to determine the impact of dysfunctional fear conditioning, and the effects of brain structure and function on these responses.

As discussed above, fear conditioning involves core reciprocal communication between the amygdala, hippocampus, and medial prefrontal cortex (PFC) (Marek, Strobel, Bredy, & Sah, 2013). In brief, the hippocampal projections to the medial PFC inform the infralimbic circuitry where convergent excitatory and inhibitory stimuli converge (Bennett, Hatton, & Lagopoulos, 2015). Oscillations in activity produce both the retrieval and extinction of fear responses in a context-dependent manner. Smaller hippocampal volumes have been consistently found in adults with chronic post-traumatic stress disorder (PTSD) but not in children with PTSD (Woon & Hedges, 2008). Smaller whole-brain, prefrontal cortical, and right temporal lobe volumes are observed in children with PTSD and are associated with an earlier age of onset and longer duration of abuse (De Bellis et al., 2002). Given the mixed evidence, discrete neurobiological profiles may be presented in pediatric versus adult patients with PTSD. Longitudinal studies are needed to better characterize the developmental neurobiology of PTSD. Careful assessment for comorbid disorders—ie, anxiety and depression—is also essential to determine unique neurobiological pathways among different anxiety disorders and depression.

ASD

Autism spectrum disorder (ASD) describes an array of conditions characterized by impairments in communication, social interaction, and relationships, involving restricted and repetitive interests and behaviors. This disorder is reported in 1% of the population, and manifests both verbally and non-verbally as intellectual deficits, language impairments, and dysfunctional motor control. The spectrum aspect of ASD indicates that the manifestation and severity of symptoms can vary greatly among individuals. However, differential diagnostic criteria for ASD do require symptoms to be present from early childhood and to impair daily functioning. It is important to note that some individuals with ASD are not diagnosed until later in life, when social demands begin to exceed their capacity. The social impairment associated with ASD can have negative effects on learning and academic achievement. Other consequences include difficulty coping with change, organization, or planning. In adulthood, many individuals with ASD struggle with independent living, poor communication, and social isolation.

Research into the underlying neurobiology of ASD has been rapidly increasing over the last decade. The number of imaging studies investigating ASD has increased four-fold since 2003. This remarkable growth occurred despite limitations that plagued the study of ASD. Early studies into ASD were hampered by participant bias and majority inclusion of high-functioning adult populations. When considering the age of onset for ASD, this distal approach was limiting. There have been several advances made in scanning young children, such as the use of mock scanners and thoughtful approaches to scanning procedures that have allowed very young children, as well as individuals with complex deficits attributed to ASD, to contribute to research (Barnea-Goraly et al., 2014). The diverse genetic and environmental factors that have been identified as risk factors for ASD converge to generate multiple phenotypes through multiple pathogenic mechanisms. One growing consensus on the neurobiological model for ASD reflects widespread and diffuse alterations in connectivity, volume, and chemistry (Pardo & Eberhart, 2007). Although genetic variations contribute to over half the incidence of ASD, differing forms of heterozygosity, frequency, inheritance, and copy number variations combine to add to the complexity of the genetic pattern (Anney et al., 2012; Gaugler et al., 2014). Structural neuropathologies of ASD and autism are equally complex, involving multiple cortical and subcortical domains, and variant biomarkers including thickened gray matter, irregular lamination, and poor gray-white boundaries (Casanova, 2006). Alterations in brain growth trajectories are involved in the pathogenesis of ASD. The growth curve of whole brain volume demonstrated larger volumes in young children with autism that subsequently decreased during adolescence to meet the typically developing control curve between the ages of 10 and 15 years (Lange et al., 2015). In the ASD group, the volume of many structures continued to decline atypically into adulthood.

These diffuse and global changes suggest dynamic and complex alterations in whole and regional brain volumes in ASD over development from childhood into adulthood (Lange et al., 2015). In the frontal lobe, older age in ASD was associated with reductions in the putative neuronal health marker N-acetyl-aspartate (Aoki, Kasai, & Yamasue, 2012). Large cohort studies have revealed that very young children (6–10 years) with higher autistic traits (scores on the social responsiveness scale) showed extensive areas of decreased gyrification (Blanken et al., 2015). Functional connectivity is reduced in adult populations, while younger individuals with ASD reflect increases in intrinsic functional connectivity (Cerliani et al., 2015; Khan et al., 2015; Murdaugh, Maximo, & Kana, 2015). Using PET technologies, deficits in serotonin synthesis were observed in children with ASD compared to their siblings and children with epilepsy (Chugani et al., 1999). In typically developing children, whole-brain serotonin synthesis capacity is greater than 200% of adult capacity until 5 years of age, and then it declines to adult levels. In children with ASD however, serotonin synthesis capacity increased very gradually from age 2 to 15 years to levels 1 to 1.5 times adult normal values. These functional findings may reflect the altered anatomical trajectories, and complex alterations associated with ASD.

Childhood-Onset Schizophrenia

Childhood-onset schizophrenia is a chronic, severe form of schizophrenia, which is often presented as treatment-resistant (Nicolson & Rapoport, 1999). In order to be diagnosed with schizophrenia, delusions, hallucinations, and/or disorganized speech must be present for a period of at least one month, accompanied by grossly disorganized or catatonic behavior, or diminished emotional expression or avolition. A child diagnosed with childhood-onset schizophrenia may experience depersonalization or derealization, as well as inappropriate affect, a dysphoric mood, somatic complaints, and sleep disturbances. There may be a lack of awareness of symptoms associated with the disorder, which can further complicate treatment and prognosis. These individuals may experience persistent cognitive impairments and severe negative symptoms. Earlier onset schizophrenia is associated with poorer prognosis, therefore those diagnosed in childhood are more likely to experience academic difficulties, problems maintaining employment, and limited social contact later in life.

Animal and post-mortem studies have revealed multidimensional brain alterations that give rise to the biological mechanisms underlying psychosis. Modeling studies have found contributing factors in the form of neuronal migration, intracellular transport, neurogenesis, synaptic regulation, and current responses (Samsom & Wong, 2015). One consistent finding in adult schizophrenia is smaller total brain volume accompanied by larger ventricles. The decrease in brain volume is even more dramatic in childhood-onset schizophrenia (Sowell, Toga, & Asarnow, 2000) and is accompanied by ventriculomegaly. Lower concentrations of the neuronal marker N-acetyl-aspartate and frontal/anterior cingulate gray matter volumes are observed in both patients with childhood-onset schizophrenia and unaffected offspring of patients with schizophrenia at increased risk for developing schizophrenia when compared to controls (Seese et al., 2011). This is suggestive of an amplified pruning of neurons that may be involved in the pathogenesis of schizophrenia. The smaller amount of brain tissue in childhood-onset schizophrenia may be the result of a progressive loss of both gray and white matter in periventricular regions. Slower growth rates were found in parietal white matter in young patients with childhood-onset schizophrenia (Gogtay et al., 2008), but conversely, the corpus callosum did not demonstrate any deviations in volume or growth trajectory (Keller et al., 2003). Additionally, fractional anisotropy in the cuneus is reduced in childhood-onset schizophrenia in comparison to healthy controls (Moran et al., 2015). Disruption in cuneus cohesiveness was also seen in healthy siblings of childhood-onset schizophrenia patients. Younger, healthy siblings of patients with childhood-onset schizophrenia showed gray matter deficits in bilateral prefrontal, bilateral temporal, and inferior parietal cortices when compared with controls (Mattai et al., 2011). A loss in prefrontal and temporal gray matter in childhood-onset schizophrenia may be a familial/trait marker of the illness. These results suggest some shared genetic risk.

Smaller right and left insula volumes were noted in childhood-onset schizophrenia patients compared to controls (Moran et al., 2014). Right insula volume was correlated inversely with positive symptoms in patients. Patients with childhood-onset schizophrenia have previously demonstrated bilateral deficits in hippocampal volume (Nugent et al., 2007). The smaller volume observed in patients remained consistent from age 9 through 26 years. Subregional maps showed heterogeneous changes. There was a smaller hippocampal volume in both the anterior and posterior ends, while the body of the hippocampus was larger in volume. This indicates that the subunits of the hippocampus are differentially affected in childhood-onset schizophrenia (Johnson et al., 2013). Shape analysis discovered an inward deformation in the anterior hippocampus in patients with childhood-onset schizophrenia (Johnson et al., 2013). These inward hippocampal deformations were associated with positive symptoms.

Subcortically, larger caudate volume has been observed in childhood-onset schizophrenia, though this might be the result of neuroleptic exposure (Frazier et al., 1996). Once typical neuroleptics were replaced with clozapine, caudate size decreased to normal within 2 years in patients. Smaller caudate volumes have been reported in neuroleptic-naive adults with schizophrenia. Hence, an initial alteration in caudate volume cannot be ruled out. A shape analysis of the caudate in patients found an outward displacement in the dorsal aspect of the body of the caudate (Chakravarty et al., 2015). Finally, one of the most consistent findings in medication-naive young adults with schizophrenia and childhood-onset schizophrenia is a smaller volume of the thalamus (Sowell et al., 2000). In addition to structural changes, functional characteristics of both schizophrenic patients and their close family members are also observed. During a weather prediction fMRI task, siblings of childhood-onset schizophrenia patients showed less activation of the frontal and striatal regions when compared to controls (Wagshal et al., 2014). In the weather prediction task, participants were told to predict the weather (sun or rain) based on cues. Participants must learn the associations between cues and outcomes and are provided feedback on the correctness of their response. This suggests that impairments in cortical-striatal function may play a role in the liability of schizophrenia.

In a promising move toward the use of imaging to improve diagnostics, machine-learning methods, using brain region data as input, were able to correctly classify subjects in either childhood-onset schizophrenia or healthy control groups with 73.7% accuracy (Greenstein, Malley, Weisinger, Clasen, & Gogtay, 2012).

Eating Disorders

Feeding and eating disorders involve the persistent disturbance of eating or eating-related behavior that results in the alteration of consumption or absorption of food. Feeding and eating disorders can significantly impair psychosocial functioning as well as physical health. Anorexia nervosa is an eating disorder that commonly begins in adolescence and involves the restriction of energy intake leading to significantly low body weight, in conjunction with an intense fear of gaining weight or becoming fat, and marked disturbances in the way in which the individual's body weight is experienced. Anorexia nervosa can present as a restricting type, where the individual accomplishes weight loss through fasting, dieting and/or excessive exercise during the past three months, or in binge-eating/purging type, where the individual has engaged in binge-eating and purging behavior for the last three months. Individuals suffering from anorexia nervosa maintain a body weight that is below the minimal normal level for age, sex, developmental trajectory, and physical health, or, in the case of some children and adolescents, fail to make expected weight gain or maintain a normal developmental trajectory. Anorexia nervosa can result in significant and potentially life-threatening medical conditions, depression, an increased risk of suicide completion, and suicidal ideation, as well as social withdrawal, isolation, and reduced academic and occupational outcomes.

Bulimia nervosa involves recurrent episodes of binge-eating accompanied by inappropriate compensatory strategies to prevent weight gain at least once per week for 3 months. An individual diagnosed with bulimia nervosa will also have a self-evaluation that is unduly influenced by body weight and shape. Like anorexia nervosa, bulimia nervosa commonly begins in adolescence. Consequences of this disorder may include significant and life-threatening medical conditions, increased risk of suicide ideation and suicide completion, and functional impairments, specifically in social domains.

Anorexia nervosa is associated smaller global brain volume in children and adolescents, however this appears somewhat reversible. This large-scale volume loss is more likely to be caused by malnutrition than the underlying neurobiology of anorexia nervosa, rather than neuronal loss. In adolescents with anorexia nervosa, a smaller concentration of frontal N-acetyl-aspartate has been found than in comparison to controls

(Castro-Fornieles et al., 2007). In addition, smaller concentrations of frontal phosphodiesters were reported as well, indicating a decrease in membrane phospholipids (Rzanny et al., 2003). Functional studies have shown that patients with anorexia nervosa have deficits when processing reward, including disruption of dopamine circuitry (Frank et al., 2012). During working memory tasks, greater activation of temporal and parietal regions is noted in adolescents with anorexia nervosa that resolved with treatment (Castro-Fornieles et al., 2010). In bulimia nervosa, greater gray matter volumes in frontal and ventral striatal areas have been found, perhaps indicating a differential trajectory of frontal executive-reward development (Van den Eynde et al., 2012). Additionally, fMRI data indicates that adolescents with bulimia nervosa demonstrate abnormal activation during tasks tapping into regulatory control and conflict resolution, with frontal and striatal regions failing to activate (Marsh et al., 2011). Further studies of eating disorders are needed, but navigating the effect of nutritional influences represent a significant confound.

Mood Disorders

Major depressive disorder (MDD) is a major public health problem, with the greatest likelihood of experiencing symptoms occurring during puberty. MDD affects approximately 15% of adolescents, and is associated with impairments in social, familial, occupational, and academic functioning. Additionally, MDD poses a major risk factor for suicide—a leading cause of death in adolescents. MDD is characterized by depressed mood, markedly diminished interest or pleasure in activities, significant weight loss or weight gain, sleep disturbances, psychomotor agitation or retardation, fatigue or loss of energy, feelings of guilt or worthlessness, a diminished ability to concentrate, and recurrent thoughts of suicide or death.

Bipolar I disorder is characterized by a manic episode—a period of abnormally and persistently elevated, expansive, or irritable mood and persistent goal-directed activity and increased energy for a period of at least one week for most of the day, every day. Manic episodes often involve pressured speech, distractibility, and increased self-esteem, decreased the need for sleep, the flight of activities, and excessive involvement in activities that are likely to have painful consequences. This disturbance causes marked impairment in social and occupational functioning and may require hospitalization to prevent harm to self or others. A hypomanic or major depressive episode may follow a manic episode, although a depressive episode is not required for a diagnosis of bipolar I. The mean age of onset for an episode of bipolar I is 18 years. Bipolar I carries a high risk of suicide, and can impair occupational function, social activity, cognitive function, and result in lower socio-economic status. Bipolar II disorder is characterized by a hypomanic episode—a less intense elevated mood or period of irritability lasting at least four consecutive days, coupled with a depressive episode. No manic episodes are present in bipolar II, however hypomanic episodes can involve increased grandiosity, a decreased need for sleep, pressured speech, distractibility, flight of ideas, increased goal-directed activity, and involvement in activities that have a high potential for painful consequences. Often, these episodes are not severe enough to impair social or occupational functioning or to require hospitalization. Like bipolar I, individuals diagnosed with bipolar II are at increased risk of suicide, unemployment, cognitive deficits, and lower socio-economic status.

Neuroimaging studies of MDD and bipolar disorder are finding increasingly converging evidence that focuses on alterations in medial temporal (eg, amygdala, hippocampus) and prefrontal structures. Smaller orbital frontal lobe volumes have been found in structural neuroimaging studies of youth with MDD (Steingard et al., 2002). Interestingly, in non-familial patients with MDD, larger left prefrontal volumes were found (Nolan et al., 2002). Consonant with that finding, greater cortical thickness in the right and left middle frontal gyrus and the left caudal anterior cingulate was found in adolescents with major depressive disorder as compared to healthy controls (Reynolds et al., 2014). In addition, the left middle frontal gyrus was inversely correlated with age in the subjects with MDD, suggesting an altered developmental trajectory in youth (Reynolds et al., 2014). Thicker caudal anterior cingulate was also found with first-episode MDD, replicating and extending this finding (van Eijndhoven et al., 2013). Imaging studies in adults with MDD and bipolar disorder have reported abnormalities of the subgenual prefrontal cortex (Botteron, Raichle, Drevets, Heath, & Todd, 2002; Drevets, Ongur, & Price, 1998; Drevets, Savitz, & Trimble, 2008; Ongur, Drevets, & Price, 1998). Recently, it was observed that pediatric-onset patients with MDD did not show this effect when compared to adult-onset patients (Jaworska et al., 2014). This finding supports the age of onset as a critical factor in the pathophysiology of MDD and provides further credence to an influence on developmental trajectories for the subregions of the frontal lobe.

Smaller hippocampal volumes have been consistently noted in pediatric MDD patients (MacMaster et al., 2014; MacMaster & Kusumakar, 2004a; MacMaster et al., 2008). Neuronal viability, as indexed by N-acetyl-aspartate, is reduced in the left but not right hippocampus (MacMaster et al., 2008). Hippocampal volume did not differentiate pediatric bipolar disorder patients from those with MDD (MacMaster et al., 2014). Smaller hippocampal volumes were also observed independently in pediatric bipolar disorder (Inal-Emiroglu et al., 2015). In lithium-treated youth with bipolar disorder, larger hippocampal volumes were found (Baykara et al., 2012). Lithium is considered neuroprotective and may prevent volume loss in the hippocampus (Manji, Moore, & Chen, 1999).

Studies in adults implicate the striatum in the pathophysiology of depressive disorders. Youth with MDD have significantly smaller bilateral striatal volumes (Matsuo et al., 2008). Additionally, right striatum volumes were negatively correlated with severity of depressive symptoms. Conversely, pediatric bipolar disorder was associated with larger caudate, putamen, and globus pallidus volumes (Liu et al., 2011). The amygdala plays a critical role in emotional arousal and the processing of emotionally salient stimuli. Ratios of amygdala to hippocampal volume were significantly larger in treatment-naive pediatric patients with MDD compared to age- and sex-matched controls (MacMillan et al., 2003). In youth with MDD, the ratios of amygdala to hippocampal volume were correlated with severity of anxiety but not depression or duration of depressive illness. With regard to amygdala volume in pediatric major depressive disorder conflicting reports exist, with some finding a smaller amygdala (Rosso et al., 2005) and others finding no difference in volume (MacMaster et al., 2008). In pediatric bipolar disorder, reductions in amygdala gray matter have been noted (Chang et al., 2005; Dickstein et al., 2005), both in children diagnosed, and at risk of developing bipolar disorder (Karchemskiy et al., 2011). Taken together, these findings could provide a pre-clinical model for diagnosis and early intervention for at-risk youth.

A larger pituitary gland has been found in several pediatric mood disorders (MacMaster & Kusumakar, 2004b; MacMaster, Leslie, Rosenberg, & Kusumakar, 2008; MacMaster et al., 2006). The pituitary gland is morphologically reactive to changes in hormone concentration and as such is a useful marker of differences in hormone activity like cortisol. MacMaster et al. (2006) found participants with non-familial MDD drove the observed difference in volume. This suggests that family history may be reflected in differences in the underlying neurobiology of depression. In the study of depressed youth with bipolar disorder, again a larger pituitary gland was found when compared to controls (MacMaster et al., 2008). This result was not in agreement with an adult study of bipolar disorder (Sassi et al., 2001) and a pediatric bipolar disorder sample (Chen et al., 2004; Sassi et al., 2001), which independently found no differences in pituitary size. One explanation can be found in the prevailing mood of the participants (depressed vs mainly euthymic). This emphasizes the need for studies of bipolar disorder across illness course.

Diffusion studies have also uncovered reduced frontal white matter integrity in pediatric bipolar disorder (Kafantaris et al., 2009; Pavuluri et al., 2009). Ventrolateral and rostral prefrontal, along with rostral anterior cingulated, demonstrate progressive volume loss in adolescents and young adults with bipolar disorder (Kalmar et al., 2009). Such accelerated gray matter loss would be indicative of an altered developmental trajectory in pediatric bipolar disorder. Functional studies in these areas also reveal increased activation in response to fearful faces (Chai et al., 2015). The left amygdala was more active in pediatric bipolar disorder when rating fearful faces in fMRI tasks (Rich et al., 2006).

MR spectroscopy has begun to unravel the specific alterations in brain chemistry and neurotransmitter concentrations in specific brain regions related to emotional regulation and higher-order processing. Changes in choline as measured by ^{1}H-MRS are thought to result from changes in signal transduction involving phosphatidylcholine second messenger cascades. Greater left orbitofrontal choline levels have been observed in adolescents with MDD as compared to healthy controls (Steingard et al., 2000). In the left DLPFC, greater choline concentrations were also observed in pediatric MDD, most commonly in individuals with family histories of mood disorders, suggesting a genetic contribution to these differences (Farchione, Moore, & Rosenberg, 2002). Increased choline concentrations could be reflective of changes in glucose metabolic rates and/or neuroendocrine function. Greater prefrontal choline levels may also be consistent with functional imaging studies that show reduced prefrontal cortical metabolism in adults with MDD. Conversely, lower choline concentrations were observed in the right anterior cingulate (MacMaster & Kusumakar, 2006) suggesting differential changes in choline concentration subregions of the frontal lobe. Lower choline-to-creatine ratios were noted in the left amygdala in pediatric MDD patients compared to controls (Kusumakar, MacMaster, Gates, Sparkes, & Khan, 2001). This alteration in cytosolic choline may be resultant from cortisol-driven changes, as increases in cortisol can result in lower choline concentrations. The functional and behavioral consequences of reduced choline are yet unexplored, however, this biochemical abnormality has been associated with impaired signal transduction systems in MDD patients (Jia et al., 2015). Building on the finding of elevated anterior cingulate choline in MDD (MacMaster & Kusumakar, 2006), a replication study found that anterior cingulate choline may distinguish unipolar from bipolar depression in females (Shi et al., 2014).

The anterior cingulate region, as discussed previously, represents a major site of chemical alterations in MDD. In addition to reduced choline concentrations, lower anterior cingulate glutamate and glutamine concentrations were found among pediatric MDD patients compared to healthy controls (Rosenberg et al., 2004, 2005), consistent with findings in adults (Auer et al., 2000). Lower anterior cingulate GABA concentrations were also observed as compared to healthy controls, with this difference being more pronounced in those youth with MDD with pronounced anhedonia (Gabbay et al., 2012). With regard to intervention, a small case series in adolescents with MDD recently replicated a finding in adults that showed an increase on DLPFC glutamate in response to repetitive transcranial magnetic stimulation treatment (Yang et al., 2014). In pediatric bipolar disorder, greater glutamate and glutamine concentrations were found in the bilateral frontal lobes and basal ganglia (Moore et al., 2007). With regard to treatment, lithium did not increase concentration of the neuronal marker N-acetyl-aspartate in youth with bipolar disorder, a finding that is not consistent with adult studies demonstrating biochemical response to medication (Patel et al., 2008).

Obsessive-Compulsive Disorder

Obsessive-compulsive disorder (OCD) is characterized by (1) obsessions—recurrent and persistent thoughts, urges, and images that are unwanted and intrusive and (2) compulsions—repetitive behaviors performed according to the rigid rules in response to the obsession. Obsessions and compulsions are time-consuming and cause significant distress in social, occupational, or other areas of functioning. In young children, compulsions can be particularly distressing as they are often not able to identify the aims of the behavior. Onset in childhood or adolescence can lead to a lifetime of OCD, with associated increased risk of suicide, family dysfunction, developmental difficulties, social impairments, and challenges for independent living. Pediatric OCD is an ideal candidate for neurodevelopmental studies as the phenomenology, nosology, and empirical treatment are well-established. Compared to mood disorders, OCD is more consistent in its expression across the lifespan. This allows researchers to study OCD at illness onset and apply findings across the lifespan. Critically, many studies in pediatric OCD have focused on treatment-naive populations. This reduces potential confounds like duration of illness and exposure to medication.

In pediatric OCD, evidence suggests dysfunction in the ventral prefrontal-striatal-thalamic and medial temporal circuits. Larger anterior cingulate volumes are a consistent finding in pediatric OCD (Rosenberg & Keshavan, 1998; Szeszko et al., 2008; Szeszko et al., 2004). OCD symptom severity was associated with larger anterior cingulate volumes. Developmentally, pediatric OCD patients did not have the normal age-related growth in anterior cingulate volume observed in healthy controls, however, the use of different modalities to examine structural abnormalities in these regions can produce conflicting results. For example, manually-traced volumetric studies in pediatric OCD have shown smaller basal ganglia volumes in patients that were associated with OCD symptom severity but not illness duration (Rosenberg et al., 1997). Using an automated method (voxel-based morphometry) to study adolescents with OCD and healthy controls, greater gray matter signal intensity in the bilateral caudate was observed (Zarei et al., 2011). This reflects fundamental differences in what properties are measured using voxel-based morphometry as compared to the manual tracing technique and highlights the need for the standardized application of objective, validated techniques (Thacker, 2005).

Biochemical models of OCD using proton magnetic resonance spectroscopy (1H-MRS), have focused on disruptions in concentrations of glutamate-glutamine. Although alterations in these metabolites may reflect changes in core physiological processes, the effects of these imbalances on neuronal–glial cycling, cell metabolism, or activity regulation is unclear (Magistretti & Pellerin, 1999). A greater concentration of glutamate and glutamine were found in the caudate in pediatric OCD patients compared to age- and sex-matched healthy controls (Rosenberg et al., 2000). No neurochemical differences were noted in the occipital lobe—which is a brain region not associated with OCD. Twelve weeks of selective serotonin reuptake inhibitor (SSRI) treatment decreased caudate glutamate and glutamine concentration, and predicted better response to paroxetine in OCD patients (Rosenberg et al., 2000). More recent investigations have suggested that caudate glutamatergic concentrations may persist even after discontinuation of medication in pediatric OCD (Bolton, Moore, MacMillan, Stewart, & Rosenberg, 2001), as well as ongoing decreased glutamate and glutamine concentrations (Rosenberg et al., 2004). This change in glutamatergic concentration was associated with the G/G genotype of the glutamate receptor gene polymorphism GRIN2B-rs1019385 in OCD patients (Arnold et al., 2009). Cognitive behavioral therapy, however, despite having a positive effect on OCD symptoms, did not change caudate glutamate and glutamine concentration (Benazon, Moore, & Rosenberg, 2003). Choline concentrations in the thalamus were greater in pediatric OCD patients compared to healthy controls (Smith et al., 2003). Choline concentrations are derived from membrane synthesis and breakdown components. Similar to the effect noted with caudate glutamatergic concentrations, cognitive behavior therapy did not change thalamic volume. This suggests that the two interventions use differing means to alter neurobiology and relieve symptoms.

Changes in functional connectivity indicate alterations in cognitive control and error monitoring in pediatric OCD (Fitzgerald et al., 2011). The genu of the corpus callosum connects left and right ventral prefrontal cortical regions such as the anterior cingulate cortex. Studies of the corpus callosum found both a larger area and lower signal intensity of the genu in treatment-naive pediatric OCD patients compared to controls (MacMaster, Keshavan, Dick, & Rosenberg, 1999; Rosenberg et al., 1997). Taken together, these studies provide evidence supporting developmental alterations in the anterior cingulate that is reflected in the symptomatology of pediatric OCD. A volumetric MRI study of pediatric OCD found larger thalamic volumes compared to controls (Gilbert et al., 2000). After SSRI treatment, thalamic volumes decreased to normalize to that of controls. The change in thalamic volume correlated robustly with the reduction in symptom severity. Furthermore, larger thalamic volume was associated with a better response to SSRI treatment. The amygdala plays a significant role in arousal and fear, and is associated with the pathophysiology of OCD. With SSRI treatment, the volume of the left amygdala decreased significantly in pediatric OCD subjects (Szeszko et al., 2004). This change in volume was associated with the SSRI dose at the time of the follow-up scan and cumulative SSRI exposure.

Tourette Sydrome

Tourette syndrome (TS) affects approximately 0.3 to 1% of the population, and is characterized by tics—repetitive, sudden, semi-voluntary sounds and movements. TS negatively affects children's quality of life in multiple domains (at home, school, and with friends and family). In approximately 15% of children with Tourette syndrome, tics can be especially disabling, corresponding with poor outcomes across physical, psychological, and cognitive domains in youth. Although the neurobiology of TS is unclear, the overarching etiological model is thought to involve disinhibition of cortico-thalamo-cortical circuits, responsible for the planning and execution of movement, and habitual behavior (Graybiel, 2008). Microstructural alterations including decreased FA and increased radial diffusivity have been detected by tract-based spatial statistics (TBSS) in the corticospinal tract and the posterior internal capsule (Neuner et al., 2010; Smith et al., 2006). White matter underlying motor control areas of the pre- and postcentral gyri, as well as connections to the anterior cingulate, are also implicated in TS pathology (Muller-Vahl et al., 2009). Significant area increases in four major subdivisions of the corpus callosum have also been identified in male TS patients (Baumgardner et al., 1996). However, this was not replicated in girls (Mostofsky, Wendlandt, Cutting, Denckla, & Singer, 1999). Smaller basal ganglia volumes are associated with Tourette syndrome in both children and adults (Peterson et al., 1993; Singer et al., 1993). Smaller volumes were found to be particularly prominent in the globus pallidus and putamen in patients with Tourette syndrome, implicating the motor pathways within cortical-subcortical circuitry—consistent with the motor phenomena of tics. Greater thalamic volumes have also been noted in Tourette syndrome as compared to healthy comparison subjects (Lee et al., 2006). Greater apparent diffusion coefficient (ADC) in cortico-striatal projection pathways has also been noted in children with Tourette syndrome (Govindan, Makki, Wilson, Behen, & Chugani, 2010).

In adults and children with TS, interhemispheric transfer is impaired in both performance and structure (Margolis, Donkervoort, Kinsbourne, & Peterson, 2006; Plessen et al., 2006, 2007). A recent structural MRI investigation evaluated the association between the size of the cavum septi pellucidi and a diagnosis of Tourette syndrome (Kim & Peterson, 2003). Linked to the development of the corpus callosum, a smaller cavum septi pellucidi was observed in children with Tourette syndrome compared to healthy pediatric controls.

Neuroimaging has provided clues as to developmental changes in TS brain structure. In a large-scale volumetric imaging study of children and adults with TS, striking abnormalities of cortical development in the parieto-occipital region was observed (Peterson et al., 2001), with a larger volume observed in children with TS. This age-associated developmental reduction in parieto-occipital volumes occurred predominantly in females. In contrast, larger parieto-occipital volumes were observed in older men with TS, suggesting a sexually dimorphic neurodevelopmental trajectory that may contribute to the greater prevalence of TS in males. Frontal lobe changes have also been associated with age. In the frontal lobe, larger DLPFC volumes were found in younger patients with TS, but volumes decreased toward adulthood (Gerard & Peterson, 2003). Reduction in tics is correlated with smaller dorsolateral prefrontal cortical volumes in older patients with TS. In the temporal lobe, the volume of the hippocampus and amygdala was found to be significantly larger in TS patients than in controls (Peterson et al., 2007). Upon closer inspection using a surface analysis, it was found that the larger volumes in the Tourette syndrome patients were derived primarily from the head and medial surface of the hippocampus and the dorsal and ventral surfaces of the amygdala. With age, the volumes of these subregions declined in TS patients but not in controls. Consequently, these subregions were significantly larger in children with TS but significantly smaller in adults with Tourette syndrome than in controls—a striking developmental change. With regard to clinical symptom scores, volumes in these subregions correlated inversely with the severity of tics, OCD, and ADHD symptoms in patients. This is suggestive that the enlargement of these subregions is a compensatory mechanism.

As fMRI studies show increased activation of the prefrontal cortex during tic suppression, one hypothesis suggests that the greater prefrontal cortical volumes observed in children with TS may be compensatory in order to allow for tic suppression (Roessner et al., 2013). However, some have hypothesized that increased prefrontal cortex volumes are not related to inhibition but instead contribute to hyper-excitability observed in TS (Jung, Jackson, Parkinson, & Jackson, 2013). Taken together, these preliminary findings support the premise of abnormal brain development in Tourette syndrome in key brain regions and connections.

Pediatric Autoimmune Neuropsychiatric Disorders Associated With Group A β-Hemolytic Streptococcal Infection

In pediatric autoimmune neuropsychiatric disorders associated with group A β-hemolytic streptococcal (GABHS) infection (PANDAS), it is hypothesized that GABHS-associated antibodies cross-react with neurons in the basal ganglia. This results in symptoms akin to that of OCD, as well as tics/Tourette syndrome and ADHD in susceptible children. Indeed, increased neuroinflammation has been observed in children with PANDAS compared to controls (Kumar, Williams, & Chugani, 2015). In contrast to pediatric OCD observations, greater basal ganglia volume has been identified in a subset of patients with PANDAS (Giedd, Rapoport, Leonard, Richter, & Swedo, 1996). Immunotherapy (ie, plasmapheresis) reduces symptoms in some PANDAS patients with marked OCD symptoms. However additional studies are needed in order to develop better differentiation from pediatric OCD and to develop targeted interventions (Arnold & Richter, 2001).

Substance and Addictive Disorders

Substance-use disorders involve cognitive, behavioral, and physiological symptoms where the individual continues the use of an addictive substance despite significant health and social problems. An individual with a substance use disorder may abuse prescription drugs in larger amounts and for longer time periods that originally intended, spend significant time or resources obtaining illicit substances, experience cravings, and be unable to discontinue use of the substance. Additionally, the use of the substance often results in failure to fulfill major role obligations at home, school or work. The individual may also use the substance in physically hazardous situations, develop a tolerance to the effects of the substance, and experience symptoms of withdrawal.

Alcohol use disorder involves a problematic pattern of use of alcohol within a 12-month period. The use of alcohol causes significant impairment or distress to the individual. Alcohol use disorder can affect school, work, interpersonal relationships, health, and driving. Alcohol use disorder contributes to absenteeism from work and school, accidents, low productivity, homelessness, and an increased risk of suicide. Feelings of sadness and irritability, as well as disinhibition, are often related to alcohol use disorder. As binge-drinking among adolescents is common, the need to understand the neurobiological underpinnings and effects of consumption are needed. In keeping with studies of adults who abuse alcohol, a significant volume reduction in bilateral hippocampi was found in adolescents who abused alcohol as compared to healthy pediatric controls (De Bellis et al., 2000). Hippocampal volume reduction correlated positively with the age of onset and negatively with duration of alcohol use. This suggests that alcohol may interfere with normal growth of the hippocampus. In youth at high risk for alcoholism, smaller amygdala volumes were noted (Hill et al., 2001), indicating a possible abnormality in the processing of emotional stimuli, and providing the first evidence that risk of alcohol abuse may be partly predicated on early alterations in brain structure. Consistent with this model, youth at risk displayed differences in resting state synchrony between left nucleus accumbens, bilateral inferior frontal gyri and the left postcentral gyrus (Weiland et al., 2012), suggesting a disconnectivity between executive and reward brain areas. In a longitudinal morphometric study (Squeglia et al., 2014), adolescents were followed over 3 years, during which 50% started drinking heavily. This cohort displayed smaller left cingulate, pars triangularis, and rostral anterior cingulate volumes as compared to the remaining participants. With time, reductions in left inferior and middle temporal gyri, left caudate and brain stem were also noted as compared to the substance naïve controls. This suggests that there are pre-existing markers that predict future drinkers and a further volume reduction over time after alcohol abuse commenced.

Cannabis use disorder, similar to alcohol use disorder, involves a problematic pattern of cannabis use involving at least two of the following over a 12-month period: using larger amounts or over a longer period of time than intended, unsuccessful efforts to cut down on use, a great deal of time spent obtaining, using or recovering from the effects of cannabis, the failure to fulfill major role obligations, continued cannabis use despite persistent problems, exposure to physically hazardous situations, tolerance to the effects of cannabis, and withdrawal. Onset of cannabis use disorder is most common during adolescence and young adulthood, resulting in family, academic, or employment difficulties. Additionally, young users experience changes in mood stability, energy, and eating patterns. School performance and motivation is often negatively affected by cannabis use disorder, and psychosocial, cognitive, and health functioning is often compromised. Cannabis use can contribute to the onset of acute psychotic episodes, or exacerbate or adversely affect treatment of psychotic illness.

Substantial cannabis use is often associated with increased rates of mental illness and cognitive impairment in adolescent users. The underlying neurobiology of this effect is not well understood. Prolonged use is thought to interfere with the normal development of endocannabinoid system with further ramifications distally. Heavy cannabis use during adolescence and into young adulthood is associated with altered brain development that can have neurobehavioral consequences (Jacobus et al., 2015). Specifically, cannabis users demonstrate decreased concavity and thickness of the sulci in the right frontal lobe compared to non-users

(Mata et al., 2010). Critically, the developmental association of gyrification with age was absent in heavy cannabis users. Additionally, adolescents with cannabis use disorder demonstrated greater concentrations of N-acetyl aspartate that were positively associated with the amount of cannabis used (Bitter et al., 2014). A systematic review of diffusion-weighted imaging studies found abnormal white matter microstructure in neocortical association pathways as well as in projection and thalamic pathways with cannabis use in adolescence (Baker, Yucel, Fornito, Allen, & Lubman, 2013). In a resting state connectivity study, heavy cannabis use in adolescents was also associated with reduced interhemispheric connectivity, further supporting possible alterations in white matter (Orr et al., 2013). A fundamental confound in the study of cannabis use in adolescents is the limited ability to quantify and control for exposure. Almost all studies rely on self-report of use with little data on the strength of cannabis used to quantify the dose. Neuroimaging studies provide objective and categorical data on brain alterations associated with heavy use of cannabis.

FUTURE DIRECTIONS

Conducting brain-imaging studies of neuropsychiatric disease in children and adolescents poses special challenges. However, this important work is poised to provide critical neurobiological understanding of the mechanisms underlying neuropathologies and the effect of interventions. Neuroimaging biomarkers that serve as both moderator (present at baseline) and mediator (changing with treatment) variables should provide an improved mechanistic understanding of the pathogenesis and maintenance of mental illness in children and adolescents. Adoption of neuroimaging as standard practice in suspected and diagnosed mental illness will lead to individualized treatment approaches and improved patient advocacy. The call for rational therapeutics demands that treatments are based on the underlying neurobiology, something traditionally lacking in psychiatry as a field (Insel & Quirion, 2005; Insel & Scolnick, 2006). Furthermore, neuroimaging is also well matched with research domain criteria approaches where targets are based more on function rather than a named disorder (Insel, 2014). Practically, MRI methods are particularly useful in children and adolescents, as they pose no threat to safety with radiation and hence lend themselves naturally to longitudinal studies. As the technology continues to evolve, resolution (spatial and temporal) will improve, novel methods will emerge, and consensuses in application will develop. This will allow for even greater progress in understanding and more effective treatments of mental illness in youth.

References

Almeida, L. G., Ricardo-Garcell, J., Prado, H., Barajas, L., Fernandez-Bouzas, A., Avila, D., & Martinez, R. B. (2010). Reduced right frontal cortical thickness in children, adolescents and adults with ADHD and its correlation to clinical variables: a cross-sectional study. *Journal of Psychiatric Research, 44*(16), 1214–1223. http://dx.doi.org/10.1016/j.jpsychires.2010.04.026.

Anney, R., Klei, L., Pinto, D., Almeida, J., Bacchelli, E., Baird, G., … Devlin, B. (2012). Individual common variants exert weak effects on the risk for autism spectrum disorderspi. *Human Molecular Genetics, 21*(21), 4781–4792. http://dx.doi.org/10.1093/hmg/dds301.

Aoki, Y., Kasai, K., & Yamasue, H. (2012). Age-related change in brain metabolite abnormalities in autism: a meta-analysis of proton magnetic resonance spectroscopy studies. *Translational Psychiatry, 2*, e69. http://dx.doi.org/10.1038/tp.2011.65.

Arnold, P. D., Macmaster, F. P., Richter, M. A., Hanna, G. L., Sicard, T., Burroughs, E., … Rosenberg, D. R. (2009). Glutamate receptor gene (GRIN2B) associated with reduced anterior cingulate glutamatergic concentration in pediatric obsessive-compulsive disorder. *Psychiatry Research, 172*(2), 136–139. http://dx.doi.org/10.1016/j.pscychresns.2009.02.005, pii:S0925-4927(09)00052-3.

Arnold, P. D., & Richter, M. A. (2001). Is obsessive-compulsive disorder an autoimmune disease? *Canadian Medical Association Journal, 165*(10), 1353–1358.

Auer, D. P., Putz, B., Kraft, E., Lipinski, B., Schill, J., & Holsboer, F. (2000). Reduced glutamate in the anterior cingulate cortex in depression: an in vivo proton magnetic resonance spectroscopy study. *Biological Psychiatry, 47*(4), 305–313.

Baker, S. T., Yucel, M., Fornito, A., Allen, N. B., & Lubman, D. I. (2013). A systematic review of diffusion weighted MRI studies of white matter microstructure in adolescent substance users. *Neuroscience and Biobehavioral Reviews, 37*(8), 1713–1723. http://dx.doi.org/10.1016/j.neubiorev.2013.06.015.

Barnea-Goraly, N., Weinzimer, S. A., Ruedy, K. J., Mauras, N., Beck, R. W., Marzelli, M. J., … Diabetes Research in Children Network (DirecNet) (2014). High success rates of sedation-free brain MRI scanning in young children using simple subject preparation protocols with and without a commercial mock scanner–the Diabetes Research in Children Network (DirecNet) experience. *Pediatric Radiology, 44*(2), 181–186. http://dx.doi.org/10.1007/s00247-013-2798-7.

Baumgardner, T. L., Singer, H. S., Denckla, M. B., Rubin, M. A., Abrams, M. T., Colli, M. J., & Reiss, A. L. (1996). Corpus callosum morphology in children with Tourette syndrome and attention deficit hyperactivity disorder. *Neurology, 47*(2), 477–482.

Baykara, B., Inal-Emiroglu, N., Karabay, N., Cakmakci, H., Cevher, N., Senturk Pilan, B., & Alsen, S. (2012). Increased hippocampal volumes in lithium treated adolescents with bipolar disorders: a structural MRI study. *Journal of Affective Disorders, 138*(3), 433–439. http://dx.doi.org/10.1016/j.jad.2011.12.047.

Benazon, N. R., Moore, G. J., & Rosenberg, D. R. (2003). Neurochemical analyses in pediatric obsessive-compulsive disorder in patients treated with cognitive-behavioral therapy. *Journal of the American Academy of Child and Adolescent Psychiatry, 42*(11), 1279–1285. http://dx.doi.org/10.1097/01.chi.0000087562.01900.de.

Bennett, M. R., Hatton, S. N., & Lagopoulos, J. (2015). Stress, trauma and PTSD: translational insights into the core synaptic circuitry and its modulation. *Brain Structure & Function.* http://dx.doi.org/10.1007/s00429-015-1056-1.

Bitter, S. M., Weber, W. A., Chu, W. J., Adler, C. M., Eliassen, J. C., Strakowski, S. M., & DelBello, M. P. (2014). N-acetyl aspartate levels in adolescents with bipolar and/or cannabis use disorders. *Journal of Dual Diagnosis, 10*(1), 39–43. http://dx.doi.org/10.1080/15504263.2013.869077.

Blanken, L. M., Mous, S. E., Ghassabian, A., Muetzel, R. L., Schoemaker, N. K., El Marroun, H., … White, T. (2015). Cortical morphology in 6- to 10-year old children with autistic traits: a population-based neuroimaging study. *The American Journal of Psychiatry, 172*(5), 479–486. http://dx.doi.org/10.1176/appi.ajp.2014.14040482.

Bolton, J., Moore, G. J., MacMillan, S., Stewart, C. M., & Rosenberg, D. R. (2001). Case study: caudate glutamatergic changes with paroxetine persist after medication discontinuation in pediatric OCD. *Journal of the American Academy of Child and Adolescent Psychiatry, 40*(8), 903–906.

Botteron, K. N., Raichle, M. E., Drevets, W. C., Heath, A. C., & Todd, R. D. (2002). Volumetric reduction in left subgenual prefrontal cortex in early onset depression. *Biological Psychiatry, 51*(4), 342–344.

Carrey, N., Bernier, D., Emms, M., Gunde, E., Sparkes, S., Macmaster, F. P., & Rusak, B. (2012). Smaller volumes of caudate nuclei in prepubertal children with ADHD: impact of age. *Journal of Psychiatric Research, 46*(8), 1066–1072. http://dx.doi.org/10.1016/j.jpsychires.2012.04.025.

Carrey, N., MacMaster, F. P., Fogel, J., Sparkes, S., Waschbusch, D., Sullivan, S., & Schmidt, M. (2003). Metabolite changes resulting from treatment in children with ADHD: a 1H-MRS study. *Clinical Neuropharmacology, 26*(4), 218–221.

Carrey, N., MacMaster, F. P., Sparkes, S. J., Khan, S. C., & Kusumakar, V. (2002). Glutamatergic changes with treatment in attention deficit hyperactivity disorder: a preliminary case series. *Journal of Child and Adolescent Psychopharmacology, 12*(4), 331–336. http://dx.doi.org/10.1089/104454602762599871.

Casanova, M. F. (2006). Neuropathological and genetic findings in autism: the significance of a putative minicolumnopathy. *Neuroscientist, 12*(5), 435–441. http://dx.doi.org/10.1177/1073858406290375.

Castellanos, F. X., Giedd, J. N., Eckburg, P., Marsh, W. L., Vaituzis, A. C., Kaysen, D., … Rapoport, J. L. (1994). Quantitative morphology of the caudate nucleus in attention deficit hyperactivity disorder. *The American Journal of Psychiatry, 151*(12), 1791–1796.

Castro-Fornieles, J., Bargallo, N., Lazaro, L., Andres, S., Falcon, C., Plana, M. T., & Junque, C. (2007). Adolescent anorexia nervosa: cross-sectional and follow-up frontal gray matter disturbances detected with proton magnetic resonance spectroscopy. *Journal of Psychiatric Research, 41*(11), 952–958. http://dx.doi.org/10.1016/j.jpsychires.2006.09.013.

Castro-Fornieles, J., Caldu, X., Andres-Perpina, S., Lazaro, L., Bargallo, N., Falcon, C., … Junque, C. (2010). A cross-sectional and follow-up functional MRI study with a working memory task in adolescent anorexia nervosa. *Neuropsychologia, 48*(14), 4111–4116. http://dx.doi.org/10.1016/j.neuropsychologia.2010.10.003.

Cerliani, L., Mennes, M., Thomas, R. M., Di Martino, A., Thioux, M., & Keysers, C. (2015). Increased functional connectivity between subcortical and cortical resting-state networks in autism spectrum disorder. *JAMA Psychiatry*. http://dx.doi.org/10.1001/jamapsychiatry.2015.0101.

Chai, X. J., Hirshfeld-Becker, D., Biederman, J., Uchida, M., Doehrmann, O., Leonard, J. A., … Gabrieli, J. D. (2015). Functional and structural brain correlates of risk for major depression in children with familial depression. *Neuroimage: Clinical, 8*, 398–407. http://dx.doi.org/10.1016/j.nicl.2015.05.004.

Chakravarty, M. M., Rapoport, J. L., Giedd, J. N., Raznahan, A., Shaw, P., Collins, D. L., … Gogtay, N. (2015). Striatal shape abnormalities as novel neurodevelopmental endophenotypes in schizophrenia: a longitudinal study. *Human Brain Mapping, 36*(4), 1458–1469. http://dx.doi.org/10.1002/hbm.22715.

Chandana, S. R., Behen, M. E., Juhasz, C., Muzik, O., Rothermel, R. D., Mangner, T. J., … Chugani, D. C. (2005). Significance of abnormalities in developmental trajectory and asymmetry of cortical serotonin synthesis in autism. *International Journal of Developmental Neuroscience, 23*(2–3), 171–182. http://dx.doi.org/10.1016/j.ijdevneu.2004.08.002, pii:S0736-5748(04)00109-1.

Chang, K., Karchemskiy, A., Barnea-Goraly, N., Garrett, A., Simeonova, D. I., & Reiss, A. (2005). Reduced amygdalar gray matter volume in familial pediatric bipolar disorder. *Journal of the American Academy of Child and Adolescent Psychiatry, 44*(6), 565–573, pii:00004583-200506000-00011.

Chen, H. H., Nicoletti, M., Sanches, M., Hatch, J. P., Sassi, R. B., Axelson, D., … Soares, J. C. (2004). Normal pituitary volumes in children and adolescents with bipolar disorder: a magnetic resonance imaging study. *Depression and Anxiety, 20*(4), 182–186.

Chugani, H. T. (1998). Biological basis of emotions: brain systems and brain development. *Pediatrics, 102*(5 Suppl. E), 1225–1229.

Chugani, D. C., Muzik, O., Behen, M., Rothermel, R., Janisse, J. J., Lee, J., & Chugani, H. T. (1999). Developmental changes in brain serotonin synthesis capacity in autistic and non-autistic children. *Annals of Neurology, 45*(3), 287–295.

Courchesne, E., Chisum, H. J., Townsend, J., Cowles, A., Covington, J., Egaas, B., ... Press, G. A. (2000). Normal brain development and aging: quantitative analysis at in vivo MR imaging in healthy volunteers. *Radiology, 216*(3), 672–682. http://dx.doi.org/10.1148/radiology.216.3.r00au37672.

De Bellis, M. D., Clark, D. B., Beers, S. R., Soloff, P. H., Boring, A. M., Hall, J., ... Keshavan, M. S. (2000). Hippocampal volume in adolescent-onset alcohol use disorders. *The American Journal of Psychiatry, 157*(5), 737–744.

De Bellis, M. D., Keshavan, M. S., Shifflett, H., Iyengar, S., Beers, S. R., Hall, J., & Moritz, G. (2002). Brain structures in pediatric maltreatment-related posttraumatic stress disorder: a sociodemographically matched study. *Biological Psychiatry, 52*(11), 1066–1078.

Dickstein, D. P., Milham, M. P., Nugent, A. C., Drevets, W. C., Charney, D. S., Pine, D. S., & Leibenluft, E. (2005). Frontotemporal alterations in pediatric bipolar disorder: results of a voxel-based morphometry study. *Archives of General Psychiatry, 62*(7), 734–741. http://dx.doi.org/10.1001/archpsyc.62.7.734, pii:62/7/734.

Drevets, W. C., Ongur, D., & Price, J. L. (1998). Neuroimaging abnormalities in the subgenual prefrontal cortex: implications for the pathophysiology of familial mood disorders. *Molecular Psychiatry, 3*(3), 220–226 190–221.

Drevets, W. C., Savitz, J., & Trimble, M. (2008). The subgenual anterior cingulate cortex in mood disorders. *CNS Spectrums, 13*(8), 663–681.

Durston, S., Pol, H. E. H., Casey, B. J., Giedd, J. N., Buitelaar, J. K., & van Engeland, H. (2001). Anatomical MRI of the developing human brain: what have we learned? *Journal of the American Academy of Child and Adolescent Psychiatry, 40*(9), 1012–1020.

van Eijndhoven, P., van Wingen, G., Katzenbauer, M., Groen, W., Tepest, R., Fernandez, G., ... Tendolkar, I. (2013). Paralimbic cortical thickness in first-episode depression: evidence for trait-related differences in mood regulation. *The American Journal of Psychiatry, 170*(12), 1477–1486. http://dx.doi.org/10.1176/appi.ajp.2013.12121504.

Ernst, M. (1999). PET in child psychiatry: the risks and benefits of studying normal healthy children. *Progress in Neuro-Psychopharmacology & Biological Psychiatry, 23*(4), 561–570.

Farchione, T. R., Moore, G. J., & Rosenberg, D. R. (2002). Proton magnetic resonance spectroscopic imaging in pediatric major depression. *Biological Psychiatry, 52*(2), 86–92, pii:S0006322302013409.

Fitzgerald, K. D., Welsh, R. C., Stern, E. R., Angstadt, M., Hanna, G. L., Abelson, J. L., & Taylor, S. F. (2011). Developmental alterations of frontal-striatal-thalamic connectivity in obsessive-compulsive disorder. *Journal of the American Academy of Child and Adolescent Psychiatry, 50*(9), 938–948. http://dx.doi.org/10.1016/j.jaac.2011.06.011 e933.

Frank, G. K., Reynolds, J. R., Shott, M. E., Jappe, L., Yang, T. T., Tregellas, J. R., & O'Reilly, R. C. (2012). Anorexia nervosa and obesity are associated with opposite brain reward response. *Neuropsychopharmacology, 37*(9), 2031–2046. http://dx.doi.org/10.1038/npp.2012.51.

Frazier, J. A., Giedd, J. N., Kaysen, D., Albus, K., Hamburger, S., Alaghband-Rad, J., ... Rapoport, J. L. (1996). Childhood-onset schizophrenia: brain MRI rescan after 2 years of clozapine maintenance treatment. *The American Journal of Psychiatry, 153*(4), 564–566.

Gabbay, V., Mao, X., Klein, R. G., Ely, B. A., Babb, J. S., Panzer, A. M., ... Shungu, D. C. (2012). Anterior cingulate cortex gamma-aminobutyric acid in depressed adolescents: relationship to anhedonia. *Archives of General Psychiatry, 69*(2), 139–149. http://dx.doi.org/10.1001/archgenpsychiatry.2011.131.

Gaugler, T., Klei, L., Sanders, S. J., Bodea, C. A., Goldberg, A. P., Lee, A. B., ... Buxbaum, J. D. (2014). Most genetic risk for autism resides with common variation. *Nature Genetics, 46*(8), 881–885. http://dx.doi.org/10.1038/ng.3039.

Gerard, E., & Peterson, B. S. (2003). Developmental processes and brain imaging studies in Tourette syndrome. *Journal of Psychosomatic Research, 55*(1), 13–22.

Giedd, J. N., Blumenthal, J., Jeffries, N. O., Castellanos, F. X., Liu, H., Zijdenbos, A., ... Rapoport, J. L. (1999). Brain development during childhood and adolescence: a longitudinal MRI study. *Nature Neuroscience, 2*(10), 861–863. http://dx.doi.org/10.1038/13158.

Giedd, J. N., Rapoport, J. L., Leonard, H. L., Richter, D., & Swedo, S. E. (1996). Case study: acute basal ganglia enlargement and obsessive-compulsive symptoms in an adolescent boy. *Journal of the American Academy of Child and Adolescent Psychiatry, 35*(7), 913–915.

Gilbert, A. R., Moore, G. J., Keshavan, M. S., Paulson, L. A., Narula, V., Mac Master, F. P., ... Rosenberg, D. R. (2000). Decrease in thalamic volumes of pediatric patients with obsessive-compulsive disorder who are taking paroxetine. *Archives of General Psychiatry, 57*(5), 449–456.

Gogtay, N., Lu, A., Leow, A. D., Klunder, A. D., Lee, A. D., Chavez, A., ... Thompson, P. M. (2008). Three-dimensional brain growth abnormalities in childhood-onset schizophrenia visualized by using tensor-based morphometry. *Proceedings of the National Academy of Sciences of the United States of America, 105*(41), 15979–15984. http://dx.doi.org/10.1073/pnas.0806485105.

Govindan, R. M., Makki, M. I., Wilson, B. J., Behen, M. E., & Chugani, H. T. (2010). Abnormal water diffusivity in corticostriatal projections in children with Tourette syndrome. *Human Brain Mapping, 31*(11), 1665–1674. http://dx.doi.org/10.1002/hbm.20970.

Graybiel, A. M. (2008). Habits, rituals, and the evaluative brain. *Annual Review of Neuroscience, 31*, 359–387. http://dx.doi.org/10.1146/annurev.neuro.29.051605.112851.

Greenstein, D., Malley, J. D., Weisinger, B., Clasen, L., & Gogtay, N. (2012). Using multivariate machine learning methods and structural MRI to classify childhood onset schizophrenia and healthy controls. *Front Psychiatry, 3*, 53. http://dx.doi.org/10.3389/fpsyt.2012.00053.

Hamm, L. L., Jacobs, R. H., Johnson, M. W., Fitzgerald, D. A., Fitzgerald, K. D., Langenecker, S. A., ... Phan, K. L. (2014). Aberrant amygdala functional connectivity at rest in pediatric anxiety disorders. *Biology of Mood & Anxiety Disorders, 4*(1), 15. http://dx.doi.org/10.1186/s13587-014-0015-4.

Hill, S. Y., De Bellis, M. D., Keshavan, M. S., Lowers, L., Shen, S., Hall, J., & Pitts, T. (2001). Right amygdala volume in adolescent and young adult offspring from families at high risk for developing alcoholism. *Biological Psychiatry, 49*(11), 894–905.

Inal-Emiroglu, F. N., Resmi, H., Karabay, N., Guleryuz, H., Baykara, B., Cevher, N., & Akay, A. (2015). Decreased right hippocampal volumes and neuroprogression markers in adolescents with bipolar disorder. *Neuropsychobiology, 71*(3), 140–148. http://dx.doi.org/10.1159/000375311.

Insel, T. R. (2014). The NIMH research domain criteria (RDoC) project: precision medicine for psychiatry. *The American Journal of Psychiatry, 171*(4), 395–397. http://dx.doi.org/10.1176/appi.ajp.2014.14020138.

Insel, T. R., & Quirion, R. (2005). Psychiatry as a clinical neuroscience discipline. *The Journal of the American Medical Association, 294*(17), 2221–2224. http://dx.doi.org/10.1001/jama.294.17.2221, pii:294/17/2221.

Insel, T. R., & Scolnick, E. M. (2006). Cure therapeutics and strategic prevention: raising the bar for mental health research. *Molecular Psychiatry, 11*(1), 11–17. http://dx.doi.org/10.1038/sj.mp.4001777, pii:4001777.

Jacobus, J., Squeglia, L. M., Meruelo, A. D., Castro, N., Brumback, T., Giedd, J. N., & Tapert, S. F. (2015). Cortical thickness in adolescent marijuana and alcohol users: a three-year prospective study from adolescence to young adulthood. *Developmental Cognitive Neuroscience*. http://dx.doi.org/10.1016/j.dcn.2015.04.006.

Jaworska, N., MacMaster, F. P., Yang, X. R., Courtright, A., Pradhan, S., Gaxiola, I., ... Ramasubbu, R. (2014). Influence of age of onset on limbic and paralimbic structures in depression. *Psychiatry and Clinical Neurosciences*. http://dx.doi.org/10.1111/pcn.12197.

Jia, Y., Zhong, S., Wang, Y., Liu, T., Liao, X., & Huang, L. (2015). The correlation between biochemical abnormalities in frontal white matter, hippocampus and serum thyroid hormone levels in first-episode patients with major depressive disorder. *Journal of Affective Disorders, 180*, 162–169. http://dx.doi.org/10.1016/j.jad.2015.04.005.

Johnson, S. L., Wang, L., Alpert, K. I., Greenstein, D., Clasen, L., Lalonde, F., ... Gogtay, N. (2013). Hippocampal shape abnormalities of patients with childhood-onset schizophrenia and their unaffected siblings. *Journal of the American Academy of Child and Adolescent Psychiatry, 52*(5), 527–536. http://dx.doi.org/10.1016/j.jaac.2013.02.003 e522.

Jung, J., Jackson, S. R., Parkinson, A., & Jackson, G. M. (2013). Cognitive control over motor output in Tourette syndrome. *Neuroscience and Biobehavioral Reviews, 37*(6), 1016–1025. http://dx.doi.org/10.1016/j.neubiorev.2012.08.009.

Kafantaris, V., Kingsley, P., Ardekani, B., Saito, E., Lencz, T., Lim, K., & Szeszko, P. (2009). Lower orbital frontal white matter integrity in adolescents with bipolar I disorder. *Journal of the American Academy of Child and Adolescent Psychiatry, 48*(1), 79–86. http://dx.doi.org/10.1097/CHI.0b013e3181900421.

Kalmar, J. H., Wang, F., Spencer, L., Edmiston, E., Lacadie, C. M., Martin, A., ... Blumberg, H. P. (2009). Preliminary evidence for progressive prefrontal abnormalities in adolescents and young adults with bipolar disorder. *Journal of the International Neuropsychological Society, 15*(3), 476–481. http://dx.doi.org/10.1017/S1355617709090584, pii:S1355617709090584.

Karchemskiy, A., Garrett, A., Howe, M., Adleman, N., Simeonova, D. I., Alegria, D., ... Chang, K. (2011). Amygdalar, hippocampal, and thalamic volumes in youth at high risk for development of bipolar disorder. *Psychiatry Research, 194*(3), 319–325. http://dx.doi.org/10.1016/j.pscychresns.2011.03.006.

Keller, A., Jeffries, N. O., Blumenthal, J., Clasen, L. S., Liu, H., Giedd, J. N., & Rapoport, J. L. (2003). Corpus callosum development in childhood-onset schizophrenia. *Schizophrenia Research, 62*(1–2), 105–114, pii:S0920996402003547.

Khan, A. J., Nair, A., Keown, C. L., Datko, M. C., Lincoln, A. J., & Muller, R. A. (2015). Cerebro-cerebellar resting-state functional connectivity in children and adolescents with autism spectrum disorder. *Biological Psychiatry*. http://dx.doi.org/10.1016/j.biopsych.2015.03.024.

Kim, K. J., & Peterson, B. S. (2003). Cavum septi pellucidi in Tourette syndrome. *Biological Psychiatry, 54*(1), 76–85.

Kumar, A., Williams, M. T., & Chugani, H. T. (2015). Evaluation of basal ganglia and thalamic inflammation in children with pediatric autoimmune neuropsychiatric disorders associated with streptococcal infection and Tourette syndrome: a positron emission tomographic (PET) study using 11C-[R]-PK11195. *Journal of Child Neurology, 30*(6), 749–756. http://dx.doi.org/10.1177/0883073814543303.

Kusumakar, V., MacMaster, F. P., Gates, L., Sparkes, S. J., & Khan, S. C. (2001). Left medial temporal cytosolic choline in early onset depression. *Canadian Journal of Psychiatry Revue Canadienne de Psychiatrie, 46*(10), 959–964.

Lange, N., Travers, B. G., Bigler, E. D., Prigge, M. B., Froehlich, A. L., Nielsen, J. A., ... Lainhart, J. E. (2015). Longitudinal volumetric brain changes in autism spectrum disorder ages 6-35 years. *Autism Research, 8*(1), 82–93. http://dx.doi.org/10.1002/aur.1427.

Langevin, L. M., MacMaster, F. P., Crawford, S., Lebel, C., & Dewey, D. (2014). Common white matter microstructure alterations in pediatric motor and attention disorders. *The Journal of Pediatrics, 164*(5), 1157–1164. http://dx.doi.org/10.1016/j.jpeds.2014.01.018 e1151.

Langevin, L. M., MacMaster, F. P., & Dewey, D. (2014). Distinct patterns of cortical thinning in concurrent motor and attention disorders. *Developmental Medicine and Child Neurology*. http://dx.doi.org/10.1111/dmcn.12561.

Lebel, C., Walker, L., Leemans, A., Phillips, L., & Beaulieu, C. (2008). Microstructural maturation of the human brain from childhood to adulthood. *Neuroimage, 40*(3), 1044–1055. http://dx.doi.org/10.1016/j.neuroimage.2007.12.053, pii:S1053-8119(07)01177-9.

Lee, J. S., Yoo, S. S., Cho, S. Y., Ock, S. M., Lim, M. K., & Panych, L. P. (2006). Abnormal thalamic volume in treatment-naive boys with Tourette syndrome. *Acta Psychiatrica Scandinavica, 113*(1), 64–67. http://dx.doi.org/10.1111/j.1600-0447.2005.00666.x.

Liao, M., Yang, F., Zhang, Y., He, Z., Su, L., & Li, L. (2014). Lack of gender effects on gray matter volumes in adolescent generalized anxiety disorder. *Journal of Affective Disorders, 155*, 278–282. http://dx.doi.org/10.1016/j.jad.2013.10.049.

Liu, I. Y., Howe, M., Garrett, A., Karchemskiy, A., Kelley, R., Alegria, D., … Chang, K. (2011). Striatal volumes in pediatric bipolar patients with and without comorbid ADHD. *Psychiatry Research, 194*(1), 14–20. http://dx.doi.org/10.1016/j.pscychresns.2011.06.008.

MacMaster, F. P., Carrey, N., Langevin, L. M., Jaworska, N., & Crawford, S. (2014). Disorder-specific volumetric brain difference in adolescent major depressive disorder and bipolar depression. *Brain Imaging and Behavior, 8*(1), 119–127. http://dx.doi.org/10.1007/s11682-013-9264-x.

MacMaster, F. P., Carrey, N., Sparkes, S., & Kusumakar, V. (2003). Proton spectroscopy in medication-free pediatric attention-deficit/hyperactivity disorder. *Biological Psychiatry, 53*(2), 184–187, pii:S0006322302014014.

MacMaster, F. P., Keshavan, M. S., Dick, E. L., & Rosenberg, D. R. (1999). Corpus callosal signal intensity in treatment-naive pediatric obsessive compulsive disorders. *Progress in Neuro-Psychopharmacology & Biological Psychiatry, 23*(4), 601–612, pii:S0278584699000196.

MacMaster, F. P., Keshavan, M., Mirza, Y., Carrey, N., Upadhyaya, A. R., El-Sheikh, R., … Rosenberg, D. R. (2007). Development and sexual dimorphism of the pituitary gland. *Life Sciences, 80*(10), 940–944. http://dx.doi.org/10.1016/j.lfs.2006.11.040, pii:S0024-3205(06)00894-0.

MacMaster, F. P., & Kusumakar, V. (2004a). Hippocampal volume in early onset depression. *BMC Medicine, 2*, 2. http://dx.doi.org/10.1186/1741-7015-2-2, pii:1741-7015-2-2.

MacMaster, F. P., & Kusumakar, V. (2004b). MRI study of the pituitary gland in adolescent depression. *Journal of Psychiatric Research, 38*(3), 231–236. http://dx.doi.org/10.1016/j.jpsychires.2003.11.001, pii:S002239560300150X.

MacMaster, F. P., & Kusumakar, V. (2006). Choline in pediatric depression. *Mcgill Journal of Medicine, 9*(1), 24–27.

MacMaster, F. P., Leslie, R., Rosenberg, D. R., & Kusumakar, V. (2008). Pituitary gland volume in adolescent and young adult bipolar and unipolar depression. *Bipolar Disorders, 10*(1), 101–104. http://dx.doi.org/10.1111/j.1399-5618.2008.00476.x, pii:BDI476.

MacMaster, F. P., Mirza, Y., Szeszko, P. R., Kmiecik, L. E., Easter, P. C., Taormina, S. P., … Rosenberg, D. R. (2008). Amygdala and hippocampal volumes in familial early onset major depressive disorder. *Biological Psychiatry, 63*(4), 385–390. http://dx.doi.org/10.1016/j.biopsych.2007.05.005, pii:S0006-3223(07)00461-1.

MacMaster, F. P., Moore, G. J., Russell, A., Mirza, Y., Taormina, S. P., Buhagiar, C., & Rosenberg, D. R. (2008). Medial temporal N-acetyl-aspartate in pediatric major depression. *Psychiatry Research, 164*(1), 86–89. http://dx.doi.org/10.1016/j.pscychresns.2007.12.022, pii:S0925-4927(08)00002-4.

MacMaster, F. P., Russell, A., Mirza, Y., Keshavan, M. S., Taormina, S. P., Bhandari, R., … Rosenberg, D. R. (2006). Pituitary volume in treatment-naive pediatric major depressive disorder. *Biological Psychiatry, 60*(8), 862–866. http://dx.doi.org/10.1016/j.biopsych.2006.04.013, pii:S0006-3223(06)00491-4.

MacMillan, S., Szeszko, P. R., Moore, G. J., Madden, R., Lorch, E., Ivey, J., … Rosenberg, D. R. (2003). Increased amygdala: hippocampal volume ratios associated with severity of anxiety in pediatric major depression. *Journal of Child and Adolescent Psychopharmacology, 13*(1), 65–73. http://dx.doi.org/10.1089/104454603321666207.

MacQueen, G., & Frodl, T. (2011). The hippocampus in major depression: evidence for the convergence of the bench and bedside in psychiatric research? *Molecular Psychiatry, 16*(3), 252–264. http://dx.doi.org/10.1038/mp.2010.80, pii:mp201080.

MacQueen, G. M., Yucel, K., Taylor, V. H., Macdonald, K., & Joffe, R. (2008). Posterior hippocampal volumes are associated with remission rates in patients with major depressive disorder. *Biological Psychiatry, 64*(10), 880–883. http://dx.doi.org/10.1016/j.biopsych.2008.06.027, pii:S0006-3223(08)00830-5.

Magistretti, P. J., & Pellerin, L. (1999). Cellular mechanisms of brain energy metabolism and their relevance to functional brain imaging. *Philosophical Transactions of the Royal Society B: Biological Sciences, 354*(1387), 1155–1163. http://dx.doi.org/10.1098/rstb.1999.0471.

Manji, H. K., Moore, G. J., & Chen, G. (1999). Lithium at 50: have the neuroprotective effects of this unique cation been overlooked? *Biological Psychiatry, 46*(7), 929–940.

Marek, R., Strobel, C., Bredy, T. W., & Sah, P. (2013). The amygdala and medial prefrontal cortex: partners in the fear circuit. *The Journal of Physiology, 591*(Pt 10), 2381–2391. http://dx.doi.org/10.1113/jphysiol.2012.248575.

Margolis, A., Donkervoort, M., Kinsbourne, M., & Peterson, B. S. (2006). Interhemispheric connectivity and executive functioning in adults with Tourette syndrome. *Neuropsychology, 20*(1), 66–76.

Marsh, R., Horga, G., Wang, Z., Wang, P., Klahr, K. W., Berner, L. A., ... Peterson, B. S. (2011). An FMRI study of self-regulatory control and conflict resolution in adolescents with bulimia nervosa. *The American Journal of Psychiatry, 168*(11), 1210–1220. http://dx.doi.org/10.1176/appi.ajp.2011.11010094.

Maslowsky, J., Mogg, K., Bradley, B. P., McClure-Tone, E., Ernst, M., Pine, D. S., & Monk, C. S. (2010). A preliminary investigation of neural correlates of treatment in adolescents with generalized anxiety disorder. *Journal of Child and Adolescent Psychopharmacology, 20*(2), 105–111. http://dx.doi.org/10.1089/cap.2009.0049.

Mata, I., Perez-Iglesias, R., Roiz-Santianez, R., Tordesillas-Gutierrez, D., Pazos, A., Gutierrez, A., ... Crespo-Facorro, B. (2010). Gyrification brain abnormalities associated with adolescence and early-adulthood cannabis use. *Brain Research, 1317,* 297–304. http://dx.doi.org/10.1016/j.brainres.2009.12.069.

Matsuo, K., Rosenberg, D. R., Easter, P. C., MacMaster, F. P., Chen, H. H., Nicoletti, M., ... Soares, J. C. (2008). Striatal volume abnormalities in treatment-naive patients diagnosed with pediatric major depressive disorder. *Journal of Child and Adolescent Psychopharmacology, 18*(2), 121–131. http://dx.doi.org/10.1089/cap.2007.0026.

Mattai, A., Hosanagar, A., Weisinger, B., Greenstein, D., Stidd, R., Clasen, L., ... Gogtay, N. (2011). Hippocampal volume development in healthy siblings of childhood-onset schizophrenia patients. *The American Journal of Psychiatry, 168*(4), 427–435. http://dx.doi.org/10.1176/appi.ajp.2010.10050681.

McClure, E. B., Monk, C. S., Nelson, E. E., Parrish, J. M., Adler, A., Blair, R. J., ... Pine, D. S. (2007). Abnormal attention modulation of fear circuit function in pediatric generalized anxiety disorder. *Archives of General Psychiatry, 64*(1), 97–106. http://dx.doi.org/10.1001/archpsyc.64.1.97.

Moore, C. M., Frazier, J. A., Glod, C. A., Breeze, J. L., Dieterich, M., Finn, C. T., ... Renshaw, P. F. (2007). Glutamine and glutamate levels in children and adolescents with bipolar disorder: a 4.0-T proton magnetic resonance spectroscopy study of the anterior cingulate cortex. *Journal of the American Academy of Child and Adolescent Psychiatry, 46*(4), 524–534. http://dx.doi.org/10.1097/chi.0b013e31802f5f2c, pii:00004583-200704000-00015.

Moran, M. E., Luscher, Z. I., McAdams, H., Hsu, J. T., Greenstein, D., Clasen, L., ... Gogtay, N. (2015). Comparing fractional anisotropy in patients with childhood-onset schizophrenia, their healthy siblings, and normal volunteers through DTI. *Schizophrenia Bulletin, 41*(1), 66–73. http://dx.doi.org/10.1093/schbul/sbu123.

Moran, M. E., Weisinger, B., Ludovici, K., McAdams, H., Greenstein, D., Gochman, P., ... Gogtay, N. (2014). At the boundary of the self: the insular cortex in patients with childhood-onset schizophrenia, their healthy siblings, and normal volunteers. *International Journal of Developmental Neuroscience, 32,* 58–63. http://dx.doi.org/10.1016/j.ijdevneu.2013.05.010.

Moreno, A., Duno, L., Hoekzema, E., Picado, M., Martin, L. M., Fauquet, J., … Vilarroya, O. (2014). Striatal volume deficits in children with ADHD who present a poor response to methylphenidate. *European Child & Adolescent Psychiatry, 23*(9), 805–812. http://dx.doi. org/10.1007/s00787-013-0510-y.

Mostofsky, S. H., Wendlandt, J., Cutting, L., Denckla, M. B., & Singer, H. S. (1999). Corpus callosum measurements in girls with Tourette syndrome. *Neurology, 53*(6), 1345–1347.

Muller-Vahl, K. R., Kaufmann, J., Grosskreutz, J., Dengler, R., Emrich, H. M., & Peschel, T. (2009). Prefrontal and anterior cingulate cortex abnormalities in Tourette Syndrome: evidence from voxel-based morphometry and magnetization transfer imaging. *BMC Neuroscience, 10*, 47. http://dx.doi.org/10.1186/1471-2202-10-47.

Murdaugh, D. L., Maximo, J. O., & Kana, R. K. (2015). Changes in intrinsic connectivity of the brain's reading network following intervention in children with autism. *Human Brain Mapping.* http://dx.doi.org/10.1002/hbm.22821.

Neuner, I., Kupriyanova, Y., Stocker, T., Huang, R., Posnansky, O., Schneider, F., … Shah, N. J. (2010). White-matter abnormalities in Tourette syndrome extend beyond motor pathways. *Neuroimage, 51*(3), 1184–1193. http://dx.doi.org/10.1016/j.neuroimage.2010.02.049.

Nicolson, R., & Rapoport, J. L. (1999). Childhood-onset schizophrenia: rare but worth studying. *Biological Psychiatry, 46*(10), 1418–1428.

Nolan, C. L., Moore, G. J., Madden, R., Farchione, T., Bartoi, M., Lorch, E., … Rosenberg, D. R. (2002). Prefrontal cortical volume in childhood-onset major depression: preliminary findings. *Archives of General Psychiatry, 59*(2), 173–179.

Nugent, T. F., 3rd, Herman, D. H., Ordonez, A., Greenstein, D., Hayashi, K. M., Lenane, M., … Gogtay, N. (2007). Dynamic mapping of hippocampal development in childhood onset schizophrenia. *Schizophrenia Research, 90*(1–3), 62–70. http://dx.doi.org/10.1016/j. schres.2006.10.014.

Ongur, D., Drevets, W. C., & Price, J. L. (1998). Glial reduction in the subgenual prefrontal cortex in mood disorders. *Proceedings of the National Academy of Sciences of the United States of America, 95*(22), 13290–13295.

Orr, C., Morioka, R., Behan, B., Datwani, S., Doucet, M., Ivanovic, J., … Garavan, H. (2013). Altered resting-state connectivity in adolescent cannabis users. *The American Journal of Drug and Alcohol Abuse, 39*(6), 372–381. http://dx.doi.org/10.3109/00952990.2013.848213.

Pardo, C. A., & Eberhart, C. G. (2007). The neurobiology of autism. *Brain Pathology, 17*(4), 434–447. http://dx.doi.org/10.1750-3639.2007.00102.x.

Patel, N. C., DelBello, M. P., Cecil, K. M., Stanford, K. E., Adler, C. M., & Strakowski, S. M. (2008). Temporal change in N-acetyl-aspartate concentrations in adolescents with bipolar depression treated with lithium. *Journal of Child and Adolescent Psychopharmacology, 18*(2), 132–139. http://dx.doi.org/10.1089/cap.2007.0088.

Pavuluri, M. N., Yang, S., Kamineni, K., Passarotti, A. M., Srinivasan, G., Harral, E. M., … Zhou, X. J. (2009). Diffusion tensor imaging study of white matter fiber tracts in pediatric bipolar disorder and attention-deficit/hyperactivity disorder. *Biological Psychiatry, 65*(7), 586–593. http://dx.doi.org/10.1016/j.biopsych.2008.10.015, pii:S0006-3223(08)01247-X.

Peterson, B. S., Choi, H. A., Hao, X., Amat, J. A., Zhu, H., Whiteman, R., … Bansal, R. (2007). Morphologic features of the amygdala and hippocampus in children and adults with Tourette syndrome. *Archives of General Psychiatry, 64*(11), 1281–1291. http://dx.doi. org/10.1001/archpsyc.64.11.1281.

Peterson, B., Riddle, M. A., Cohen, D. J., Katz, L. D., Smith, J. C., Hardin, M. T., & Leckman, J. F. (1993). Reduced basal ganglia volumes in Tourette's syndrome using three-dimensional reconstruction techniques from magnetic resonance images. *Neurology, 43*(5), 941–949.

Peterson, B. S., Staib, L., Scahill, L., Zhang, H., Anderson, C., Leckman, J. F., … Webster, R. (2001). Regional brain and ventricular volumes in Tourette syndrome. *Archives of General Psychiatry, 58*(5), 427–440.

Plessen, K. J., Gruner, R., Lundervold, A., Hirsch, J. G., Xu, D., Bansal, R., ... Hugdahl, K. (2006). Reduced white matter connectivity in the corpus callosum of children with Tourette syndrome. *Journal of Child Psychology and Psychiatry, and Allied Disciplines, 47*(10), 1013–1022.

Plessen, K. J., Lundervold, A., Gruner, R., Hammar, A., Lundervold, A., Peterson, B. S., & Hugdahl, K. (2007). Functional brain asymmetry, attentional modulation, and interhemispheric transfer in boys with Tourette syndrome. *Neuropsychologia, 45*(4), 767–774.

Reynolds, S., Carrey, N., Jaworska, N., Langevin, L. M., Yang, X. R., & Macmaster, F. P. (2014). Cortical thickness in youth with major depressive disorder. *BMC Psychiatry, 14*, 83. http://dx.doi.org/10.1186/1471-244X-14-83.

Rich, B. A., Vinton, D. T., Roberson-Nay, R., Hommer, R. E., Berghorst, L. H., McClure, E. B., ... Leibenluft, E. (2006). Limbic hyperactivation during processing of neutral facial expressions in children with bipolar disorder. *Proceedings of the National Academy of Sciences of the United States of America, 103*(23), 8900–8905. http://dx.doi.org/10.1073/pnas.0603246103.

Roessner, V., Wittfoth, M., August, J. M., Rothenberger, A., Baudewig, J., & Dechent, P. (2013). Finger tapping-related activation differences in treatment-naive pediatric Tourette syndrome: a comparison of the preferred and nonpreferred hand. *Journal of Child Psychology and Psychiatry, and Allied Disciplines, 54*(3), 273–279. http://dx.doi.org/10.1111/j.1469-7610.2012.02584.x.

Rosenberg, D. R., & Keshavan, M. S. (1998). A.E. Bennett Research Award. Toward a neurodevelopmental model of of obsessive–compulsive disorder. *Biological Psychiatry, 43*(9), 623–640.

Rosenberg, D. R., Keshavan, M. S., Dick, E. L., Bagwell, W. W., MacMaster, F. P., & Birmaher, B. (1997). Corpus callosal morphology in treatment-naive pediatric obsessive compulsive disorder. *Progress in Neuro-Psychopharmacology & Biological Psychiatry, 21*(8), 1269–1283, pii:S0278584697001632.

Rosenberg, D. R., Keshavan, M. S., O'Hearn, K. M., Dick, E. L., Bagwell, W. W., Seymour, A. B., ... Birmaher, B. (1997). Frontostriatal measurement in treatment-naive children with obsessive-compulsive disorder. *Archives of General Psychiatry, 54*(9), 824–830.

Rosenberg, D. R., MacMaster, F. P., Keshavan, M. S., Fitzgerald, K. D., Stewart, C. M., & Moore, G. J. (2000). Decrease in caudate glutamatergic concentrations in pediatric obsessive-compulsive disorder patients taking paroxetine. *Journal of the American Academy of Child and Adolescent Psychiatry, 39*(9), 1096–1103. http://dx.doi.org/10.1097/00004583-200009000-00008, pii:S0890-8567(09)66322-X.

Rosenberg, D. R., Macmaster, F. P., Mirza, Y., Smith, J. M., Easter, P. C., Banerjee, S. P., ... Renshaw, P. (2005). Reduced anterior cingulate glutamate in pediatric major depression: a magnetic resonance spectroscopy study. *Biological Psychiatry, 58*(9), 700–704. http://dx.doi.org/10.1016/j.biopsych.2005.05.007, pii:S0006-3223(05)00583-4.

Rosenberg, D. R., Mirza, Y., Russell, A., Tang, J., Smith, J. M., Banerjee, S. P., ... Moore, G. J. (2004). Reduced anterior cingulate glutamatergic concentrations in childhood OCD and major depression versus healthy controls. *Journal of the American Academy of Child and Adolescent Psychiatry, 43*(9), 1146–1153. http://dx.doi.org/10.1097/01.chi.0000132812.44664.2d, pii:S0890-8567(09)61449-0.

Rosso, I. M., Cintron, C. M., Steingard, R. J., Renshaw, P. F., Young, A. D., & Yurgelun-Todd, D. A. (2005). Amygdala and hippocampus volumes in pediatric major depression. *Biological Psychiatry, 57*(1), 21–26.

Rubia, K., Alegria, A. A., Cubillo, A. I., Smith, A. B., Brammer, M. J., & Radua, J. (2014). Effects of stimulants on brain function in attention-deficit/hyperactivity disorder: a systematic review and meta-analysis. *Biological Psychiatry, 76*(8), 616–628. http://dx.doi.org/10.1016/j.biopsych.2013.10.016.

Rzanny, R., Freesmeyer, D., Reichenbach, J. R., Mentzel, H. J., Pfleiderer, S. O., Klemm, S., ... Kaiser, W. A. (2003). 31P-MR spectroscopy of the brain in patients with anorexia nervosa: characteristic differences in the spectra between patients and healthy control subjects. *Rofo, 175*(1), 75–82. http://dx.doi.org/10.1055/s-2003-36611.

Samsom, J. N., & Wong, A. H. (2015). Schizophrenia and depression co-morbidity: what we have learned from animal models. *Front Psychiatry, 6,* 13. http://dx.doi.org/10.3389/fpsyt.2015.00013.

Sassi, R. B., Nicoletti, M., Brambilla, P., Harenski, K., Mallinger, A. G., Frank, E., ... Soares, J. C. (2001). Decreased pituitary volume in patients with bipolar disorder. *Biological Psychiatry, 50*(4), 271–280.

Seese, R. R., O'Neill, J., Hudkins, M., Siddarth, P., Levitt, J., Tseng, B., ... Caplan, R. (2011). Proton magnetic resonance spectroscopy and thought disorder in childhood schizophrenia. *Schizophrenia Research, 133*(1–3), 82–90. http://dx.doi.org/10.1016/j.schres.2011.07.011.

Shaw, P., Eckstrand, K., Sharp, W., Blumenthal, J., Lerch, J. P., Greenstein, D., ... Rapoport, J. L. (2007). Attention-deficit/hyperactivity disorder is characterized by a delay in cortical maturation. *Proceedings of the National Academy of Sciences of the United States of America, 104*(49), 19649–19654. http://dx.doi.org/10.1073/pnas.0707741104.

Shi, X. F., Forrest, L. N., Kuykendall, M. D., Prescot, A. P., Sung, Y. H., Huber, R. S., ... Kondo, D. G. (2014). Anterior cingulate cortex choline levels in female adolescents with unipolar versus bipolar depression: a potential new tool for diagnosis. *Journal of Affective Disorders, 167,* 25–29. http://dx.doi.org/10.1016/j.jad.2014.05.051.

Singer, H. S., Reiss, A. L., Brown, J. E., Aylward, E. H., Shih, B., Chee, E., ... Bryan, R. N. (1993). Volumetric MRI changes in basal ganglia of children with Tourette's syndrome. *Neurology, 43*(5), 950–956.

Smith, S. M., Jenkinson, M., Johansen-Berg, H., Rueckert, D., Nichols, T. E., Mackay, C. E., ... Behrens, T. E. (2006). Tract-based spatial statistics: voxelwise analysis of multi-subject diffusion data. *Neuroimage, 31*(4), 1487–1505. http://dx.doi.org/10.1016/j.neuroimage.2006.02.024.

Smith, E. A., Russell, A., Lorch, E., Banerjee, S. P., Rose, M., Ivey, J., ... Rosenberg, D. R. (2003). Increased medial thalamic choline found in pediatric patients with obsessive-compulsive disorder versus major depression or healthy control subjects: a magnetic resonance spectroscopy study. *Biological Psychiatry, 54*(12), 1399–1405.

Soliva, J. C., Fauquet, J., Bielsa, A., Rovira, M., Carmona, S., Ramos-Quiroga, J. A., & Vilarroya, O. (2010). Quantitative MR analysis of caudate abnormalities in pediatric ADHD: proposal for a diagnostic test. *Psychiatry Research, 182*(3), 238–243. http://dx.doi.org/10.1016/j.pscychresns.2010.01.013, pii:S0925-4927(10)00038-7.

Sowell, E. R., Toga, A. W., & Asarnow, R. (2000). Brain abnormalities observed in childhood-onset schizophrenia: a review of the structural magnetic resonance imaging literature. *Mental Retardation and Developmental Disabilities Research Reviews, 6*(3), 180–185. http://dx.doi.org/10.1002/1098-2779(2000)6:3<180::AID-MRDD5>3.0.CO;2-I.

Squeglia, L. M., Rinker, D. A., Bartsch, H., Castro, N., Chung, Y., Dale, A. M., ... Tapert, S. F. (2014). Brain volume reductions in adolescent heavy drinkers. *Developmental Cognitive Neuroscience, 9,* 117–125. http://dx.doi.org/10.1016/j.dcn.2014.02.005.

Stanley, J. A., Kipp, H., Greisenegger, E., MacMaster, F. P., Panchalingam, K., Keshavan, M. S., ... Pettegrew, J. W. (2008). Evidence of developmental alterations in cortical and subcortical regions of children with attention-deficit/hyperactivity disorder: a multivoxel in vivo phosphorus 31 spectroscopy study. *Archives of General Psychiatry, 65*(12), 1419–1428. http://dx.doi.org/10.1001/archgenpsychiatry.2008.503, pii:65/12/1419.

Stanley, J. A., Kipp, H., Greisenegger, E., MacMaster, F. P., Panchalingam, K., Pettegrew, J. W., ... Bukstein, O. G. (2006). Regionally specific alterations in membrane phospholipids in children with ADHD: an in vivo 31P spectroscopy study. *Psychiatry Research, 148*(2–3), 217–221. http://dx.doi.org/10.1016/j.pscychresns.2006.08.003, pii:S0925-4927(06)00126-0.

Steingard, R. J., Renshaw, P. F., Hennen, J., Lenox, M., Cintron, C. B., Young, A. D., ... Yurgelun-Todd, D. A. (2002). Smaller frontal lobe white matter volumes in depressed adolescents. *Biological Psychiatry, 52*(5), 413–417.

Steingard, R. J., Yurgelun-Todd, D. A., Hennen, J., Moore, J. C., Moore, C. M., Vakili, K., ... Renshaw, P. F. (2000). Increased orbitofrontal cortex levels of choline in depressed adolescents as detected by in vivo proton magnetic resonance spectroscopy. *Biological Psychiatry, 48*(11), 1053–1061, pii:S0006-3223(00)00942-2.

Strawn, J. R., Bitter, S. M., Weber, W. A., Chu, W. J., Whitsel, R. M., Adler, C., ... DelBello, M. P. (2012). Neurocircuitry of generalized anxiety disorder in adolescents: a pilot functional neuroimaging and functional connectivity study. *Depression and Anxiety, 29*(11), 939–947. http://dx.doi.org/10.1002/da.21961.

Strawn, J. R., John Wegman, C., Dominick, K. C., Swartz, M. S., Wehry, A. M., Patino, L. R., ... DelBello, M. P. (2014). Cortical surface anatomy in pediatric patients with generalized anxiety disorder. *Journal of Anxiety Disorders, 28*(7), 717–723. http://dx.doi.org/10.1016/j. janxdis.2014.07.012.

Szeszko, P. R., Christian, C., Macmaster, F., Lencz, T., Mirza, Y., Taormina, S. P., ... Rosenberg, D. R. (2008). Gray matter structural alterations in psychotropic drug-naive pediatric obsessive-compulsive disorder: an optimized voxel-based morphometry study. *The American Journal of Psychiatry, 165*(10), 1299–1307. http://dx.doi.org/10.1176/appi. ajp.2008.08010033, pii:appi.ajp.2008.08010033.

Szeszko, P. R., MacMillan, S., McMeniman, M., Chen, S., Baribault, K., Lim, K. O., ... Rosenberg, D. R. (2004). Brain structural abnormalities in psychotropic drug-naive pediatric patients with obsessive-compulsive disorder. *The American Journal of Psychiatry, 161*(6), 1049–1056.

Szeszko, P. R., MacMillan, S., McMeniman, M., Lorch, E., Madden, R., Ivey, J., ... Rosenberg, D. R. (2004). Amygdala volume reductions in pediatric patients with obsessive-compulsive disorder treated with paroxetine: preliminary findings. *Neuropsychopharmacology, 29*(4), 826–832. http://dx.doi.org/10.1038/sj.npp.1300399, pii:1300399.

Thacker, N. A. (2005). *Tutorial: A critical analysis of voxel based morphometry (VBM)*. Manchester: University of Manchester.

Thompson, P. M., Giedd, J. N., Woods, R. P., MacDonald, D., Evans, A. C., & Toga, A. W. (2000). Growth patterns in the developing brain detected by using continuum mechanical tensor maps. *Nature, 404*(6774), 190–193. http://dx.doi.org/10.1038/35004593.

Van den Eynde, F., Suda, M., Broadbent, H., Guillaume, S., Van den Eynde, M., Steiger, H., ... Schmidt, U. (2012). Structural magnetic resonance imaging in eating disorders: a systematic review of voxel-based morphometry studies. *European Eating Disorders Review, 20*(2), 94–105. http://dx.doi.org/10.1002/erv.1163.

Vinette, S. A., & Bray, S. (2015). Variation in functional connectivity along anterior-to-posterior intraparietal sulcus, and relationship with age across late childhood and adolescence. *Developmental Cognitive Neuroscience, 13*, 32–42. http://dx.doi.org/10.1016/j. dcn.2015.04.004.

Wagshal, D., Knowlton, B. J., Suthana, N. A., Cohen, J. R., Poldrack, R. A., Bookheimer, S. Y., ... Asarnow, R. F. (2014). Evidence for corticostriatal dysfunction during cognitive skill learning in adolescent siblings of patients with childhood-onset schizophrenia. *Schizophrenia Bulletin, 40*(5), 1030–1039. http://dx.doi.org/10.1093/schbul/sbt147.

Weiland, B. J., Nigg, J. T., Welsh, R. C., Yau, W. Y., Zubieta, J. K., Zucker, R. A., & Heitzeg, M. M. (2012). Resiliency in adolescents at high risk for substance abuse: flexible adaptation via subthalamic nucleus and linkage to drinking and drug use in early adulthood. *Alcoholism, Clinical and Experimental Research, 36*(8), 1355–1364. http://dx.doi. org/10.1111/j.1530-0277.2012.01741.x.

Woolley, J., Heyman, I., Brammer, M., Frampton, I., McGuire, P. K., & Rubia, K. (2008). Brain activation in paediatric obsessive compulsive disorder during tasks of inhibitory control. *The British Journal of Psychiatry, 192*(1), 25–31. http://dx.doi.org/10.1192/bjp. bp.107.036558, pii:192/1/25.

Woon, F. L., & Hedges, D. W. (2008). Hippocampal and amygdala volumes in children and adults with childhood maltreatment-related posttraumatic stress disorder: a meta-analysis. *Hippocampus, 18*(8), 729–736. http://dx.doi.org/10.1002/hipo.20437.

Yang, X. R., Carrey, N., Bernier, D., & MacMaster, F. P. (2012). Cortical thickness in young treatment-naive children with ADHD. *Journal of Attention Disorders.* http://dx.doi.org/10.1177/1087054712455501.

Yang, X. R., Kirton, A., Wilkes, T. C., Pradhan, S., Liu, I., Jaworska, N., ... MacMaster, F. P. (2014). Glutamate alterations associated with transcranial magnetic stimulation in youth depression: a case series. *The Journal of ECT, 30*(3), 242–247. http://dx.doi.org/10.1097/YCT.0000000000000094.

Zarei, M., Mataix-Cols, D., Heyman, I., Hough, M., Doherty, J., Burge, L., ... James, A. (2011). Changes in gray matter volume and white matter microstructure in adolescents with obsessive-compulsive disorder. *Biological Psychiatry, 70*(11), 1083–1090. http://dx.doi.org/10.1016/j.biopsych.2011.06.032.

Genetic Process in Resilience and Vulnerability and the Consequence of Abuse

M. Peskin[1], G. Zalsman[1,2]

[1]Tel Aviv University, Tel Aviv, Israel; [2]Columbia University, New York, NY, United States

VULNERABILITY AND RESILIENCE

Maltreatment and Psychopathology

Child maltreatment has been conceptualized as a pathogenic relational experience that represents one of the most adverse and stressful challenges that confronts children in all societies that have been studied (Cicchetti & Lynch, 1995). Abuse, neglect, and family violence have been described as toxic conditions that expose children to chronic, severe, and prolonged stress (Shonkoff, Boyce, & McEven, 2009). Child maltreatment is the best-established risk factor that may have a negative impact on numerous domains of child functioning by leading to adaptive interconnected and interacting biological systems to become chronically dysregulated. Repeated disruptions in developmental processes and failure of the adaptive system can cascade or spread its effects even across other systems (Cicchetti & Tucker, 1994; Masten & Cicchetti, 2010). Maladaptive physiological and psychological consequences are likely to persist throughout the lifespan (Juster, McEwen, & Lupien, 2010; Karatsoreos & McEwen, 2012).

Stress is an ambiguous concept, with subjective and negative connotations making it less useful in strict scientific approaches. A more recent, better-defined, neutral view of stress, has been provided by the concept of allostasis and allostatic load and overload (McEwen & Stellar, 1993; McEwen & Wingfield, 2003). "Allostatic responses are

Positive Mental Health, Fighting Stigma and Promoting Resiliency for Children and Adolescents
http://dx.doi.org/10.1016/B978-0-12-804394-3.00004-8

those physiological changes that occur in response to environmental perturbations" (Karatsoreos & McEwen, 2011). The concept is related to homeostasis. Homeostasis can be described as the way the body maintains and returns to stability. Allostasis is concerned with the whole dynamic process of achieving this balance. Homeostasis implies remaining stable by being the same, while allostasis suggests remaining stable by changing. Thus, allostasis reflects the fact that unavoidable environmental perturbations awake essential responses for survival. "These responses are not negative in-and-of-themselves, but instead play an important positive role in helping an organism adapt to a changing environment" (Karatsoreos & McEwen, 2011). Biological mechanisms turn on to achieve stability of homeostatic systems. Allostatic load refers to the condition in which these activated neurobiological adaptation processes are insufficient or poorly organized resulting in pathology or chronic illness. In this conceptualization, allostatic load is "the price the individual pays for being forced to adapt to adverse psychosocial or physical situations" (McEwen, 1998). In other words, allostatic load may represent either the exposure to too much stress or the inefficient operation of the adaptive systems. Allostatic load can be measured by biological biomarkers.

The vast majority of maltreated children are adversely affected by their experiences (Cicchetti, 2012). Child maltreatment challenges the subject capacity to adapt to adversity, and may provide an allostatic load (or overload) since this chronic exposure heightens and sustains neural and neuroendocrine responsiveness (Ganzel, Morris, & Wethington, 2010; Juster et al., 2011). Over time, allostatic load can accumulate and have adverse effects on various organ systems (McEwen, 1998).

However, not all maltreated children develop psychopathology. Garmezy claimed that most children maintain the ability to display some resilience even in the presence of chronic and serious adversity (Garmezy, 1974). Research has shown that some children who have been exposed to harsh and inadequate caretaking succeed in dealing with adversity and exhibit resilient functioning (Haskett, Nears, Ward, & McPherson, 2006). The outcome of child maltreatment does not always bring about psychopathology, and whether or not it occurs will depend on the balance between the allostatic load and the severity of the homeostatic disturbance. Child maltreatment provides a great example of multifinality: various outcomes may stem from similar beginnings (Cicchetti & Rogosch, 1996).

Resilience

It is crucial to examine and understand the factors and mechanisms that promote positive adaptation when experiencing significant adversity (Rutter, 2012). Resilience is a power instilled in the individual, the capacity for successful adaptation, positive functioning, and competence despite high-risk conditions, chronic stress, or following prolonged or severe trauma (Egeland, Carlson, & Sroufe, 1993). Since the dynamic neurobiological adaptation system has the faculty to withstand or recover from significant challenges, like early maltreatment, that has threatened its stability, viability, or development (Masten, 2011), child abuse and neglect is a framework for the study of resilience. The fact is that resilience cannot be directly measured; rather, it is inferred by examining positive adaptation in conjunction with adversity (Edmond, Auslander, Elze, & Bowland, 2006). The widespread and potentially devastating phenomenon of child maltreatment has become an opportunity for a naturalistic study of human resilience.

Developmental outcomes are conceived as the result of interactions and transactions among genetic and environmental factors (Sroufe, 1997; Sroufe, Egeland, Carlson, & Collins 2005). The developmental process is characterized by a hierarchical integration of the systems that may be considered as holons (Bowman, 2009). Children maltreatment has become also an opportunity for the study of the resilience/vulnerability developmental pathway.

GENETIC FACTORS

Until the last decade, most of the studies have been focused on the effects of psychosocial-cultural-environmental factors in adults who were exposed to maltreatment and this has also been the case with most of the studies on resilient maltreated children (Edwards, Holden, Felitti, & Anda, 2003; Luthar, 2006). Advances in molecular technology and knowledge in the field of genetics have given rise to "the fourth wave of resilience science" (Masten, 2014), which is characterized by dynamic, system-oriented approaches, with a focus on the interaction of genes with experience, connecting levels of analysis and multidisciplinary integration. Particular genetic variants may serve a protective function against environmental risks for some individuals (Belsky et al., 2009). In this context, a summary of the studies and findings of the genetic factors operating under the resilience/vulnerability response spectrum of maltreated children will be provided.

The Monoamine Oxidase A Gene uVNTR Polymorphism

Caspi et al. (2002), in their well-known study published in 2002, found that a functional polymorphism in the promoter region of the monoamine oxidase A gene (MAOA-uVNTR polymorphism) moderated the impact of child maltreatment on the development of antisocial behavior in adult male subjects. The effect of child maltreatment on antisocial behavior in adulthood was significantly less among males with high MAOA activity than among those with low MAOA activity. Replication studies results stressed the need for a more sophisticated design in trying to understand the role of the MAOA in the outcome of maltreated children (Foley et al., 2004; Haberstick et al., 2005; Nilsson et al., 2005; Young et al., 2005). New research conducted by Kim-Cohen et al. (2006) evaluated the cumulative evidence regarding MAOA activity in the context of childhood adversity via meta-analysis. It was demonstrated that across studies the association between maltreatment and mental health problems was significantly stronger in the group of males with the genotype conferring low versus high MAOA activity. The authors concluded that the findings "provide the strongest evidence to date suggesting that the MAOA gene influences vulnerability to environmental stress, and that this biological process can be initiated early in life." In the light of resilience framework, the finding suggests an association between high MAOA activity and resilient outcomes, with more active MAOA leading to better management of the maltreatment-induced changes in the catecholaminergic neurotransmitter system. Subsequent, additional studies found significant interaction between child maltreatment and the MAOA genotype on aggressive/antisocial behavior in maltreated children (eg, Weder et al., 2009), adolescents (eg, Aslund et al., 2009), and adults (eg, Ferguson, Boden, Horwood, Miller, & Kennedy, 2011).

Cicchetti, Rogosch, and Thibodeau (2012) conducted the first multi-genetic study to examine $G \times E$ interaction on antisocial behavior in maltreated children with a large number of maltreated children ($N = 349$) including the MAOAuVNTR polymorphism and also the tryptophan hydroxylase gene (TPH1) gene and the serotonin transporter promoter (5-HTLPR) gene. With respect to the MAOAuVNTR, they concluded, "the risk for antisocial behavior associated with maltreatment is reduced among children with high MAOA activity genotypes."

However, in a very recent study, childhood maltreatment in a large sample ($N = 4316$) participating in the National Longitudinal Study of Adolescent Health, MAOA genotype was not a significant moderator of the relationship between maltreatment and antisocial behaviors (Haberstick et al., 2014).

The TAT Haplotype in the Corticotropin-Releasing Hormone Type 1 Receptor Gene

The hypothalamic-pituitary-adrenal axis is the main mediator of the stress response. Bradley et al. (2008) investigated probable association between child physical, sexual, and emotional abuse and a TAT haplotype of the corticotropin-releasing hormone type 1 receptor gene (TAT CRHR1) on adult depressive symptoms. They found significant association between the gene and diminished effects of the abuse in the population studied. Polanczyk et al. (2009), in a replication study with women in the E-Risk Study and men and women of the Dunedin study, found the same association as Bradley only in the E-Risk Study.

DeYoung, Cicchetti, and Rogosch (2011) investigated probable association between child maltreatment and the TAT CRHR1 on neuroticism. The study sheds light on the crucial importance of taking into account different types of maltreatment. They found a significant association between having two copies of the TAT haplotype and higher risk of neuroticism unless the children had been sexually abused or had experienced three or four different types of maltreatment, in which case they may be protected from increased neuroticism.

The TAT CRHR1 was one of the four genes examined by Cicchetti and Rogosch (2012) in one of their $G \times E$ studies into resilient functioning in maltreated children. They compared maltreated and non-maltreated school-aged children ($N = 595$) regarding CRHR1, serotonin transporter promoter (5-HTTLPR) gene, dopamine receptor DRD4-521C/T single nucleotide polymorphism (SNP), and the oxytocin receptor gene, all "genes which have known associations with aspects of behavior found to be predictive of resilience in single level psychosocial studies." A consistent finding of the study, relevant to the four genes, was related to Belsky and Pluess (2009) differential susceptibility to environmental influence hypothesis. They highlight their influence on the reactivity to environment. Genes have an experiential-framed role. Non-maltreated children, especially those without copies of the TAT haplotype, had higher levels of resilient functioning relative to maltreated children with the same number of copies. The whole equation is "vulnerability to adverse experience versus profit from a supportive context" (Ellis, Boyce, Belsky, Bakermans-Kranenburg, & van Ijzendorn, 2011).

Tryptophan Hydroxylase 1 Gene

The tryptophan hydroxylase 1 (TPH1) gene was one of the three genes also analyzed by Cicchetti, Rogosch, and Thibodeau (2012) in a sample of maltreated and non-maltreated low-income children, along with the 5-HTTLPR gene and MAOA genes (mentioned in the previous section). The study design included three sources of evaluation of children's antisocial behavior: self-report, peer-report, and adult counselor-report; and three variables of child maltreatment: subtypes (neglect, emotional maltreatment, physical abuse, and sexual abuse), developmental timing, and chronicity. Maltreated children with the GG genotype were found to be at lower risk for antisocial behavior. This was also the case for children who experienced physical or sexual abuse and for chronically maltreated children.

Serotonin Transporter Promoter Gene (5HTTLPR)

The most studied candidate gene polymorphism in depression as an example of gene × environment interaction is the 5HTTLPR as the promotor of the serotonin transporter gene. Children, adolescents, and young adult carriers of the short (S)-allele are reported to be vulnerable to major depression when exposed to adverse events during childhood (Caspi et al., 2002; Eley et al., 2004; Kaufman et al., 2004; Zalsman et al., 2006a,b). We replicated these findings (Zalsman et al., 2006a) in terms of severity of depression. In a meta-analysis of 54 studies, Karg, Burmeister, Shedden, and Sen (2011) confirmed that the 5-HTTLPR polymorphism moderates the relationship between childhood stress and adult depression ($p = .00002$). When stratifying the analysis by the type of stressor studied, they found strong evidence for an association between the S-allele and increased stress sensitivity to childhood maltreatment ($p = .00007$), but it was early and not late stress that was pathogenic.

Li and Lee (2010) investigated the interaction between the 5-HTTLPR gene and adverse childhood experiences on the development of antisocial behavior using data from the wave one of the National Longitudinal Study of Adolescent Health, when participants were about 15 years old. No significant G × E interaction was found for boys, while maltreated girls who were homozygous for the gene were much likely to exhibit an antisocial phenotype.

Douglas et al. (2011) used in their study the same triallelic polymorphism of 5-HTTPRL as Zalsman et al. (2006a) in order to examine genetic and environmental risks for developing antisocial personality disorder in adult substance-dependent individuals. They found a higher percentage of antisocial personality disorder associated with the SS genotype in a small group of African American women.

As mentioned previously, Cicchetti and Rogosch (2012) included the 5-HTTPRL in their molecular genetic investigation of school-aged children and found that non-maltreated children with the SS genotype variant were significantly more likely to have resilient functioning, whereas maltreated children with the same variant had significantly lower resilient functioning. That is consistent with Rutter's perspective: "the genetic polymorphisms that are associated with vulnerability to adverse environments may also be associated with greater responsivity to positive environments" (Rutter, 2013).

In an additional study referenced previously, with a low-income population (Cicchetti, Rogosch, & Thibodeau, 2012), the findings suggested lower risk for antisocial behavior associated with the LL genotype, with greatest risk perceived by peers for children with the SS genotype.

Other Genes Which May Be Mediators Between Child Maltreatment, and Maladjustment and Psychopathology

In the last 2 years, numerous studies have been published which have investigated genes for possible mediation between child maltreatment and maladjustment and psychopathological conditions: additional genes related to the hypothalamic-pituitary-adrenal axis:

- polymorphisms within CRHR1/2 (Guillaume et al., 2013)
- single-nucleotide polymorphism of the FK506 binding protein 51 (FKBP5) (Tozi et al., 2015; White et al., 2012)
- neuropeptide S receptor Gene (Klauke et al., 2014)
- interleukin 1 B gene (Ridout et al., 2014)
- norepinephrine transporter (Cicchetti & Rogosch, 2014)
- Met alleles of the brain-derived neurotrophic factor (BDNF) (Brown et al., 2014)
- Val66Met polymorphism of the BDNF (Min et al., 2013)
- cholinergic receptor gene NA4 (Grazioplene, DeYoung, Rogosch, & Cicchetti, 2013)
- Val158Met catechol-O-methyltransferase gene (Goldberg et al., 2013)
- dopamine transporter (DAT1) (Li & Lee, 2012)

These emergent studies, while still awaiting replication, may be considered an indication of the increasing efforts of researchers to elucidate the genetic underpinnings of children's resilience or vulnerability following maltreatment.

Gene Environment Timing $(G \times E \times T)$ Interactions

Early stress (ES) produces alterations in brain structure and function that mediate the environment's effect on mood regulation and response to stress in adulthood (for review see Zalsman, 2010). Brain vulnerability to ES is thought to decline with age at the time of exposure, but little attention has been given to the relationship between age of ES and its impact on mood regulation and brain integrity (Baker et al., 2013).

Early stressful life events predict depression and anxiety in carriers of specific polymorphisms and alter brain responses, but brain structural phenotypes are largely unknown. We studied the interaction between short-term stress during specific time-windows and emotion-regulation using a genetic animal model of depression, the Wistar-Kyoto (WKY) rat (Zalsman et al., 2015). Brain structural alterations were analyzed using Diffusion Tensor Imaging (DTI). WKY and Wistar rats were divided into experimental groups: early stress (ES): from postnatal day (PND) 27, rats were exposed to three consecutive days of stressors; late stress (LS): from

PND 44, rats were exposed to the same protocol; control: no stressors. From PND 50, all animals were behaviorally tested for levels of anxiety- and despair-like behaviors and then scanned. Gene × Environment × Timing (G × E × T) interactions ($p = 0.00022$ after Hochberg correction) were found in ventral orbital cortex, cingulate cortex, external capsule, amygdala, dentate gyrus, and in the emotion regulation measures. WKY showed longer immobility in a forced swim test, but no effect of ES was detected. We demonstrated that stress in pre-pubertal or adolescent phases of development may influence structural integrity of specific brain regions and emotion regulation behaviors depending on genetic vulnerability, consistent with a G × E × T interaction in mood dysregulation (Zalsman et al., 2015).

SUMMARY AND FUTURE DIRECTIONS

Child maltreatment and abuse represent the most adverse and stressful challenges that confront children in all societies that have been studied. These stressful events may precede pathogenic processes for the developing brain. Genetic polymorphisms were reported to interact with environmental adverse factors to create psychopathology. New data show that the timing of the insult to the developing brain is crucial for the outcome. This effect has biological correlates in the structure of the brain in rodents and probably humans. Future studies will attempt to evaluate this in human subjects using imaging and molecular imaging techniques. This would give the potential for the development of personalized treatments.

Acknowledgments

Prof. Zalsman dedicates this chapter to the late Prof. Donald J. Cohen, former president of the IACAPAP, a mentor, a teacher, a clinician, and a great researcher who has led the way to the understanding of gene–environment interactions in early childhood.

References

Aslund, C., Nordquist, N., Comasco, E., Leppert, J., Oreland, L., & Nilsson, K. W. (2009). Maltreatment, MAOA, and delinquency: sex differences in gene-environment interaction in a large population-based cohort of adolescents. *Behavior Genetics, 41*, 262–272.

Baker, L. M., Williams, L. M., Korgaonkar, M. S., Cohen, R. A., Heaps, J. M., & Paul, R. H. (2013). Impact of early vs. late childhood early life stress on brain morphometrics. *Brain Imaging and Behavior, 7*, 196–203.

Belsky, J., Jonassaint, C., Pluess, M., Stanton, M., Brummett, B., & Williams, R. (2009). Vulnerability genes or plasticity genes? *Molecular Psychiatry, 14*, 746–754.

Belsky, J., & Pluess, M. (2009). Beyond diathesis stress: differential susceptibility to environmental influences. *Psychological Bulletin, 35*, 885–908.

Bowman, K. J. (2009). Holarchical development: discovering and applying missing drives from Den Wilber's twenty tenets. *International Journal of Transpersonal Studies, 28*, 1–24.

Bradley, R. G., Binder, E. B., Epstein, M. P., Tang, Y., Nair, H. P., Liu, W., … Ressler, K. J. (2008). Influence of child abuse on adult depression: moderation by the corticotropin-releasing hormone receptor gene. *Archives of General Psychiatry, 65*, 190–200.

Brown, G. W., Craig, T. K., Harris, T. O., Herbert, J., Hodgson, K., Tansey, K. E., & Uher, R. (2014). Functional polymorphism in the brain-derived neurotrophic factor gene interacts with stressful life events but not childhood maltreatment in the etiology of depression. *Depression and Anxiety, 31*, 326–334.

Caspi, A., McClay, J., Moffit, T. E., Mill, J., Martin, J., Craig, I. W., … Poulton, R. (2002). Role of genotype in the cycle of violence in maltreated children. *Science, 297*, 851–854.

Cicchetti, D. (2012). Annual research review: resilient functioning in maltreated children – past, present, and future perspectives. *Journal of Child Psychology and Psychiatry, 54*, 402–422.

Cicchetti, D., & Lynch, M. (1995). Failures in the expectable environment and their impact on individual development: the case of child maltreatment. In D. Cicchetti, & D. J. Cohen (Eds.), *Developmental psychopathology: Risk, disorder, and adaptation* (Vol. 2) (pp. 32–71). New York: Wiley.

Cicchetti, D., & Rogosch, F. A. (1996). Equifinality and multifinality in developmental psychopathology. *Development and Psychopathology, 8*, 597–600.

Cicchetti, D., & Rogosch, F. A. (2012). Gene × Environment interaction and resilience: effects of child maltreatment and serotonin, corticotropin releasing hormone, dopamine, and oxytocin genes. *Development and Psychopathology, 24*, 411–427.

Cicchetti, D., & Rogosch, F. A. (2014). Genetic moderation of child maltreatment effects on depression and internalizing symptoms by serotonin transporter linked polymorphic region (5-HTTLPR), brain-derived neurotrophic factor (BDNF), norepinephrine transporter (NET), and corticotropin releasing hormone receptor 1 (CRHR1) genes in African American children. *Development and Psychopathology, 26*, 1219–1239.

Cicchetti, D., Rogosch, F. A., & Thibodeau, E. L. (2012). The effects of child maltreatment on early signs of antisocial behavior: genetic moderation by tryptophan hydroxylase, serotonin transporter, and monoamine oxidase A genes. *Development and Psychopathology, 24*, 907–928.

Cicchetti, D., & Tucker, D. (1994). Development and self-regulatory structures of the mind. *Development and Psychopathology, 6*, 533–549.

DeYoung, C., Cicchetti, D., & Rogosch, F. A. (2011). Moderation of the association between childhood maltreatment and neuroticism by the corticotropin-releasing hormone receptor 1 gene. *Journal of Child Psychology and Psychiatry, 52*, 898–906.

Douglas, K., Chan, G., Gelernter, J., Arias, A. J., Anton, R. R., Poling, J., … Kranzler, H. R. (2011). 5-HTTLPR as a potential mediator of the effects of adverse childhood experiences on risk of antisocial personality disorder. *Psychiatric Genetics, 21*, 240–248.

Edmond, T., Auslander, W., Elze, D., & Bowland, S. (2006). Signs of resilience in sexually abused adolescent girls in the foster care system. *Journal of Child Sexual Abuse, 15*, 1–28.

Edwards, V. J., Holden, G. W., Felitti, V. J., & Anda, R. F. (2003). Relationship between multiple forms of childhood maltreatment and adult mental health in community respondents: results from the adverse childhood experiences study. *American Journal of Psychiatry, 160*, 1453–1460.

Egeland, B., Carlson, E. A., & Sroufe, L. A. (1993). Resilience as process. *Development and Psychopathology, 5*, 517–528.

Eley, T. C., Sugden, K., Corsico, A., Gregory, A. M., Sham, P., McGuffin, P., … Craig, I. W. (2004). Gene-environment interaction analysis of serotonin system markers with adolescent depression. *Molecular Psychiatry, 9*, 908–915.

Ellis, B. J., Boyce, W. T., Belsky, J., Bakermans-Kranenburg, M. J., & van Ijzendorn, M. H. (2011). Differential susceptibility to the environment: an evolutionary-neurodevelopmental theory. *Development and Psychopathology, 23*, 7–28.

Ferguson, D. M., Boden, J. M., Horwood, L. J., Miller, A. L., & Kennedy, M. A. (2011). MAOA, abuse exposure and antisocial behavior: 30-year longitudinal study. *British Journal of Psychiatry, 198,* 457–463.

Foley, D. L., Eaves, L. J., Wormley, B., Silberg, J. L., Maes, H. H., Kuhn, J., & Riley, B. (2004). Childhood adversity, monoamine oxidase A genotype, and risk for conduct disorder. *Archives of General Psychiatry, 61,* 738–744.

Ganzel, B. L., Morris, P. A., & Wethington, E. (2010). Allostasis and the human brain: integrating models of stress from the social and life sciences. *Psychological Review, 117,* 134–174.

Garmezy, N. (1974). The study of competence in children at risk for severe psychopathology. In E. J. Anthony, & C. Koupernik (Eds.), *The child in his family Children at psychiatric risk: Vol. 3.* (pp. 77–97). New York: Wiley.

Goldberg, X., Fatjo-Vilas, M., Alemani, S., Nenedic, I., Gasto, C., & Fañanas, L. (2013). Gene-environment interaction on cognition: a twin study of childhood maltreatment and COMT variability. *Journal of Psychiatric Research, 47,* 989–994.

Grazioplene, R. G., DeYoung, C. G., Rogosch, F. A., & Cicchetti, D. (2013). A novel differential susceptibility gene: CHRNA4 and moderation of the effect of maltreatment on child personality. *Journal of Child Psychology and Psychiatry, 54,* 872–880.

Guillaume, S., Perroud, N., Jollant, F., Jaussent, I., Olie, E., Malafosse, A., & Courtet, P. (2013). HPA axis genes may modulate the effect of childhood adversities on decision-making in suicide attempters. *Journal of Psychiatric Research, 47,* 259–265.

Haberstick, B. C., Lessem, J. M., Hewitt, J. K., Smolen, A., Hopfer, D. J., Halpern, C. T., … Mullan Harris, K. (2014). MAOA genotype, childhood maltreatment, and their interaction in the etiology of adult antisocial behaviors. *Biological Psychiatry, 75,* 25–30.

Haberstick, B. C., Lessem, J. M., Hopfer, C. J., Smolen, A., Ehringer, M. A., Timberlakel, D., & Hewitt, J. K. (2005). Monoamine oxidase A (MAOA) and antisocial behaviors in the presence of childhood and adolescent maltreatment. *American Journal of Medical Genetics, Part B: Neuropsychiatric Genetics, 135B*(1), 59–64.

Haskett, M. E., Nears, K., Ward, C. S., & McPherson, A. V. (2006). Diversity in adjustment of maltreated children: factors associated with resilient functioning. *Clinical Psychology Review, 26,* 796–812.

Juster, R. P., Bizik, G., Picard, M., Arsenault-Lapierre, G., Sindi, S., Trepanier, L., … Lupien, S. J. (2011). A trans-disciplinary perspective of chronic stress in relation to psychopathology throughout life span development. *Development and Psychopathology, 23,* 725–776.

Juster, R. P., McEwen, B. S., & Lupien, S. J. (2010). Allostatic load biomarkers of chronic stress and impact on health and cognition. *Neuroscience and Biobehavioral Reviews, 35,* 2–16.

Karatsoreos, I. N., & McEwen, B. S. (2012). Annual research review: the neurobiology and physiology of resilience and adaptation across the life course. *Journal of Child Psychology and Psychiatry, 54,* 337–347.

Karatsoreos, I. N., & McEwen, B. S. (2011). Psychobiological allostasis: resistance, resilience and vulnerability. *Trends in Cognitive Sciences, 15,* 576–584.

Karg, K., Burmeister, M., Shedden, K., & Sen, S. (2011). The serotonin transporter promoter variant (5-HTTLPR), stress, and depression meta-analysis revisited: evidence of genetic moderation. *Archives of General Psychiatry, 68,* 444–454.

Kaufman, J., Yang, B. Z., Douglas-Palumberi, H., Houshyar, S., Lipschitz, D., Krystal, J. H., & Gelernter, J. (2004). Social supports and serotonin transporter gene moderate depression in maltreated children. *Proceedings of the National Academy of Sciences of the United States of America, 101,* 17316–17321.

Kim-Cohen, J., Caspi, A., Taylor, A., Williams, B., Newcombe, R., Craig, I. W., & Moffitt, T. E. (2006). MAOA, maltreatment, and gene-environment interaction predicting children's mental health: new evidence and a meta-analysis. *Molecular Psychiatry, 2006,* 903–913.

Klauke, B., Deckert, J., Zwanzger, P., Baumann, C., Arolt, V., Pauli, P., … Domschke, K. (2014). Neuropeptide S receptor gene (NPSR) and life events: G × E effects on anxiety sensitivity and its subdimensions. *World Journal of Biological Psychiatry, 15,* 17–25.

Li, J. J., & Lee, S. S. (2010). Latent class analysis of antisocial behavior: interaction of serotonin transporter genotype and maltreatment. *Journal of Abnormal Child Psychology, 38,* 789–801.

Li, J. J., & Lee, S. S. (2012). Interaction of dopamine transporter (DAT1) genotype and maltreatment for ADHD: a latent class analysis. *Journal of Child Psychology and Psychiatry, 53,* 997–1005.

Luthar, S. S. (2006). Resilience in development: a synthesis of research across five decades. In (2nd ed.) D. Cicchetti, & D. Cohen (Eds.), *Developmental psychopathology: Risk, disorder and adaptation* (Vol. 3) (pp. 739–795). New York: Wiley.

Masten, A. S. (2011). Resilience in children threatened by extreme adversity: frameworks for research, practice and translational synergy. *Development and Psychopathology, 19,* 921–930.

Masten, A. S. (2014). *Ordinary magic: Resilience in development.* New York, London: The Gilford Press.

Masten, A. S., & Cicchetti, D. (2010). Developmental cascades. *Development and Psychopathology, 23,* 493–506.

McEwen, B. S. (1998). Stress, adaptation, and disease. Allostasis and allostatic load. *Annals of the New York Academy of Science, 840,* 33–34.

McEwen, B. S., & Stellar, E. (1993). Stress and the individual mechanisms leading to disease. *Archives of Internal Medicine, 153*(18), 2093–2101.

McEwen, B. S., & Wingfield, J. C. (2003). The concept of allostasis in biology and biomedicine. *Hormones and Behavior, 43,* 2–15.

Min, J. A., Lee, H. J., Lee, S. H., Park, Y. M., Kang, S. G., & Chae, J. H. (2013). Gender-specific effects of brain-derived neurotrophic factor Val66Met polymorphism and childhood maltreatment on anxiety. *Neuropsychobiology, 67,* 6–13.

Nilsson, K., Sjoberg, R., Damberg, M., Leppert, J., Ohrvik, J., Alm, P., ... Oreland, L. (2005). Role of monoamine oxidase A genotype and psychosocial factors in male adolescent criminal activity. *Biological Psychiatry, 59,* 121–127.

Polanczyk, G., Caspi, A., Williams, B., Price, T. S., Danese, A., Sugen, K., ... Moffitt, T. E. (2009). Protective effects of CRHR1 gene variants on the development of adult depression following childhood maltreatment. *Archives of General Psychiatry, 66,* 978–985.

Ridout, K. K., Parade, S. H., Seifer, R., Price, L. H., Gelernter, J., Feliz, P., & Tyrka, A. R. (2014). Interleukin 1B gene (IL1B) variation and internalizing symptoms in maltreated preschoolers. *Development and Psychopathology, 26,* 1277–1287.

Rutter, M. (2012). Resilience as a dynamic concept. *Development and Psychopathology, 24,* 335–344.

Rutter, M. (2013). Annual research review: resilience – clinical implications. *Journal of Child Psychology and Psychiatry, 54,* 474–487.

Shonkoff, J. P., Boyce, W. T., & McEwen, B. S. (2009). Neuroscience, molecular biology, and the childhood roots of health disparities. Building a new framework for health promotion and disease prevention. *Journal of the American Medical Association, 301*(21), 2252–2259.

Sroufe, L. A. (1997). Psychopathology as an outcome of development. *Development and Psychopathology, 9,* 251–268.

Sroufe, L. A., Egeland, B., Carlson, E., & Collins, W. A. (2005). *The development of the person: The Minnesota study of risk and adaptation from birth to adulthood.* New York: Guilford.

Tozzi, L., Carballedo, A., Wetterling, F., McCarthy, H., O'Keane, V., Gill, M., ... Frodl, T. (July 2015). Single-nucleotide polymorphism of the FKBP5 gene and childhood maltreatment as predictors of structural changes in brain areas involved in emotional processing in depression. *Neuropsychopharmacology.* http://dx.doi.org/10.1038/npp.2015.170 Neuropsychopharmacology advance online publication.

Weder, N., Yang, B. Z., Douglas-Palumberi, H., Massey, J., Krystal, J. H., Gelernter, J., & Kaufman, J. (2009). MAOA genotype, maltreatment, and aggressive behavior: the changing impact of genotype at varying levels of trauma. *Biological Psychiatry, 65,* 417–424.

White, M. G., Bogdan, R., Fisher, P. M., Muñoz, K. E., Williamson, D. E., & Hariri, A. R. (2012). FKBP5 and emotional neglect interact to predict individual differences in amygdala reactivity. *Genes, Brain and Behavior, 11,* 869–878.

Young, S., Smolen, A., Hewitt, J., Haberstick, M., Stallings, M., Corley, R., ... Crowley, T. J. (2005). Interaction between MAO-A genotype and maltreatment in risk for conduct disorder: failure to confirm in adolescent patients. *American Journal of Psychiatry, 163,* 1019–1025.

Zalsman, G. (2010). Timing is critical: gene, environment and timing interactions in genetics of suicide in children and adolescents. *European Psychiatry, 25,* 284–286.

Zalsman, G., Gutman, A., Shbiro, L., Rosenan, R., Man, J. J., & Weller, A. (2015). Genetic vulnerability, timing of short-term stress and mood regulation: a Rodent Diffusion Tensor Imaging Study. *European Neuropsychopharmacology, 25,* 2075–2085.

Zalsman, G., Huang, Y. Y., Oquendo, M. A., Burke, A. K., Hu, X. Z., Brent, D. A., ... Mann, J. J. (2006a). Association of a triallelic serotonin transporter gene promoter region (5-HTTLPR) polymorphism with stressful life events and severity of depression. *American Journal of Psychiatry, 163,* 1588–1593.

Zalsman, G., Oquendo, M. A., Greenhill, L., Goldberg, P. H., Kamali, M., Martin, A., & Mann, J. J. (2006b). Neurobiology of depression in children and adolescents. *Child and Adolescent Psychiatric Clinics of North America, 15,* 843–868 vii–viii.

Resilience and Developmental Health in Autism Spectrum Disorder

P. Szatmari[1], L. Zwaigenbaum[2], S. Georgiades[3],
M. Elsabbagh[4], C. Waddell[5], T. Bennett[3], S.
Bryson[6], E. Duku[3], E. Fombonne[7], P. Mirenda[8],
W. Roberts[1], I. Smith[6], T. Vaillancourt[9], J. Volden[2]

[1]University of Toronto, Toronto, ON, Canada; [2]University of Alberta,
Edmonton, AB, Canada; [3]McMaster University, Hamilton, ON, Canada;
[4]McGill University, Montreal, QC, Canada; [5]Simon Fraser University,
Vancouver, BC, Canada; [6]Dalhousie University, Halifax, NS, Canada;
[7]Oregon Health & Science University (OHSU), Portland, OR, United
States; [8]University of British Columbia, Vancouver, BC, Canada;
[9]University of Ottawa, Ottawa, ON, Canada

INTRODUCTION

Autism spectrum disorder (ASD) is a neurodevelopmental disorder characterized by delays and deficits in social communication and by a pattern of repetitive stereotyped behaviors and interests. The disorder usually starts in infancy then changes as development proceeds, although the two core phenotypes in social communication and behavior generally remain. The disorder occurs in roughly 1 in 100 children, with boys outnumbering girls by approximately 3–5 to 1 (Elsabbagh et al., 2012). ASD has a very high burden of suffering because the associated difficulties are often profound, persisting into and throughout adulthood for the majority, despite the existence of many effective treatments. Economic

Positive Mental Health, Fighting Stigma and Promoting Resiliency for Children and Adolescents
http://dx.doi.org/10.1016/B978-0-12-804394-3.00005-X

costs are also high as a result—data from the US estimate that families spend a substantial amount of their annual average income on their ASD child's health care costs (Parish, Thomas, Williams, & Crossman, 2015).

There has been an explosion of research interest in the characterization of ASD over the last decade and the concept of clinical and etiologic heterogeneity has gained prominence (Willsey & State, 2015). Not only are there significant variations in social communication and repetitive behavior between individuals with ASD, but such variation also exists within the same person over time. Moreover other phenotypes also co-vary with these core phenotypes, so it is now clear that ASD is a "multivariate" phenotype rather than a single "spectrum." These comorbidities include variation in cognitive and language abilities, the presence of mental and physical health problems, and a variety of other phenotypes. The emerging clinical picture is that ASD is really an overlay of many different dimensional phenotypes in addition to social communication and repetitive behavior that change over time. It is also true that a greater understanding of the etiology of ASD has emerged. It is now clear that the disorder has a very heterogeneous genetic etiology (possibly in interaction with environmental risk factors). The nature of those genetic risk factors is also becoming clearer. Rare, potentially deleterious, genetic variants (either copy number variants, single nucleotide variants, or small insertions/deletions) occur in key genes responsible for brain development, cell adhesion, and chromatin modeling more often in those affected with ASD than in the general population (De Rubeis & Buxbaum, 2015). Environmental risk factors such as advanced paternal age, prematurity, gestational diabetes, and maternal anticonvulsants have also been identified and are worthy of further investigation especially in the context of genetic vulnerability (Tordjman et al., 2014). Unfortunately, there is little understanding of the relationship between this clinical and genetic (ie, etiologic) heterogeneity, and the interaction between genetic variants and the environment.

The objective of this chapter is to discuss the concept of "resilience" in ASD against the background of this heterogeneity. Classically, resilience refers to the occurrence of an unexpected "good outcome" in the face of adversity. In this case, adversity is the diagnosis of ASD and resilience becomes a marker of heterogeneity in prognosis in the context of that adversity. "Resilience in ASD" may seem like an odd conjunction because ASD is thought of as a "lifelong" disorder where good outcomes are not possible in the face of ongoing signs and symptoms of ASD. However, this is both a narrow view of resilience and a stigmatizing view of ASD as it implies a highly value-laden concept of what constitutes "good outcomes." So while resilience and ASD may at first seem like "odd" bedfellows, if we embrace more current concepts of resilience, it opens up new avenues for research, policy, and clinical practice—to collectively embrace a more developmentally sensitive and hopeful view of ASD and to celebrate the diversity that ASD brings.

WHAT IS RESILIENCE?

Resilience is a term that rose to prominence in psychology literature after World War II (Masten, 2014). It referred to the capacity of individuals to avoid a poor mental health outcome in the face of adversity. Historically, adversity was characterized in terms of environmental events such as war, natural disasters, extreme poverty, child abuse or neglect, or living with a mentally ill parent. The importance of highlighting resilience arose from the finding that not all children exposed to severe adversities developed a "disorder" or poor mental health outcomes (Masten, 2014). Many studies concluded there must be some characteristic of the children themselves that protected them from negative outcomes associated with adversity—outcomes such as anxiety, depression, attention-deficit/hyperactivity disorders (ADHD), and disruptive behavior disorders.

Over time the notion of resilience has been refined and now has more contextual nuance; resilience is seen not only as a characteristic of the child but also as a potential characteristic of the environment that strengthens the child's ability to cope with adversity (Ungar, Ghazinour, & Richter, 2013). Such environmental characteristics might include: a strong and supportive relationship with a caregiver; a positive school milieu; or home, school and community settings that accommodate children's needs including their social, emotional, and cognitive development. Resilience is now more accurately seen as a result of a *process*—hereby interactions between the child and the contextual characteristics of their environment can lead to good or optimal outcomes despite external adversities or risk factors (Ungar et al., 2013). The hope was that these same environmental characteristics might form the basis of systematic interventions that could influence outcomes even in those children without the "child-based" attributes of resilience. It always needs to be acknowledged that the overarching goal of policy and practice is to reduce children's exposure to avoidable adversities.

A more nuanced appreciation of resilient "outcomes" is also emerging. A child might be resilient regarding a particular outcome (eg, not developing a mental disorder) but not another (eg, poor school performance or poor ability to form social attachments) (Masten, 2014). In addition, resilience must be seen in a developmental context. A child can be resilient at one time point (eg, in early childhood) and not at another (eg, later in adolescence) (Masten, 2014). As well, mental health comprises social and emotional wellbeing—just two of the crucial domains of children's development. The cognitive and physical developmental domains are also associated with success in childhood and adulthood, such that these domains, too, must be taken into account—to broaden the notion of resilience beyond mental health alone (Ungar et al., 2013).

To apply this more nuanced concept of resilience to ASD, one must agree that the initial adversity is a risk genotype that predisposes the individual to develop ASD. There may be other adversities that are either biological (such as epilepsy) or environmental (such as limited family income and support, or lack of access to evidence-based services) that influence development for child with ASD, but the initial and most prominent adversities are the biological (in this case genetic) and environmental mechanisms (which are not yet known) that lead to ASD. If a child with ASD "recovers" from the diagnosis, does well in school, makes friends, or has a good quality of life, that child can be said to be "resilient." Put simply, resilience is a "good" outcome in the face of ASD.

Yet a literature search in PubMed (done in September 2015, key words "resilience," "autism," "autism spectrum disorder"; details available from the author) did not uncover a *single* publication that discussed resilience in children with ASD. There are several publications on resilience in *parents* of children with ASD, but none that focus on the children. In contrast, there is substantial literature on the poor outcomes associated with ASD, much of it focused on variation in the persistence of autistic symptoms, intellectual disability, or language impairments over time (Magiati, Tay, & Howlin, 2014). In other words, the outcome literature in ASD has been largely concerned with the prevalence and risk factors associated with "poor" outcomes. More recently there has been some research on "optimal" outcomes, but this literature is much smaller and largely from one research group (see next section).

DEFINING "OPTIMAL OUTCOMES"

In this section, we will share the findings from a critical review of the literature focusing on "optimal outcomes" in children with ASD. In particular, we focused on definitions of optimal outcomes used in the literature, then sought all the published papers on these optimal outcomes.

The term "optimal outcome" was introduced by Fein and colleagues to characterize children with a past diagnosis of ASD whose symptoms later fell below thresholds for the diagnosis and who no longer showed evidence of delays in intellectual and adaptive functioning (Fein, Dixon, Paul, & Levin, 2005; Kelly, Paul, Fein, & Naigles, 2006; Sutera et al., 2007). Their work built upon past research examining predictors of outcomes in ASD, and specifically, efforts to characterize autistic individuals who ceased to meet criteria for the diagnosis. Much of this research was done in the context of natural history studies (eg, Rutter, Greenfeld, & Lockyer, 1967; Sigman et al., 1999). However, Lovaas (1987) described a group of children with autism who—following 2 years of intensive early intervention—had "recovered" from ASD, as evidenced by improvement in intellectual functioning (with IQs moving into the average range) and educational mainstreaming in the first grade. Gresham and MacMillan (1998) and others have argued that having an IQ in the average range and functioning in a regular grade one classroom, or even resolution of ASD symptoms does not constitute "recovery"—as this does not preclude the persistence of comorbidities requiring support and intervention. As such, Fein's group, even with a stricter case definition (relative to Lovaas, 1987) has been cautious not to equate "optimal outcome" with "recovery" (Ozonoff, 2013).

Fein et al. (2013) defined optimal outcome (OO) as the presence of a documented ASD diagnosis by age 5 years (including speech delay), coupled with: (1) not meeting criteria for ASD; (2) not showing evidence of social impairments "of an autistic quality" on the Autism Diagnostic Observation Schedule (ADOS); (3) having communication and socialization skills within 1.5 SD of the mean on the Vineland Adaptive Behavioral Scales (VABS); (4) being in a regular classroom placement with no special education services specific to ASD (eg, social skills group); and (5) having relationships with typically developing friends according to parent reports. Notably, Fein's group used a simpler, less restrictive definition (ASD symptoms becoming subthreshold for diagnosis coupled with average cognitive and adaptive skills) to estimate the OO rate in a defined prospective cohort—finding that 13 of 73 or 18% of children met these OO criteria (Sutera et al., 2007). Subsequent studies using the Fein et al. (2013) case definition have used a case–control design, such that rates of OO cannot be estimated. However, recent studies have examined OO during late childhood and adolescence, providing a unique window into how resilience in ASD may be expressed at this critical stage of development.

Fein et al. (2013) also studied a group of 34 individuals aged 8 to 21 years who had a history of early ASD and later OO, comparing them to an age, sex, and nonverbal-IQ-matched group with a current diagnosis of continuing ASD, as well as to typically developing (TD) peers. Although 7 of 34 (20.6%) in the OO group were rated on the ADOS as having mild social impairments interpreted as being unrelated to ASD (eg, reduced eye contact due to shyness, or inappropriate social overtures due to poor impulse control), there were no significant differences in social or communication or adaptive skills between the OO and TD groups, both of which were rated as more advanced than the ASD group. Orinstein et al. (2015a) reported on mental health outcomes in the same sample, finding that both the OO and ASD groups had higher rates of ADHD symptoms and diagnoses as well as specific phobias, relative to the TD group. Notably, Fein et al. (2005) had previously reported a case series of children whose diagnoses had shifted from ASD to ADHD. In a complementary study based on secondary coding of behaviors observed during the ADOS, Orinstein et al. (2015b), reported mild social impairments in the OO group relative to TD peers, with difficulties with attention, self-control (eg, giggling), and general immaturity; signs and symptoms more consistent with a diagnosis of ADHD than ASD. Interestingly, despite these social difficulties, the OO group was rated as more "likable" (albeit by undergraduate university students' ratings from videos, rather than by peers) than both the TD and ASD groups, on the basis of their social engagement, friendliness, and approachability. However, the OO group gave a less sophisticated description of "friendship" than the TD group (eg, less likely to discuss the importance of trust and reliability). Finally, no differences between OO and TD groups were reported on current ratings of repetitive interests and behavior (Troyb et al., 2014), nor narrative performance (Suh et al., 2014). An earlier report identified subtle pragmatic language deficits in 5- to 8-year-old children with OO, including difficulty identifying the goals and motivations of story characters and misinterpretation of story events (Kelly et al. 2006), although follow-up at age 8 to 13 years suggested that these deficits were no longer present (Suh et al., 2014). Notably, children with OO also had a history of earlier referral to services and more intensive intervention (particularly prior to age 3) than the ASD comparison group (Orinstein et al., 2014).

This focus on optimal outcomes generated much interest both academically and publically by providing a more optimistic view of ASD (Helt et al., 2008). The idea that upwards of 18% of ASD individuals might have *an* "optimal outcome" was quite surprising and encouraging. The hope was that by identifying the characteristics associated with "optimal outcomes" novel interventions could be developed that would promote such "resilient" outcomes for children with ASD more generally.

While interesting, these findings are nevertheless accompanied by three methodological concerns. First, the studies were largely retrospective and sampling was completed by advertising for volunteers who were now "free" of their ASD diagnosis. As a result, the generalizability of the findings is unclear. The control groups were often children with ASD who did not have optimal outcomes so the design was effectively case–control. As with many case–control studies, there may be biases where subjects with optimal outcomes who volunteer may differ in systematic ways from those having optimal outcomes sampled longitudinally, or those without an optimal outcome sampled in other ways. The retrospective collection of predictor variables may also be biased by recall differences between the cases and controls. Nevertheless, this was an efficient design given the rarity of optimal outcomes in children with ASD. It therefore provided a useful start to this line of inquiry.

A second methodological concern lies with the definition of optimal outcomes. "Optimal" is a value-laden concept mainly defined to date by researchers as the absence of an ASD diagnosis with "typical" intellectual and adaptive functioning. Yet others may have a different perspective. Many people with ASD, especially those who identify as part of the "neuro-diversity movement," challenge the idea that having an ASD diagnosis is incompatible with "optimal" outcomes (Kapp, Gillespie-Lynch, Sherman, & Hutman, 2013). Many adults with ASD are "proud" of their diagnosis and in fact celebrate the talents and strengths that are unique to the condition. In turn, many parents of children with ASD are more concerned with mental health or adaptive functioning than with the persistence, or not, of an ASD diagnosis. Recognizing that it is possible to have many autistic symptoms and still have good mental health and adaptive functioning, many parents might consider these particular outcomes as markers of success to be celebrated as well. Therefore definitions of optimal outcomes should include the perspectives of people with ASD (including those who are "lower functioning"), and parents, as well as the perspective of researchers. All three perspectives should be valued with none having obvious primacy over the others. The importance of including multiple perspectives in the definition of "optimal" outcomes is also consistent with the recent movement worldwide to incorporate "patient-oriented outcomes" in clinical trials and by extension in longitudinal studies (www.picori.org). Furthermore, this more inclusive approach is consistent with longstanding movements to celebrate developmental disability, while also working toward creating more supportive environments for all children (Nussbaum, 2011; Shinn, 2015). The perspectives of two other groups could also be considered in this mix, particularly regarding practical applications for new concepts of resilience: policymakers who plan services for populations of people with ASD and their families; and clinicians who care for individuals with autism and their families.

Third, not only should multiple perspectives be incorporated into the definition of "optimal outcomes," but the very notion of an "optimal outcome" in the singular also ignores the multivariate nature of the ASD phenotype. As noted above, it is important to take a lifespan perspective so that a good outcome may occur at one point in development but not necessarily at another. The multivariate nature of ASD also means that an optimal outcome may be present for one phenotype but not necessarily for another. Again, a child with ASD may have an optimal mental health outcome but not necessarily lose their ASD diagnosis. The same may hold true for other aspects of development that are associated with ASD, eg, language and educational achievement, or medical symptoms. But the definitions currently used suggest that a person with ASD who has an intellectual disability cannot have an optimal outcome. What if that person retains their intellectual disability as they develop—but also realize their full potential and have a good quality of life? Is that not an optimal outcome given the extent and severity of the adversity? The key is to see resilience as a process whereby the child may avoid poor health outcomes associated with a specific adversity, in this case the ASD genotype. This perspective allows for a much more nuanced concept of "optimal" outcomes in ASD.

In short, we need a more comprehensive concept of resilience that can accommodate this multivariate-developmental perspective for ASD. Here, we therefore argue that the concept of "developmental health" appears to fit well within this framework, while still allowing a consideration of "optimal outcomes" in ASD.

WHAT IS DEVELOPMENTAL HEALTH?

Havighurst (1972) proposed that the stages of human development may be best conceptualized as a series of integrated tasks. Examples of these tasks include: developing speech; developing the ability to regulate emotions and behavior; being ready to attend school; and adjusting to a changing physical sense of self, to new intellectual abilities, and to increased academic demands. "Developmental health" in turn can be defined as the physical and mental health status of an individual coupled with coping and competence at particular developmental stages—whether infancy, childhood, adolescence, or young adulthood (Keating & Hertzman, 1999). Within this framework, a "resilient" individual is one who has good developmental health and who, having experienced some adversity, is still able to meet the demands of a specific developmental stage.

While the early years have been the main focus of ASD research to date, adolescence is also a crucial developmental stage—in that skills developed and mastered during this period have important implications for making a successful transition to adulthood, including independent living for some people with ASD. However, the tasks associated with developmental health for "typical" adolescents need to be conceptualized, taking into account the specific strengths and challenges associated with ASD. An important goal for our research team has been to operationalize the domain of developmental health for adolescents with ASD in a way that ensures high relevance for youth and families. Following the "patient-oriented research agenda" mandate, we held focus groups and conducted web surveys with parents involved in our Pathways study (Szatmari et al. 2015). We asked participants what issues were most pertinent to them as their children with ASD moved into adolescence (we plan to interview youth in the current phase of the study). The results of these focus groups were remarkably consistent and are reflected in the following five themes that we propose as key aspects of developmental health in ASD during adolescence.

1. **Socialization**: positive peer and family relationships, sexually healthy behavior, and full community participation.
2. **Functional independence**: competent at activities of daily living, functioning safely in the community, and taking responsibility to manage life tasks relevant to adolescence.

3. **Self-determination**: setting appropriate goals, problem solving, making good choices, and engaged in vocational planning.
4. **Educational achievement**: good academic achievement, positive relationships with teachers and school peers, a feeling of connectedness to school, and full participation in school-related activates.
5. **Emotional/behavioral regulation**: good self-regulation of anxiety and mood, low frequency of challenging behaviors.

REVIEW OF STUDIES OF DEVELOPMENTAL HEALTH IN ASD

To focus on resilience in one or more aspects of developmental health in childhood and adolescence, it is important to first understand the variation in competence observed in ASD across the five domains listed in the previous section. We conducted a literature review (key words: autism, ASD, prospective, longitudinal, and terms for each of the domains of developmental health) that focused primarily on identifying longitudinal studies that crossed into adolescence, or in the absence of prospective data, cross-sectional studies that investigated child-level and "contextual" (ie, family, school, and community) variables associated with variation in developmental health (as defined above) from childhood through adolescence. We were interested in the prevalence and correlates of "better-than-expected" outcomes (a term we prefer to "optimal" outcomes) in this population for the various aspects of developmental health identified by our parent-informed focus groups. Due to space restrictions, we exclude studies of developmental health that were restricted to childhood alone—but it cannot be forgotten that health in adolescence builds on the developmental foundations laid in childhood. We also need to be aware that the perspectives of youth with ASD must be included in a comprehensive view of developmental health in ASD and we hope to conduct this when a greater proportion of youth in our Pathways study are verbal or able to use assistive technology.

SOCIALIZATION

On average, children with ASD do make gains in social development during the preschool and childhood years, but most remain significantly impaired overall relative to same-aged peers during adolescence (Anderson, Oti, Lord, & Welch, 2009; McGovern & Sigman, 2005). Even though many participate in social activities, most individuals with ASD also remain relatively isolated from family and friends despite their desire for meaningful friendships and other relationships (Bauminger & Kasari, 2000; Cottenceau et al., 2012; Humphrey & Lewis, 2008; Whitehouse, Watt, Line, & Bishop, 2009). Verbal or cognitively capable children with ASD also report higher rates of loneliness (Bauminger & Kasari, 2000; Cottenceau et al., 2012). Being bullied is a common experience for youth with ASD with rates as high as 46% (Schroeder, Cappadocia, Bebko, Pepler, & Weiss, 2014; Shattuck, Orsmond, Wagner, & Cooper, 2011; Van Roekel & Scholte, 2010). Finally, several studies indicate that adolescents with ASD have similar levels of sexual interest but less knowledge about sexual development compared to typically developing peers, which increases their vulnerability to exploitation and to the development of problematic sexual behavior (Hénault & Attwood, 2002; Nichols & Blakeley-Smith, 2010).

Despite the importance of socialization for young people with ASD, few longitudinal studies have tracked trajectories of socialization through adolescence. Szatmari, Bryson, Boyle, Streiner, and Duku (2003) and Szatmari et al. (2009) followed 68 children, with "high-functioning" ASD from diagnosis at 4 to 6 years to early (10 to 13 years) and late (17 to 19 years) adolescence. Overall, age-equivalent scores on social adaptive functioning scores improved over time, but the rate of improvement slowed later in adolescence (Szatmari et al., 2009). McGovern and Sigman (2005) followed 48 children with ASD across three time points: childhood, middle school/early adolescence, and adolescence/adulthood. They found that social communication, social adaptive skills, and responsiveness improved at each time point. Time spent in peer interaction in middle school was also significantly inversely related to the degree of social impairment in late adolescence/early adulthood (McGovern & Sigman, 2005). More recently, Liptak, Kennedy, and Dosa (2011) analyzed data on community participation for 725 youth with ASD from the National Longitudinal Transition Study-2. Participants were assessed at ages 15.4 (range 13 to 17) and 19.2 (range 17 to 21) years. Early predictors of greater participation were the ability to communicate more effectively, having fewer autistic symptoms, higher family income, and having parents who advocated for their children within the school system (Liptak et al., 2011). It is noteworthy that several contextual variables (such as family social supports and living with two parents) at 13 to 17 years were also associated with greater participation in social activities at 17 to 21 years.

FUNCTIONAL INDEPENDENCE

Currently there is no commonly accepted definition of functional independence, or of related terms such as "activities of daily living" and "adaptive functioning." One useful definition conceptualizes functional independence as a mastery of skills that involve coping with the demands of daily activities in the everyday environment (Liss et al., 2001). Functional-independence abilities (eg, taking care of health, grooming, and domestic needs) prepare children with ASD for an increase in responsibility, and are often emphasized in interventions from early childhood into adolescence. In the limited literature on adolescents with ASD, child-related variables have been described as potential predictors of independent performance of daily living skills (Smith, Maenner, & Seltzer, 2012). This longitudinal study of functional independence in ASD reported improvements in daily living skills during adolescence, plateauing in the late 20s and a decline in the early 30s.

In a review, Hume, Loftin, and Lantz (2009) described predictors and variables associated with greater functional independence for adolescents with ASD based on cross-sectional studies. This review described child-level predictors such as joint attention, imitation, and executive functioning. These difficulties presumably interfere with the capacity to learn daily living skills. The development of functional independence may also be negatively affected by over-reliance on adult support (eg, caregivers or school and employment supports). It should be highlighted that in the current literature, according to our review, there are no data on contextual variables influencing this aspect of developmental health.

SELF-DETERMINATION

The concept of self-determination refers to the development of skills, attitudes, and beliefs that enable individuals to exercise control over their own lives (Wehmeyer, Abery, Mithaug, & Stancliffe, 2003). Exercising self-determination has emerged, particularly in special education literature, as an important goal for people with developmental disabilities (Wehmeyer et al., 2003). Developing these skills and attitudes is now seen as an important educational target for youth with disabilities associated with a better transition to adulthood outcomes (Schall, Wehman, & McDonough, 2012), and higher quality of life (Shogren, Lopez, Wehmeyer, Little, & Pressgrove, 2006). In a recent randomized control trial (RCT), students with intellectual disability (ID) or learning disabilities (LD) who received instruction promoting self-determination showed significantly greater growth in self-determination over 3 years than students exposed to a control intervention (Wehmeyer, Palmer, Shogren, Williams-Diehm, & Soukop, 2013). In addition, contextual factors such as instructional history, rather than child-level characteristics such as sex or IQ, are associated with enhanced capacity for self-determination (Lee & Carter, 2012). Most self-determination research has studied adolescents and young adults with a range of developmental disabilities, and their teachers. To our knowledge, only one (cross-sectional) study of self-determination has included a group specifically identified as having ASD (Carter et al., 2013). In this study, parents reported that skills related to self-determination were important for their adolescent children, but also reported that performance of these skills was poor. Children's self-determination capacity by their parents were mainly predicted by the perceived level of their disabilities ("severe to profound" vs "mild to moderate"). Other recent findings also reflect issues pertaining to sense of identity and self-awareness among adolescents with ASD. For example, some authors have reported discrepancies between self- and parent-judgments of the severity of adolescents' ASD symptoms (Johnson, Filliter, & Murphy, 2009), as well as a tendency among those with ASD to be less able to report their own competence and personality traits (Koning & Magill-Evans, 2001; Schriber, Robins, & Solomon, 2014).

EDUCATIONAL ACHIEVEMENT

Academic functioning is a broad concept and includes not only actual achievement in reading and arithmetic but also student–teacher relationships, and school connectedness. Achievement for students with ASD in subjects such as math or language and arts has received little research attention until quite recently. In a 2009 review, Schaefer Whitby and Mancil identified only six studies examining academic achievement in ASD, all focused on "high-functioning" individuals. Of these, only two included adolescents (Goldstein, Minshew, & Siegal, 1994; Minshew, Goldstein, Taylor, & Siegel, 1994). Schaefer et al. concluded that children and adolescents with ASD were frequently performing lower than expected in academic subjects, but the pattern of achievement was inconsistent (2009). In another study of 100 adolescents with ASD, almost three-quarters had at least one area of significant strength or weakness in reading and math achievement, compared to expectations based on IQ scores (Jones et al., 2009). With regard to educational placement, almost all students in the "high math" group were in "mainstream schools" (the study was conducted in the United Kingdom), while students in the other three groups were enrolled in both special education and mainstream schools. A smaller study ($N=15$) from the United States also suggested that school placement may be directly related to academic achievement (Keen, Webster, & Ridley, 2015).

In both typically developing teens and those with intellectual disability, positive teacher–student relationships has helped improve behavioral trajectories in adolescents with low self-regulatory abilities (Wang, Brinkworth, & Eccles, 2013). But studies examining this topic in children with ASD have been confined to younger ages. In children, there appear to be reciprocal relationships involving children's problem behavior, time spent in mainstream classes, and quality of the student–teacher relationship (Robertson, Chambers, & Kasari, 2003). Despite its importance, student–teacher relationships have yet to be examined in adolescents with ASD, or in a longitudinal study including this population.

EMOTIONAL AND BEHAVIORAL REGULATION

Emotional problems (anxiety and mood difficulties) and behavioral problems (oppositional defiant disorder or ODD, conduct disorder, and ADHD) are common in individuals with ASD. For example, Kim, Szatmari, Bryson, Streiner, and Wilson (2000) reported that rates of these mental health disorders were three times the population rate among higher-functioning children with ASD. Leyfer et al. (2006) examined the prevalence of emotional and behavioral problems in 5- to 17-year-olds with ASD (mean age = 9.2) and found that 72% had at least one psychiatric disorder. The most common psychiatric disorders were: specific phobias (44.3%), obsessive-compulsive disorder (37.5%), ADHD (30.6%), separation anxiety (11.9%), depression (10.1%), and ODD (7%). Using a population-derived sample, Simonoff et al. (2008) reported similar findings; 70% of children with ASD aged 10 to 14 had at least one comorbid mental health condition, with 41% having two or more. The most common co-occurring disorders were: social anxiety disorder (29.2%), ADHD (28.2%), and ODD (29.2%) (Simonoff et al., 2008). These rates are much higher than in the general population, and underscore the extent of the burden carried by children with ASD and their families when considering this aspect of developmental health.

Despite these findings from cross-sectional studies, few longitudinal studies exist on emotional and behavioral regulation for children with ASD. Ballaban-Gil, Rapin, Tuchman, and Shinnar (1996) examined behavioral, language, and social changes in 102 adolescents and young adults with ASD. Participants were re-assessed on average 11.3 years (range 3.2 to 22.7 years) after their initial clinical visit. Internalizing difficulties were not assessed but externalizing problems were—including temper tantrums, rages, and aggression. Results indicated that problem behavior improved for 18% of the adolescent sample and worsened for 44%. For adults, improvement was seen in 16% and decline in 49%. Shattuck et al. (2007) also examined changes in maladaptive behavior (ie, internalizing, externalizing, and asocial behavior) across 4.5 years in a sample of 241 adolescents and adults with ASD (ages ranged from 10 to 52 with a mean of 22 years) and found significant improvement in internalizing behavior for 39.4% of participants and in externalizing behavior for 30.7%. Consistent with studies of typically developing children, there was considerable heterogeneity internalizing and externalizing behavior worsened for 11.2% and 17.4% of the sample, respectively. More recently, Gray et al. (2012) followed a sample of 119 children and adolescents with ASD across five time points (Time 1 mean age = 8.7 years and Time 5 mean age = 24.8 years) and found that behavioral (eg, disruptive) and emotional (eg, anxiety) problems tended to improve slightly over time.

CONCLUSION ON LITERATURE REVIEW OF RESILIENCE IN DEVELOPMENTAL HEALTH

This brief review confirms that there is considerable variation in developmental health during adolescence for people with ASD. By implication, this means that some young people with ASD do "better-than-expected" in at least one aspect of developmental health at a point in time in the context of their diagnosis. The proportion of resilient individuals with ASD depends on the specific aspect of developmental health under investigation and the developmental stage of the individual. "Resilience" is not a stable characteristic for anyone, let alone someone with ASD. Nevertheless, the fact that resilience exists in an ASD population is important because it shows that there is good evidence for taking a hopeful, "strengths-based" approach to children with ASD in research, policy, and practice endeavors. This will have implications on how we communicate about the diagnosis, what we can strive for in our interventions, and how important it is to take a life span perspective in assessing developmental health in individuals with ASD.

Another finding and important conclusion from the literature review pertains to the nature and extent of the influence of contextual or *environmental* factors in encouraging resiliency for children with ASD. Correlates associated with "better than expected outcomes" include not only variation in the ASD phenotype such as higher IQ or greater language abilities, but also environmental factors—including higher family socioeconomic status, good child and family supports, and accommodating schools. Crucially, these environmental factors are amenable to change—thereby opening new opportunities for favorably altering developmental trajectories for children with ASD. In short, collectively, we need to create and sustain environments that accommodate children with ASD, so they and their families can flourish and live with dignity (Nussbaum, 2011). This important area merits considerably more attention in research, policy and practice, both clinical and educational. Resilience needs to be seen in the context of creating accommodating and supportive environments—for *all* children with ASD.

FUTURE DIRECTIONS FOR RESEARCH, POLICY, AND PRACTICE

Resilience is not possible if children with ASD and their families are not adequately supported so that children can flourish. But in operationalizing this principle, we must also engage young people with ASD and their families in an empowering paradigm. For those who cannot directly participate in such engagement, careful attention needs to be paid to ascertaining and addressing the needs—and to ascertaining and celebrating their achievements, too. Beyond important environmental impediments such as socioeconomic status and supports, people with ASD can also experience adversities such as stigmatization and marginalization as a result of their diagnoses or perceived disabilities. Stigmatization and marginalization therefore also need to be addressed, as they, too, affect wellbeing and outcomes, potentially preventing people with ASD from expressing their resilience. As a start, to help address these issues, researchers, policymakers and practitioners could embrace youth and family engagement in conducting studies, and in planning and implementing new (clinical and educational) services—the goal being to empower children and families to be hopeful and to meet positive goals, as many are already doing (Shepherd & Waddell, 2015).

Resilience means having good developmental health in the face of adversity—in this case, a diagnosis of ASD. "Good developmental health" in turn is a function of the interactions between a person with ASD and his/her environments. The concept of resilience therefore has an important role in ASD research, policy, and practice—in moving toward a "strengths-based" approach in understanding children with ASD and in intervening to honor their contributions to society and to improve their lives, throughout their lives.

References

Anderson, D. K., Oti, R. S., Lord, C., & Welch, K. (2009). Patterns of growth in adaptive social abilities among children with autism spectrum disorders. *Journal of Abnormal Child Psychology, 37*(7), 1019–1034.

Ballaban-Gil, K., Rapin, I., Tuchman, R., & Shinnar, S. (1996). Longitudinal examination of the behavioral, language, and social changes in a population of adolescents and young adults with autistic disorder. *Pediatric Neurology, 15*(3), 217–223.

Bauminger, N., & Kasari, C. (2000). Loneliness and friendship in high-functioning children with autism. *Child Development, 71*, 447–456.

Carter, E. W., Lane, K. L., Cooney, M., Weir, K., Moss, C. K., & Machalicek, W. (2013). Parent assessments of self-determination importance and performance for students with autism or intellectual disability. *American Journal on Intellectual and Developmental Disabilities, 118*, 16–31.

Cottenceau, H., Roux, S., Blanc, R., Lenoir, P., Bonnet-Brilhault, F., & Barthelemy, C. (2012). Quality of life of adolescents with autism spectrum disorders: comparison to adolescents with diabetes. *European Journal of Child and Adolescent Psychiatry, 21*, 289–296.

De Rubeis, S., & Buxbaum, J. D. (2015). Genetics and genomics of autism spectrum disorder: embracing complexity. *Human Molecular Genetics*, 24(R1).

Elsabbagh, M., Divan, G., Koh, Y. J., Kim, Y. S., Kauchali, S., Marcín, C., ... Fombonne, E. (2012). Global prevalence of autism and other pervasive developmental disorders. *Autism Research: Official Journal of the International Society for Autism Research*, 5(3), 160–179.

Fein, D., Barton, M., Eigsti, I. M., Kelley, E., Naigles, L., Schultz, R. T., ... Tyson, K. (2013). Optimal outcome in individuals with a history of autism. *Journal of Child Psychology and Psychiatry, and Allied Disciplines*, 54(2), 195–205.

Fein, D., Dixon, P., Paul, J., & Levin, H. (2005). Brief report: pervasive developmental disorder can evolve into ADHD: case illustrations. *Journal of Autism and Developmental Disorders*, 35(4), 525–534.

Goldstein, G., Minshew, N. J., & Siegal, D. J. (1994). Age differences in academic achievement in high-functioning autistic individuals. *Journal of Clinical and Experimental Neuropsychology*, 16, 671–680.

Gray, K., Keating, C., Taffe, J., Brereton, A., Einfeld, S., & Tonge, B. (2012). Trajectory of behavior and emotional problems in autism. *American Journal on Intellectual and Developmental Disabilities*, 117(2), 121–133.

Gresham, F. M., & MacMillan, D. L. (1998). Early intervention project: can its claims be substantiated and its effects replicated? *Journal of Autism and Developmental Disorders*, 28(1), 5–13.

Havighurst, R. J. (1972). *Developmental tasks and education* (3rd ed.). New York: McKay.

Helt, M., Kelley, E., Kinsbourne, M., Pandey, J., Boorstein, H., Herbert, M., & Fein, D. (2008). Can children with autism recover? If so, how? *Neuropsychology Review*, 18(4), 339–366.

Hénault, I., & Attwood, T. (2002). *The sexual profile of individuals with Asperger's syndrome: The need for comprehension, support and education*. Melbourne: World Inaugural Autism Congress Publication.

Hume, K., Loftin, R., & Lantz, J. (2009). Increasing independence in autism spectrum disorders: a review of three focused interventions. *Journal of Autism and Developmental Disorders*, 39(9), 1329–1338.

Humphrey, N., & Lewis, S. (2008). 'Make me normal': the views and experiences of pupils on the autistic spectrum in mainstream secondary schools. *Autism: The International Journal of Research and Practice*, 12, 23–46.

Johnson, S. A., Filliter, J. H., & Murphy, R. R. (2009). Discrepancies between self- and parent-perceptions of autistic traits and empathy in high functioning children and adolescents on the autism spectrum. *Journal of Autism and Developmental Disorders*, 39, 1706–1714.

Jones, C., Happe, F., Golden, H., Marsden, A., Tregay, J., Simonoff, E., ... Charman, T. (2009). Reading and arithmetic in adolescents with autism spectrum disorders: peaks and dips in attainment. *Neuropsychology*, 23, 718–728.

Kapp, S. K., Gillespie-Lynch, K., Sherman, L. E., & Hutman, T. (2013). Deficit, difference, or both? Autism and neurodiversity. *Developmental Psychology*, 49(1), 59–71.

Keating, D. P., & Hertzman, C. (1999). *Developmental health and the wealth of nations: Social, biological, and educational dynamics*. New York: Guilford Press.

Keen, D., Webster, A., & Ridley, G. (2015). How well are children with autism spectrum disorder doing academically at school? An overview of the literature. *Autism: The International Journal of Research and Practice*, 20(3), 276–294.

Kelley, E., Paul, J. J., Fein, D., & Naigles, L. R. (2006). Residual language deficits in optimal outcome children with a history of autism. *Journal of Autism and Developmental Disorders*, 36(6), 807–828.

Kim, J. A., Szatmari, P., Bryson, S. E., Streiner, D. L., & Wilson, F. J. (2000). The prevalence of anxiety and mood problems among children with autism and Asperger syndrome. *Autism: The International Journal of Research and Practice*, 4, 117–132.

Koning, C., & Magill-Evans, J. (2001). Social and language skills in adolescent boys with Asperger syndrome. *Autism: The International Journal of Research and Practice*, 5, 23–36.

Lee, G. K., & Carter, E. W. (2012). Preparing transition-age students with high-functioning autism spectrum disorders for meaningful work. *Psychology in the Schools, 49,* 988–1000.

Leyfer, O., Folstein, S., Bacalman, S., Davis, N., Dinh, E., Morgan, J., ... Lainhart, J. (2006). Comorbid psychiatric disorders in children with autism: interview development and rates of disorders. *Journal of Autism and Developmental Disorders, 36,* 849–861.

Liptak, G. S., Kennedy, J. A., & Dosa, N. P. (2011). Social participation in a nationally representative sample of older youth and young adults with autism. *Journal of Developmental and Behavioral Pediatrics, 32,* 277–283.

Liss, M., Harel, B., Fein, D., Allen, D., Dunn, M., Feinstein, C., ... Rapin, I. (2001). Predictors and correlates of adaptive functioning in children with developmental disorders. *Journal of Autism and Developmental Disorders, 31,* 219–230.

Lovaas, O. I. (1987). Behavioral treatment and normal educational and intellectual functioning in young autistic children. *Journal of Consulting and Clinical Psychology, 55*(1), 3–9.

Magiati, I., Tay, X. W., & Howlin, P. (2014). Cognitive, language, social and behavioural outcomes in adults with autism spectrum disorders: a systematic review of longitudinal follow-up studies in adulthood. *Clinical Psychology Review, 34*(1), 73–86.

Masten, A. (2014). Global perspectives on resilience in children and youth. *Child Development, 85*(1), 6–20.

McGovern, C. W., & Sigman, M. (2005). Continuity and change from early childhood to adolescence in autism. *Journal of Child Psychology and Psychiatry, 46,* 401–408.

Minshew, N. J., Goldstein, G., Taylor, H. G., & Siegel, D. J. (1994). Academic achievement in high functioning autistic individuals. *Journal of Clinical and Experimental Neuropsychology, 16,* 261–270.

Nichols, S., & Blakeley-Smith, A. (2010). "I'm not sure we're ready for this...": working with families toward facilitating healthy sexuality for individuals with autism spectrum disorders. *Social Work in Mental Health, 8,* 72–91.

Nussbaum, M. C. (2011). *Creating capabilities.* Cambridge, MA: Harvard University Press.

Orinstein, A. J., Helt, M., Troyb, E., Tyson, K. E., Barton, M. L., Eigsti, I. M., ... Fein, D. A. (2014). Intervention for optimal outcome in children and adolescents with a history of autism. *Journal of Developmental and Behavioral Pediatrics, 35*(4), 247–256.

Orinstein, A. J., Suh, J., Porter, K., De Yoe, K. A., Tyson, K. E., Troyb, E., ... Fein, D. A. (2015b). Social function and communication in optimal outcome children and adolescents with an autism history on structured test measures. *Journal of Autism and Developmental Disorders, 45*(8), 2443–2463.

Orinstein, A., Tyson, K. E., Suh, J., Troyb, E., Helt, M., Rosenthal, M., ... Fein, D. A. (2015a). Psychiatric symptoms in youth with a history of autism and optimal outcome. *Journal of Autism and Developmental Disorders, 45* [Epub ahead of print].

Ozonoff, S. (2013). Editorial: recovery from autism spectrum disorder (ASD) and the science of hope. *Journal of Child Psychology and Psychiatry, 54*(2), 113–114.

Parish, S. L., Thomas, K. C., Williams, C. S., & Crossman, M. K. (2015). Autism and families' financial burden: the association with health insurance coverage. *American Journal on Intellectual and Developmental Disabilities, 120*(2), 166–175.

Robertson, K., Chamberlain, B., & Kasari, C. (2003). General education teachers' relationships with included students with autism. *Journal of Autism and Developmental Disorders, 33*(2), 123–130.

Rutter, M., Greenfeld, D., & Lockyer, L. (1967). A five to fifteen year follow-up study of infantile psychosis. II. Social and behavioural outcome. *The British Journal of Psychiatry, 113*(504), 1183–1199.

Schaefer Whitby, P., & Mancil, G. R. (2009). Academic achievement profiles of children with high functioning autism and Asperger syndrome: a review of the literature. *Education and Training in Developmental Disabilities, 44,* 551–560.

II. RISK AND RESILIENCE

Schall, C., Wehman, P., & McDonough, J. (2012). Transition from school to work for students with autism spectrum disorders: understanding the process and achieving better outcomes. *Pediatric Clinics of North America, 59*, 189–202.

Schriber, R. A., Robins, R. W., & Solomon, M. (2014). Personality and self-insight in individuals with autism spectrum disorder. *The Journal of Social Psychology, 106*, 112–130.

Schroeder, J. H., Cappadocia, M. C., Bebko, J. M., Pepler, D. J., & Weiss, J. A. (2014). Shedding light on a pervasive problem: a review of research on bullying experiences among children with autism spectrum disorders. *Journal of Autism and Developmental Disorders, 44*, 1520–1534.

Shattuck, P. T., Orsmond, G. I., Wagner, M., & Cooper, B. P. (2011). Participation in social activities among adolescents with an autism spectrum disorder. *PLoS One, 6*(11), e27176.

Shattuck, P. T., Seltzer, M. M., Greenberg, J. S., Orsmond, G. I., Bolt, D., Kring, S., ... Lord, C. (2007). Change in autism symptoms and maladaptive behaviors in adolescents and adults with an autism spectrum disorder. *Journal of Autism and Developmental Disorders, 37*(9), 1735–1747.

Shepherd, C. A., & Waddell, C. (2015). A qualitative study of autism policy in Canada: seeking consensus on children's services. *Journal of Autism and Developmental Disorders, 45*(11), 3550–3564.

Shinn, M. (2015). Community psychology and the capabilities approach. *American Journal of Community Psychology, 55*(3–4), 243–252.

Shogren, K. A., Lopez, S. J., Wehmeyer, M. L., Little, T. D., & Pressgrove, C. L. (2006). The role of positive psychology constructs in predicting life satisfaction in adolescents with and without cognitive disabilities: an exploratory study. *Journal of Positive Psychology, 1*, 37–52.

Sigman, M., Ruskin, E., Arbeile, S., Corona, R., Dissanayake, C., Espinosa, M., ... Zierhut, C. (1999). Continuity and change in the social competence of children with autism, Down syndrome, and developmental delays. *Monographs of the Society for Research in Child Development, 64*(1), 1–114.

Simonoff, E., Pickles, A., Charman, T., Chandler, S., Loucas, T., & Baird, G. (2008). Psychiatric disorders in children with autism spectrum disorders: prevalence, comorbidity, and associated factors in a population-derived sample. *Journal of the American Academy of Child and Adolescent Psychiatry, 47*, 921–929.

Smith, L., Maenner, M., & Seltzer, M. (2012). Developmental trajectories in adolescents and adults with autism: the case of daily living skills. *Journal of the American Academy of Child and Adolescent Psychiatry, 51*, 622–631.

Suh, J., Eigsti, I. M., Naigles, L., Barton, M., Kelley, E., & Fein, D. (2014). Narrative performance of optimal outcome children and adolescents with a history of an autism spectrum disorder (ASD). *Journal of Autism and Developmental Disorders, 44*(7), 1681–1694.

Sutera, S., Pandey, J., Esser, E. L., Rosenthal, M. A., Wilson, L. B., Barton, M., ... Fein, D. (2007). Predictors of optimal outcome in toddlers diagnosed with autism spectrum disorders. *Journal of Autism and Developmental Disorders, 37*(1), 98–107.

Szatmari, P., Bryson, S. E., Boyle, M. H., Streiner, D. L., & Duku, E. (2003). Predictors of outcome among high functioning children with autism and Asperger syndrome. *Journal of Child Psychology and Psychiatry and Allied Disciplines, 44*, 520–528.

Szatmari, P., Bryson, S., Duku, E., Vaccarella, L., Zwaigenbaum, L., Bennett, T., & Boyle, M. (2009). Similar developmental trajectories in autism and Asperger syndrome: from early childhood to adolescence. *Journal of Child Psychology and Psychiatry, 50*, 1459–1467.

Szatmari, P., Georgiades, S., Duku, E., Bennett, T. A., Bryson, S., Fombonne, E., ... Pathways in ASD Study Team (2015). Developmental trajectories of symptom severity and adaptive functioning in an inception cohort of preschool children with autism spectrum disorder. *JAMA Psychiatry, 72*(3), 276–283.

Tordjman, S., Somogyi, E., Coulon, N., Kermarrec, S., Cohen, D., Bronsard, G., ... Xavier, J. (2014). Gene × environment interactions in autism spectrum disorders: role of epigenetic mechanisms. *Frontiers in Psychiatry, 4*(5), 53–73.

Troyb, E., Orinstein, A., Tyson, K., Eigsti, I. M., Naigles, L., & Fein, D. (2014). Restricted and repetitive behaviors in individuals with a history of ASDs who have achieved optimal outcomes. *Journal of Autism and Developmental Disorders, 44*(12), 3168–3184.

Ungar, M., Ghazinour, M., & Richter, J. (2013). Annual research review: what is resilience within the social ecology of human development. *Journal of Child Psychology and Psychiatry, 54*(4), 348–366.

Van Roekel, E., & Scholte, R. H. J. (2010). Loneliness in adolescence: gene × environment interactions involving the serotonin transporter gene. *Journal of Child Psychology and Psychiatry, 51*, 747–754.

Wang, M. T., Brinkworth, M., & Eccles, J. (2013). Moderating effects of teacher-student relationship in adolescent trajectories of emotional and behavioral adjustment. *Developmental Psychology, 49*(4), 690–705.

Wehmeyer, M. L., Abery, B., Mithaug, D. E., & Stancliffe, R. J. (2003). *Theory in self-determination: Foundations for educational practice.* Springfield, IL: Charles C Thomas.

Wehmeyer, M. L., Palmer, S. B., Shogren, K., Williams-Diehm, K., & Soukop, J. H. (2013). Establishing a causal relationship between intervention to promote self-determination and enhanced student self-determination. *Journal of Special Education, 46*, 195–210.

Whitehouse, A., Watt, H., Line, E., & Bishop, D. V. M. (2009). Adult psychosocial outcomes of children with specific language impairment, pragmatic language impairment, and autism. *International Journal of Language and Communication Disorders, 44*, 511–528.

Willsey, A. J., & State, M. W. (2015). Autism spectrum disorders: from genes to neurobiology. *Current Opinion in Neurobiology, 30*, 92–99.

Mental Health Promotion for Indigenous Youth

L.J. Kirmayer[1,2], E. Sheiner[2], D. Geoffroy[2]

[1]McGill University, Montreal, QC, Canada; [2]Jewish General Hospital, Montreal, QC, Canada

INTRODUCTION

Indigenous youth in many countries face high levels of mental health problems, including suicide (Gracey & King, 2009; Stephens, Porter, Nettleton, & Willis, 2006). While many of the relevant strategies for the promotion of mental health and well-being and the prevention of mental disorders are similar to those for youth in other contexts, there are some unique challenges and opportunities for Indigenous populations and communities. These include the histories of colonization, cultural suppression, and marginalization that have profoundly affected many communities across multiple generations as well as the distinctive ways of life and current social and geographic contexts that shape the values and aspirations of youth and their families. These historical and social structural issues contribute to specific social determinants of health and illness, influence well-being and resilience, and have important implications for mental health promotion.

In this chapter, we review some of the salient features of Indigenous contexts and characteristics that affect the well-being of Indigenous youth. We outline an approach to mental health promotion that takes into account historical, transgenerational, and contemporary contexts and seeks to build on the strength and resilience of Indigenous communities and youth. Our examples come from Canada, but have broader application for Indigenous peoples in many countries as well as for youth from other marginalized communities that have faced historical loss and devaluation, and must meet the challenges of globalization and ongoing culture change. Comparisons of Canada with Australia and New Zealand, settler

Positive Mental Health, Fighting Stigma and Promoting Resiliency for Children and Adolescents
http://dx.doi.org/10.1016/B978-0-12-804394-3.00006-1

societies in which Indigenous people have faced similar historical forces, are especially instructive (Durie, Milroy, & Hunter, 2009).

INDIGENOUS YOUTH IN GLOBAL CONTEXT

The term "Indigenous" is generally applied to people who are the descendants of the pre-colonization populations of a region or who have maintained their own social, economic, cultural, and political institutions since colonization and the establishment of nation states (Sissons, 2005). As a result of colonization and the policies of settler societies, Indigenous peoples around the world have experienced great adversity, with denigration and suppression of their cultures and values, and disruption of their traditional ways of life. Occurring over many generations, these histories have impacted on the lives and well-being of contemporary Indigenous youth.

Globally, over 370 million people identify as Indigenous. There are more than 5,000 Indigenous cultures, and the largest numbers of Indigenous peoples live in Africa, Asia, and Latin America, where their struggles to maintain cultural identity and community are often eclipsed by the interests of the nation state. In many instances, governments have violently suppressed efforts of Indigenous peoples to maintain their identities and exert a measure of sovereignty (International Work Group for Indigenous Affairs, 2015). In recent years, struggles to recognize and strengthen Indigenous rights have gained political traction, which has also had important impacts on the mental health of youth in these communities (Niezen, 2009; United Nations General Assembly, 2007).

Indigeneity is not only a matter of historical priority and political recognition. In many instances, Indigenous peoples have maintained distinctive cultures, and ways of life. In Canada, Indigenous peoples constitute 4.3 percent of the population and include First Nations (who include some 650 communities with 11 major language groups), Métis (people of mixed-descent, mainly French and First Nations, who identify as a distinct people), and Inuit, the Indigenous people of the arctic. More than 50 percent of Indigenous people in Canada live in cities, while others live in diverse settings from peri-urban reserves to smaller rural and remote communities.

Around the world, a high proportion of Indigenous peoples are children and youth. The late demographic transition and rapid growth rate of many Indigenous populations has resulted in a population that is much younger than that of the general population in many societies. Along with the challenges of rapid cultural changes, socioeconomic disadvantage, geographic isolation, and political marginalization, the dynamics of the emerging cohorts of young people are important for understanding the stresses and challenges that Indigenous youth face.

SOURCES OF ADVERSITY AND YOUTH MENTAL HEALTH

Efforts to promote the well-being of Indigenous youth in settler societies like Canada must begin with an understanding of the diversity of cultures and the pervasive effects of the centuries-long process of culture change and forced assimilation.

Prior to contact with Europeans, Indigenous peoples in North America had diverse ways of life: some were agrarian and lived in larger communities or even empires; others were nomadic and lived in small bands of one or a few extended families, moving in an annual cycle across broad regions in search of game to provide sustenance. Contact brought new trade possibilities but also exposure to new infectious diseases with devastating effects. Colonization was marked by violent encounters with settlers who viewed the original inhabitants mainly as obstacles to their ever-widening claims of land and resources. Enclosure in a nation state led to profound changes in living circumstances of Indigenous peoples, with displacement from traditional lands and increasingly pervasive state control.

In Canada, the process of transformation antedated colonization, when contact with the fur trade initiated changes in the subsistence patterns of hunting peoples of the North and changes in yearly cycles of migration with the beginnings of settlements near trading posts. With the creation of the nation state, processes of sedentarization in settlements accelerated and Indigenous peoples were linked to a larger global economy. These geographic and economic changes were followed by generations of increasing government control with policies that were explicitly aimed at suppressing Indigenous languages, cultures, and relationship to the land.

For over 100 years, Indigenous children and youth in Canada were the target of large-scale efforts at forced assimilation, most notably through the government-mandated Indian Residential School system (Castellano, Archebald, & DeGagné, 2011). From the late 1800s through the 1980s, more than 150,000 Indigenous children were sent to residential schools that were usually located in rural locations distant from their home communities and were run by the churches and staffed by priests, nuns, and non-Indigenous teachers. The schools were part of an explicit federal policy of education that aimed, in the words of their chief architect, Duncan Scott Campbell, to "kill the Indian in the child" (Truth and Reconciliation Commission, 2015, p. 2). Children were forbidden to speak their languages and followed a curriculum that had no place for their own history or values and that was designed to train them for agricultural, domestic, or industrial labor. In addition to the damaging psychological effects of forced separation of parent and child, and of cultural suppression and denigration, the residential schools were sites of great privation, exposing children to physical and sexual abuse by teachers and other students.

Generations of children who passed through this oppressive system, went on to live in cities or returned to their communities with views of child-rearing and family life influenced by institutional regimes in ways that affected their own parenting skills.

In parallel with the residential schools, Canada instituted the Indian Act, legislation that made Indigenous peoples "wards of the Crown." This authorized and obligated the government to provide care and services for Indigenous peoples but also imposed bureaucratic control over myriad aspects of reserve life. The Indian Act defined who was and who was not an Indian and undermined the autonomy of communities, peoples, and nations. Subsequent legislation banned many forms of traditional communal and spiritual practices, which were viewed as antithetical to the Christian values of the dominant society as well as the interests of the state in promoting assimilation.

Other state and institutional policies also undermined the autonomy, cultural integrity, and well-being of youth, family, and communities. For example, the child protection system engaged in the widespread removal of Indigenous youth from their families. In what has been called the "Sixties Scoop," large numbers of Indigenous children were preferentially placed in non-Aboriginal homes throughout Canada, the United States, and overseas, without implementing programs or policies to preserve their cultural identities (Sinclair, 2007). Although this practice has lessened in recent years, Indigenous children continue to be greatly overrepresented in the foster care system. As of 2011, 3.6 percent of all First Nations children 14 years old and under in foster care, compared to only 0.3 percent among non-Aboriginal children (Statistics Canada, 2013).

These and other policies have had profound transgenerational effects at psychological, social, economic, and political levels, including: the disruption of parenting and family life; breakdowns in the transmission of cultural knowledge, language, and values; and the undermining of collective identity and community solidarity. Many of those who went through the residential schools have had difficulties in parenting due to their experiences in punitive institutional settings. These experiences have led to difficulties in emotion regulation and responsiveness that reflect the lack of warmth and intimacy in their own childhoods, exposure to physical and sexual abuse, loss of cultural knowledge, language and tradition, and systematic devaluing of Indigenous identity (Kirmayer, Simpson, & Cargo, 2003).

There is growing evidence for the transgenerational impact of residential schools on mental health. Retrospective studies have documented the multigenerational effects of exposure to residential schools and mental health outcomes for the descendants of residential school survivors. In a study of First Nations adults in Manitoba, having a parent or grandparent who attended a residential school was associated with increased likelihood of childhood abuse and a history of suicide ideation and attempts (Elias et al., 2012). There is evidence that multiple residential exposures across generations have cumulative negative effects on the mental health of youth and adults with reduced well-being and increased risk of suicidal behavior (Bombay, Matheson, & Anisman, 2011, 2014). The vulnerability associated with these transgenerational effects interacts with ongoing adversity to give rise to elevated rates of mental health problems.

The effects of governmental policies and cultural disruptions on Indigenous communities can also been seen in the relationship between local control of institutions and youth well-being. In an important study, Chandler and Lalonde (1998) compared rates of suicide across 29 tribal councils of First Nations communities in British Columbia with measures of what they deemed "cultural continuity." Their index of cultural continuity included six variables that were determined by contacting communities: (1) engagement in efforts to secure Aboriginal title to traditional lands; (2) a degree of self-government; some degree of community control over (3) educational services, (4) police and fire, (5) health services; and (6) cultural facilities to preserve and promote local culture. Communities that had none of these factors had very elevated suicide rates; the presence of each factor reduced the suicide rate—indeed, communities that had all of these factors had no suicides over the five-year period examined. In a later extension of the study to a 10-year time period, two additional indicators were collected that were also found to be protective: a high proportion of women in local government, and the provision of child and family services within the community (Chandler & Lalonde, 2009). Although Chandler and Lalonde termed their index "cultural continuity" because of a developmental psychological model that emphasized the central role of self-continuity as a protective factor in suicide risk, the factors they examined seem more closely related to flexible adaptation of cultural institutions to political and bureaucratic contexts in ways that allow communities to assert a sense of local control or self-determination. In support of the focus on culture, however, is evidence that efforts to retain or promote local language may be a particularly strong protective factor (Hallett, Chandler, & Lalonde, 2007). The benefits of these community factors are seen not only in lower suicide rates but also in fewer motor vehicle accidents and higher rates of school completion (Chandler, 2010). This work has been widely influential in Indigenous mental health because it links community level structural and organizational factors to individual mental health. More work is needed to replicate this in other settings and to examine the potential social and psychological mediators that link community politics to youth well-being (Tiessen, Taylor, & Kirmayer, 2010).

As a result of this history of deliberately suppressing cultural identity and practices, culture is a salient construct for Indigenous peoples, both as a site of collective wounding, trauma, and loss and as a potential vehicle of restoration and renewal. Given the evidence that disruption of cultural identity and transmission has impacted on the well-being of Indigenous communities, there is longstanding interest in notions of "culture as cure" (Brady, 1995; Dell et al., 2011; Duran, Duran, Heart, & Horse-Davis, 1998; Gone, 2013; Kirmayer, Brass, & Valaskakis, 2009). The reclamation of traditional knowledge and affirmation of collective values and restoration of cultural institutions and practices are all seen as specific medicine for the historical violence endured by Indigenous peoples.

In recent years, the events and impacts of colonization and forced assimilation have been framed in terms of historical trauma, loss, and grief (Mohatt, Thompson, Thai, & Tebes, 2014). The construct of historical trauma was influenced by studies of the psychological impact of genocide, particularly the experience of Jewish Holocaust survivors (Braveheart & DeBruyn, 1998). It serves to locate individual suffering in a larger historical frame and points toward the importance of political recognition and redress (Kirmayer, Gone, & Moses, 2014). The recent Canadian Truth and Reconciliation Commission (TRC) (2015) recognized the Indian Residential Schools and allied policies are instruments of cultural genocide. The TRC made many recommendations for insuring that future Indigenous are aware of this history and that Indigenous cultures and communities are supported in their processes of healing and strengthening their collective identities, power, and presence. Current efforts at mental health promotion for Indigenous youth in Canada occur against this backdrop of increasing political recognition and calls for restitution and reconciliation.

CULTURAL ROOTS OF WELL-BEING AND RESILIENCE

Mental health is not simply the absence of illness but includes states of well-being that encompass positive dimensions of social and psychological functioning (World Health Organization, 2011). While well-being may be widely recognized and characterized by energy or vitality, positive emotions, sense of meaning, self-efficacy, and hopefulness, the specific ways in which wellness is configured, achieved and experienced vary with particular cultural values, social contexts, and ways of life (Kral, Salusky, Inuksuk, Angutimarik, & Tulugardjuk, 2014; Ruiz-Casares, Guzder, Rousseau, & Kirmayer, 2014; Taylor, 2008).

For many Indigenous peoples, in addition to the ability to realize personal goals and capacities, relations with family and community, and with the land may be central to the experience of well-being. These modes of experiencing well-being are tied to particular cultural concepts of personhood that emphasize relational and ecocentric dimensions of the self (Kirmayer, 2007). The relational self, which has received much study in cross-cultural psychology particularly among East Asians, views the quality of connections to others in family and community not only as important for individual well-being but as, in some sense, constitutive of the person. Hence, individual and family well-being are tightly linked (Connors & Maidman, 2001). There is evidence that Indigenous well-being is closely associated with social support within family and community (Kral & Idlout, 2012; McMahon, Kenyon, & Carter, 2013; Richmond, Ross, & Egeland, 2007; Stuart & Jose, 2014). Families may also play a crucial role in helping to buffer the effects of racism and discrimination (Yasui, Dishion, Stormshak, & Ball, 2015). However, Indigenous family systems may have distinct dynamics owing to the history of living small bands or groups of one or a few extended families, particular cultural values, and the impact of new forms of community structure, with implications for efforts to promote positive parenting (Turner & Sanders, 2007). Certain cultural practices create relational bonds that supplement those of the nuclear or extended family. For example, some Inuit still practice traditional naming practices of *saunik* in which an individual who receives the name of a deceased person takes the relationships of that person (Kirmayer, Fletcher, & Watt, 2009). Thus, a child may be the grandmother, aunt, or cousin of an older person. These symbolic bonds may be given power by an ontology that sees the name as containing or transmitting a name-soul, but even without subscribing to that ontology, the everyday practice of respecting such filial relationships can contribute to well-being as well as strengthening bonds between individuals and families.

Less attention has been paid to another mode of self-construal common among people living close to the land, who may understand their self as embedded in ongoing transactions with the environment, including other animals and other non-human beings (Kingsley, Townsend, Henderson-Wilson, & Bolam, 2013; Kirmayer, 2007). These forms of selfhood are not mutually exclusive but may be evoked by specific contexts and used to make particular kinds of value judgments. For example, for the ecocentric self, damage to the environment may be experienced as direct damage to the person. In a sense, the environment may be thought of as an extension of the person, necessary for individual well-being, or as part of kinship relations, as a living being to whom one owes filial responsibility, recognition, and care. This is a radically different way of thinking about the environment than one finds in most Euro-Canadian discourse, with implications for mental health, resilience, and healing (McCormick, 2009). Although environmental conditions are among the major determinants of health for all populations—whether recognized by local knowledge or not—the integration of the environment into the concept of the person and self-construal gives relations to the land added significance for health. There is evidence that land-based activities, grounded in respect and caring for the land, correlate with indicators of health and well-being for Indigenous people (Burgess, Berry, Gunthorpe, & Bailie, 2008;

Kant, Vertinsky, Zheng, & Smith, 2013). Indeed, for many Indigenous peoples, land-based activities involve cultural practices that express core values of collective identity.

Many of the same social and environmental interactions associated with well-being may also contribute to resilience. Interest in resilience stems from the recognition that many youth deemed "at-risk" for mental health problems flourish despite adversity (Ungar, 2012). The metaphor of resilience is derived from the physical sciences, where the resilience of a material refers to its ability to maintain or return to its original shape after being exposed to a physical stressor. Although superficially apt, this metaphor fails to capture the complex nature of human resilience, in which the processes of responding to adversity are dynamic and culturally situated. Moreover, human resilience usually results in transformation rather than simply a return to an original form. Individual resilience may involve mobilizing a wide range of adaptive capacities including knowledge, skills, and attitudes that allow the person to problem solve, regulate emotions, and maintain social relations. Resilience may also occur on interpersonal, family, and community levels through the dynamics of social interactions and networks that respond to challenges by mobilizing resources and maintaining collective solidarity. Hence, resilience should not be understood only as an individual trait, but also as the result of processes that involve larger social configurations—families, communities, and entire peoples (Ungar, 2012; Kirmayer, Dandeneau, Marshall, Phillips, & Williamson, 2011). In the case of oppressed peoples and communities, resilience may also be part of active processes of empowerment and self-transformation. Table 6.1 summarizes some approaches to community resilience relevant to Indigenous youth.

The construct of resilience is especially relevant to understanding the mental health of Indigenous peoples because of their ongoing exposure to specific forms of social, cultural, and structural adversity. While Indigenous youth share many of the risk factors identified in classic studies of resilience conducted among youth with parents suffering from severe mental illnesses as well as inter-city youth facing poverty, violence, and discrimination, the distinctive stressors associated with colonization, structural disadvantage, racism and discrimination all warrant dedicated research and systematic clinical consideration (Burack, Blidner, Flores, & Fitch, 2007; Burack, Bombay, Flores, Stewart, & Ponizovsky, 2014; Currie, Wild, Schopflocher, Laing, & Veugelers, 2012; Hopkins, Zubrick, & Taylor, 2014).

Research on individual factors related to resilience among vulnerable youth suggests that self-esteem, optimism, intelligence, and certain personality traits related to sociability and perseverance, cognitive problem-solving abilities, capacity for emotion regulation, positive ethnic identity, social support, and prosocial involvement can all contribute to better ability to respond to challenges and recover from perturbations (Ames, Rawana,

TABLE 6.1   Some Dimensions of Indigenous Community Wellness and Resilience

Dimensions	Indicators/measures
Family and community connectedness	Support from relatives Intergenerational communication Positive parenting and family communication Strengths-based interactions in families
Oral tradition & storytelling	Knowledge of traditional stories Community sharing of stories
Connection to the land	Participation in land-based activities Consumption of country food
Healing traditions	Number of healers or others with healing knowledge Frequency of healing activities Number of people participating
Spirituality & ceremony	Elders and others with ceremonial knowledge Frequency of ceremonies Level of people participation
Cultural knowledge & identity	Language acquisition and use Activities to learn, honor or celebrate collective knowledge and identity Cultural heritage centers
Local control	Local control of fire, police, education, social services, and other organizations
Political Activism	Land claims, self-government, involvement of community in challenges to development

Gentile, & Morgan, 2013; Masten, 2014; Zimmerman et al., 2013). Factors that impair normal stress responses can impede the adaptive transformation of the organism in response to stressors (Cicchetti, 2013). However, the relative importance of these factors may depend on the kinds of challenges faced and the adaptive strategies feasible in a given context as well as local cultural values. Moreover, there may be tradeoffs between different resilience factors. Thus, the individual characteristics that contribute to social success may differ from those that support academic success and, depending on attitudes toward schooling and peer group dynamics in a community, these adaptive strategies may compete or reinforce each other (Iarocci, Root & Burack, 2009). For example, a study of adolescents attending a Naskapi First Nation school (grade 11) found that positive peer relationships were associated with academic success (Burack et al., 2013). Strong identification with Indigenous culture is associated with levels of physical and relational aggression among Naskapi youth as rated by their peers (Flanagan et al., 2011). There may be multiple pathways to success in school for Indigenous youth, including both conventional expectations for assertive learning and strong cultural identity (Fryberg et al., 2013). Matching style of education to culture may be especially important for Indigenous youth who are low on both assertive and cultural identification. While cultural identity can be an important source of resilience for youth, the implications of strengthening cultural identification depend on social contexts, which may valorize or denigrate Indigenous identity (Adams, Fryberg, Garcia, & Delgado-Torres, 2006).

A qualitative study of Indigenous perspectives on resilience in several First Nations, Inuit, and Métis communities identified multiple sources of strength related to culture and context, including: (1) maintenance, learning, and revitalization of language and culture; (2) participation in traditional land-based activities for subsistence, recreation, ceremony, and healing; (3) knowledge-sharing through processes of storytelling rooted in oral tradition, which foster relationships across the generations as Elders share their wisdom and experience; and (4) mobilization of the community for political action to assert Indigenous rights (Kirmayer et al., 2011, 2012). Each of these sources of strength depends not only on the individual psychological processes but also on family and community dynamics.

Thus, in addition to individual sources of resilience, there are important processes of resilience at family and community levels (Kirmayer, Sedhev, Whitley, Dandeneau, & Isaac, 2009a,b; Ungar, 2011a,b; 2015; MacDonald, Ford, Willox, & Ross, 2013; MacDonald et al., 2015; Allen et al., 2014; Nystad, Spein, & Ingstad, 2014; Ulturgasheva, Rasmus, Wexler, Nystad, & Kral, 2014; Wexler, Joule, Garoutte, Mazziotti, & Hopper, 2014). This points to the need for an ecosocial approach to resilience that examines the systemic contexts of youth development and adaptation (Kirmayer, 2015). Families can provide youth both emotional and material support. However, the nature and configurations of family and community life have changed over time. For Indigenous peoples who were nomadic hunters prior to colonization, the extended family was the basic unit of society and the larger communities created by the state to provide health care services and education have required developing new modes of living together. In some cases, there are fault lines within communities along kinship lines resulting in uneven distribution of resources and power within the community.

The literature on social capital links resilience to the nature of community structure, resources, and relations (Kirmayer et al., 2009). As an asset for resilience, social capital refers to individuals' access to social relations that can provide material, emotion and problem-solving resources, or in the case of communities, to structural strengths that can be described in terms of levels of trust, participation, reciprocity, and collective action (Ledogar & Fleming, 2008). The elements of personal and collective social capital and resilience interact with one another at both individual and community levels. For example, community social capital increases the availability of resources to youth in need.

Indigenous peoples draw from many sources of resilience some of which are rooted in their traditional cultures and ways of life (Kirmayer et al., 2011). These cultural resources include traditional land-based and domestic activities, spirituality and ceremonies, language, and healing practices (Fleming & Ledogar, 2008). Traditional activities span a range of practices that include: hunting, fishing, foraging, and trapping; beading, weaving and sewing clothing, as well as decorative and ceremonial objects; building dwellings, vehicles, and tools; as well as a variety of Indigenous sports and creative activities, such as lacrosse. Traditional spirituality encompasses knowledge, beliefs, and practices related to every aspect of life, including subsistence activities like hunting as well as life cycle rituals, such as funerary practices, food blessings, coming of age ceremonies, and celebrations related to annual seasonal cycles. The legacy of Christian missionizing as well as ongoing exposure to specific traditions and to pan-Indian spirituality has contributed to substantial diversity in attitudes and practices of spirituality within many communities. Hence, mental health promotion must accommodate a wide range of positions and levels of engagement with traditional and emerging forms of spirituality, religious practice, and ways of life.

Indigenous languages are important vehicles of cultural knowledge. In the 2011 Census, about 17 percent of Indigenous people in Canada reported they could converse in an Aboriginal language (Langlois & Turner, 2014). As the media for traditional stories and teachings as well as the lexicons used to describe the landscape and transmit ceremonial knowledge and practices, Indigenous languages remain important sites of cultural revitalization and a source of identity and pride for many Indigenous youth (Liebenberg, Ikeda, & Wood, 2015). In Australia, New Zealand, and Canada, Indigenous youth are using digital media and telecommunications technologies to learn and use their languages and cultures (Kral, 2010; Molyneaux et al., 2014).

Traditional healing practices bring together many strands of cultural identity including language, relationship to the land, family in forms of spirituality that affirm core values of recognition, and care (McCormick, 2009). Many Indigenous scholars emphasize models of holistic health healing that encompass individuals as well as communities, stressing the interconnectedness of bodily health with emotional, social, and spiritual health (Durie, 2005; Duran, 2006). The popularity of the pan-Indian symbolism of the Medicine Wheel reflects this understanding of the need for integrative healing based on finding balance among different human needs and capacities. Traditional healing activities include a wide variety of practices that draw on cultural knowledge as well as local plants and animals for their therapeutic effects. In addition to their potential beneficial effects for specific conditions, these practices also serve to affirm Indigenous identity and pride through the reclamation of activities that were prohibited by the government (Adelson, 2000). The emphasis on holistic healing within the Indigenous rhetoric of health calls for integrative solutions to issues related to mental health. This implies that remedies should not be sought only at the level of pharmacology and the brain, but must extend into domains of cognition, embodiment, and social relations.

ASSESSING YOUTH WELL-BEING AND RESILIENCE IN RESEARCH AND CLINICAL CONTEXTS

Person-centered psychiatry advocates assessing wellness as well as illness as a basic approach to understanding the patient as person and devising individual and broader public health strategies for positive mental health (Mezzich et al., 2010). Health is more than simply the absence of illness; it is an orthogonal construct (Keyes, 2012). An individual can suffer from an illness or disability, yet still thrive despite this challenge. This perspective links wellness to resilience in ways that are both universal and culture-specific (Kirmayer, Bennegadi, & Kastrup, 2016).

Positive measures of well-being are crucial to the development of mental health promotion policies and programs (Lippman, Moore, & McIntosh, 2009). Advancing the study of resilience among Indigenous youth requires individual and community level measures that reflect local structural, cultural, and practical realities. The construct of resilience can be operationalized in terms of the range of intermediate outcomes that enable people to thrive in adverse contexts. However, existing measures tend to focus on dimensions salient for non-Indigenous populations and may not sufficiently attend to the social, contextual, and political processes that are key determinants of well-being in Indigenous communities (Taylor, 2008).

A variety of culturally informed measures of Indigenous youth well-being and distress have been developed in recent years and, although none has had sufficient validation to recommend routine use, several show promise. Table 6.2 summarizes the characteristics of some of these measures. In addition to adopting local language, idioms, and symbols, the measures are distinctive for including dimensions of well-being explicitly linked to cultural identity, connection to the land, and spirituality. For comparison, one measure that aims for wide cross-cultural applicability by addressing overarching domains is also included. None of the measures have yet received sufficient validation in Indigenous populations.

Indigenous leaders, scholars, and mental health practitioners have identified the need for research that builds on community strengths and explores pathways to resilience and well-being. Central to this approach is a shift in the focus and protocols of research to address the priorities of Indigenous communities and to respect and integrate Indigenous knowledge and methodologies (Alfred, 2005; Smith, 1999). The shift toward

TABLE 6.2 Measures of Indigenous Youth Wellness, Resilience, and Distress

Measure	Population	Integration of culture	Domains	Instrument characteristics	Validation
Westerman Aboriginal symptoms checklist – Youth (Westerman, 2003)	Aboriginal peoples in Australia	New measure	Depression Suicide Alcohol/Drug usage impulsivity Anxiety Cultural resilience	53 items, multiple choice	Focus groups with Aboriginal parents, youth and mental health professionals. Factor analysis, internal reliability analysis ($n = 183$)
Strong souls (Thomas, Cairney, Gunthorpe, Paradies, & Sayers, 2010)	Aboriginal peoples in Australia	New measure	Anxiety Depression Suicide-risk Resilience	25 items, multiple choice	Pilot tested with students to assess appropriateness and initial discriminative power and internal reliability ($n = 67$) factor analysis, Internal reliability analysis ($n = 361$)
Child and Youth Resilience Measure-28 (Ungar & Liebenberg, 2011)	Diverse groups (mainly non-Indigenous, but included one First Nation in Canada)	Aims to capture global domains that apply across diverse cultures and settings	Access to material resources Relationships Identity Power and control Cultural adherence Social justice Cohesion	28 items	Validated in general population not Indigenous (Liebenberg, Ungar, & Van de Vijver, 2012)
Aboriginal Children's Health and Well-Being Measure (Young et al., 2013)	First Nations Communities in Ontario	New measure	Spiritual well-being Emotional well-being Physical well-being Mental well-being	58 items, multiple choice	Community consultation, advisory committee meetings, and focus groups. Established content validity and construct validity ($n = 18$) (Young et al., 2015a,b)

Continued

TABLE 6.2 Measures of Indigenous Youth Wellness, Resilience and Distress—cont'd

Measure	Population	Integration of culture	Domains	Instrument characteristics	Validation
Cultural Connectedness Measure (Snowshoe et al., 2015)	First Nations, Métis and Inuit youth in Saskatchewan and Southwestern Ontario	New measure, with 6 items adapted from the multigroup ethnic identity measure — Revised (Phinney & Ong, 2007)	Identity Traditions Spirituality	29 items	Key informant interviews ($n=3$) and youth focus group ($n=15$) Established criterion validity, factor analysis and scale score reliability ($n=319$)
Native Wellness Assessment (http://nnapf.com)	First Nations Communities of Canada	New measure	Spiritual wellness Emotional wellness Physical wellness Mental wellness	66 items, multiple choice, self-report and observer rated versions	Publications forthcoming

resilience and measures of positive mental health and well-being is consistent with Indigenous critiques of standard illness-based research. Research on resilience and measures of well-being can be conceptualized in ways that reflect Indigenous values and perspectives. This also has implications for the way in which research is conducted, by engaging with Indigenous perspectives on knowledge, epistemologies, and methodologies. Culturally responsive research using strength-based methodologies can support efforts to decolonize practices in health and education (Snowshoe, Crooks, Tremblay, Craig, & Hinson, 2015; Chino & Debruyn, 2006).

There is increasing recognition of the value of an ecosocial approach to research on social determinants of health, which views individuals as embedded in and in constant interaction with families, communities, and larger social and environmental systems (Krieger, 2012). Individuals live at the intersection of multiple social status, identities, and networks that configure their identity, exposures to risk factors for illness and access to protective factors that promote well-being. Analyzing the interactions of these statuses is essential to understand why Indigenous youth experience particular forms of adversity and to devise effective mental health promotion strategies (Bauer, 2014).

Research is needed in this area because of the many distinctive features of Indigenous communities and populations, which face specific social determinants of health related to culture, history, geography, and political context (Anderson, Baum & Bentley, 2007; Carson, Dunbar, Chenhall, & Bailie, 2007; Gone & Trimble, 2012; Gracey & King, 2009; King, Smith, & Gracey, 2009; Kolahdooz, Nader, Kyoung, & Sharma, 2015; Reading, 2009; Valeggia & Snodgrass, 2015; Wexler, 2014). Indigenous communities grapple with geographic, climatic, political, and economic challenges that limit educational and work opportunities for youth, and hence, may color their visions of the future (MacDonald et al., 2013). The stereotypes and negative views of Indigenous people that persist in the larger society contribute to significant levels of discrimination experienced by many Indigenous youth.

Indigenous youth living in rural and remote communities constitute relatively large local cohorts of individuals who are closely related to each other. This leads to high levels of communication and identification increasing the risk of contagion effects as seen in cluster suicides (Niezen, 2009), or serve to amplify positive health messages. At the same time, the large cohort may create intense competition for limited resources. In Indigenous communities this may be mitigated by cultural values of non-competition and cooperation, sharing, and kinship ties. In terms of delivery of prevention programs, there are challenges both for communities located in remote geographic regions and for urban populations who may be dispersed in cities with little specialized services available that recognize or strengthen Indigenous connections and identity (Wexler et al., 2015; Yi, Landais, Kolahdooz, & Sharma, 2015). Internet-based mental health promotion programs and services, which can be made available in both remote and urban settings, may provide ways to surmount some of these obstacles (Clarke, Kuosmanen, & Barry, 2015; Cotton, Nadeau, & Kirmayer, 2014).

PROMOTING POSITIVE MENTAL HEALTH AMONG INDIGENOUS YOUTH

Contemporary approaches to mental health promotion aim to mobilize all sectors of society to improve living conditions and, in the case of children and youth, support optimal development (Herrman & Jané-Llopis, 2012). While there is evidence for many effective interventions, particularly those that support healthy parenting of infants, children, and youth, (Hosman & Jané-Llopis, 2005), there are limited data on programs specifically designed for Indigenous youth that take into account their distinctive history, culture, social, and geographic contexts (Clelland, Gould, & Parker, 2007).

Mental health promotion reinforces factors that contribute to health and resilience, while working to reduce or eliminate factors related to poor mental health. In its emphasis on health and wellness, rather than illness, health promotion complements more narrowly focused prevention approaches. Mental health promotion interventions vary according to participants' age, cultural background, and socioeconomic status as well as other contextual factors (Barry & Jenkins, 2007; Barry, Clarke, Jenkins, & Patel, 2013). The contexts of Indigenous youth in rural, remote, and urban settings merit separate consideration in designing and delivering mental health promotion programs. Indigenous youth possess strengths based on competencies associated with contemporary youth in general, such as technological literacy and participation in global, web-based communities, as well as more specific coping skills and strategies grounded in cultural knowledge, values and practices.

Table 6.3 summarizes some strategies for mental health promotion for Indigenous youth and illustrative examples. These are roughly organized in terms of risk, protective, and resilience factors found to correlate with positive mental health in epidemiological and ethnographic studies, including: clear cultural identity; sense of self-efficacy and self-esteem; family interaction and communication; positive peer interactions; access to material resources and infrastructure (adequate housing, food, telecommunications, recreational opportunities, etc.); educational and vocational opportunities; tolerance and integration of diversity; and assertion of collective political agency. The list is not exhaustive and the categories are not mutually exclusively. Although assigned to one resilience factor based on

TABLE 6.3   Methods of Promoting Indigenous Youth Wellness and Resilience

Resilience Factor	Intervention	Examples
Indigenous identity Cultural revitalization Language revitalization Connection with the land	Sharing of history and tradition through storytelling Culture camps Language programs	Project Venture (Carter, Straits, & Hall, 2007) Our Life (Goodkind, LaNoue, Lee, Lance Freeland, & Freund, 2012)
Sense of self-efficacy Self-esteem Problem-solving and social skills	Programs to develop youth leadership	Uniting Our Nations Cultural Leadership Camp (youthrelationships.org/culture-camp) Outdoor Adventure Leadership Experience (Ritchie, Wabano, Russell, Enosse, & Young, 2014) Zuni Life Skills Development Curriculum (LaFromboise & Lewis, 2008)
Positive relationships with family	Parenting education Family-centered programs Prevention child maltreatment and domestic violence	PROSPER (Spoth, Greenberg, Bierman, & Redmond, 2004) Family Well-being Empowerment Program (Tsey et al., 2007) Triple P-Positive Parenting Program (Sanders, 2012) http://www.triplep.net Other programs (Connors & Maidman, 2001)
Positive relationships with peers	Relationship skills training Peer mentoring	Fourth-R (Crooks, 2009; Crooks, Chiodo, Thomas, & Hughes, 2010) Peer Mentoring Program (youthrelationships.org/peer-mentoring)
Community infrastructure	Adequate living environment Food security Recreational and leisure activities	Developing adequate housing, services, and material resources Developing recreational spaces, and communal meeting places
Educational & vocational opportunities	Increase school retention and completion Developing training and employment opportunities	School programs that integrate Indigenous knowledge and ways of knowing
Respect for diversity within community and in larger society	Inclusive community events Anti-racism and discrimination programs	Powwows and other activities that bring diverse groups together

Continued

TABLE 6.3 Methods of Promoting Indigenous Youth Wellness and Resilience — cont'd

Resilience Factor	Intervention	Examples
Collective agency, recognition, and empowerment	Political activism for social justice	Truth and reconciliation interventions, land claims, local government, legal challenges to development (Guerin, 2010; Truth and Reconciliation Commission, 2015)

Kenyon, D.B., & Hanson, J.D. (2012). Incorporating traditional culture into positive youth development programs with American Indian/Alaska Native youth. Child Development Perspectives, 6(3), 272–279; Kirmayer, L.J., Fraser, S-L., Fauras, V., Dandeneau, S., & Whitley, R. (2009). Current approaches to Aboriginal youth suicide prevention. Ottawa: Health Canada, First Nations and Inuit Health Branch; Kirmayer, L.J., Sedhev, M., Whitley, R., Dandeneau, S., & Isaac, C. (2009). Community resilience: models, metaphors and measures. Journal of Aboriginal Health, 7(1), 62–117. More programs can be found at: www.namhr.ca.

prominent components, all of the programs listed address multiple resilience factors. Mental health services can provide an important resource for the local adaption and implementation of promotion programs as well as interventions for youth experiencing crises or mental health problems.

In addition to taking into account specific risk and resilience factors associated with Indigenous experiences of colonialism and structural adversity, mental health promotion must also address differences in paradigms or perspectives on health and well-being among Indigenous peoples. Indeed, Indigenous scholars and practitioners have argued that delivering interventions predicated on Western (non-Indigenous) perspectives to Indigenous populations constitutes a form of neo-colonialism and oppression, through a failure to acknowledge Indigenous views on health and healing (Duran, 2006; Stewart, 2008). The sensitive integration of Indigenous worldviews into mental health promotion is essential both for program acceptability and effectiveness (Durie, 2005). For clinical services providing secondary and tertiary prevention, interventions tailored to Indigenous worldviews can augment access to mental health resources—historically under-utilized by Aboriginal peoples—and improve low treatment retention rates (McCormick, 2009; Wendt & Gone, 2012; Stewart, 2008).

Culturally competent mental health promotion assumes different forms depending on the priorities and perspectives of the Indigenous collaborators involved (Kirmayer, 2012; Wendt & Gone, 2012). Indigenous health practitioners in New Zealand have developed the construct of cultural safety as a complement to cultural competence which has been embraced by educators and policy makers in Canada (Brascoupé & Waters, 2009; Indigenous Physicians Association of Canada, 2009). Cultural safety emphasizes the need to recognize and address the structural violence that accounts for health disparities and that continues to make health care institutions unsafe for Indigenous peoples. To develop and implement culturally safe, responsive, and effective mental health promotion programs, mental health practitioners need to work in close partnership with Indigenous communities, with ongoing dialogue and explicit commitments to ensure that communities retain control of programs. This process can follow the principles of community-based participatory action research supplemented with explicit attention to the ethical issues raised in working with Indigenous populations and communities (Cargo & Mercer, 2008; Chino & Debruyn, 2006). Youth too can play an active role as partners in developing programs to meet their needs (Jacquez, Vaughn, & Wagner, 2013).

While the resultant programs will vary in response to particular cultures and contexts, there are commonalities among diverse Indigenous perspectives. Based on in-depth interviews with Indigenous mental health service providers in Canada, Stewart (2008) outlined four overlapping themes central to Indigenous mental health and healing: community, holistic approach, interdependence, and cultural identity. Community, as the social system of individuals who live together, sharing communal knowledge, institutions, and practices is foundational for Indigenous mental health promotion. Although Indigenous communities share a link to a specific culture, members may vary widely in how strongly they identify with particular traditions or practices. Hence, mental health promotion must allow for this diversity. The notion of a holistic approach alludes to the need for services that address the major domains or dimensions of life, including elements that are frequently paid little attention in clinical contexts, such as spirituality and nutrition. This is sometimes framed in terms of the four quadrants of the Medicine Wheel, covering mental, physical, emotional, and spiritual domains, each of which has both individual and social dimensions. The concept of interdependence suggests that healing extends beyond the individual, through strengthening connections with family members, community elders, and others. Finally, cultural identity refers to the notion that developing and maintaining a clear sense of Indigenous identity can be an integral part of the healing process, and of effective mental health promotion, as cultural marginalization is replaced by revitalization.

CULTURALLY BASED, FAMILY-CENTERED MENTAL HEALTH PROMOTION FOR INDIGENOUS YOUTH

In this section we summarize a mental health promotion program that illustrates some of the principles described above. With support from the Innovation Program of the Public Health Agency of Canada, our team has been developing and evaluating a broad mental health promotion intervention for Indigenous youth. *Listening to One Another to Grow Strong* is a 14-session program for young people (10 to 14 years of age) and their parents. The program focus on strengthening cultural identity, family life communication and support, and provides skills for problem-solving, critical thinking, and emotion regulation relevant to dealing with interpersonal conflict, bullying, discrimination, and substance use.

The program emphasizes experiential learning and group activities that strengthen cultural identity and family communication. The intervention is based on the Strengthening Families program developed by Spoth et al. (2002), which has been recognized as an evidence-based mental health promotion strategy by the US Substance Abuse and Mental Health Services Administration (SAMHSA). The original program was expanded and adapted for Native American communities in the US, and then for Anishinabe communities in Canada by Les Whitbeck and Melissa Walls (Whitbeck, Walls, & Welch, 2012, 2014).

Pilot data on the effectiveness of an initial implementation of the program with Anishinabe children in grades 5 to 8, found positive results for younger children who had not yet begun to experiment with alcohol or drugs. The study also provided support for the efficacy of the basic model for creating culturally specific prevention programs. Culturally specific content was more likely to be retained and used by both parents and children. Emphasis on traditional practices not only increased the use of the traditional family communication mechanism, it appeared to have enhanced appropriate assertiveness. The program also resulted in gains in anger management. In the pilot study, compared to community controls, participating children were seven times more likely to recognize early signs of anger. This is important, given baseline findings regarding the associations between anger, delinquency, and early onset substance abuse. Anger is also linked to impulsive behavior in the literature, which is often a precursor to suicidal behavior. There were also gains in the area of parental monitoring, with intervention mothers compared to control group mothers more likely to report that they knew when their children came in at night. Participating children also reported gains in parental monitoring when compared to control group children. At post-test, the children were more likely to report that their parents "know my friends and their families." There was a trend toward increasing traditional values of community responsibility for children.

The pilot program was further expanded to include sessions covering: learning about specific First Nation culture and community history; traditional family values, belonging and communication; knowledge and attitudes about substance abuse; help-seeking for emotional distress; coping with anger and conflict; coping with sadness and loss; peer communication and prosocial behavior; problem-solving skills; dealing with historical loss; dealing with discrimination; learning refusal skills (for substance use) and parental monitoring; and building social support networks within the community. Additional material was incorporated to address priorities identified by community partners, including cyberbullying, and new material was prepared on critical thinking about substance use to replace the outdated session on "refusal skills."

Key components of the intervention include: active community involvement in local cultural adaptation, training and delivery; engagement of elders and community knowledge holders as resource people; use of culturally-grounded language, symbols, stories, and practices to convey key components of the intervention skills; and intensive involvement of parents and caretakers. The program usually includes both male and female facilitators, who provide role modeling through activities that engage both genders. Explicit attention to local history and language and the participation of elders help bridge the gap between generations. Most sessions involve youth and parents sharing meals together and participating in talking circles, both of which facilitate communication within and between families.

The design of the intervention emphasizes cultural adaptation, which may include changes in program content, activities, scheduling, and location. Fidelity is maintained at the level of the goals of each session. A toolkit including adaptation and implementation guidelines, a facilitator's manual as well as parent and youth participant activity manuals was prepared. Participating communities use these materials as a basis to develop their own culturally localized version, incorporating Indigenous language, stories, values, ceremonies, and symbols. This process of local cultural adaptation, which may take many hours, over several weeks or months, is a crucial component of the intervention that serves to bring together an active group of advocates and resource people and ensure community "ownership" of the program.

Over the first five years of the project, the program has been culturally adapted to five different First Nations spanning 14 communities in four provinces, situated in very different geographical and social contexts. Qualitative reports collected as part of ongoing program evaluation from participants, facilitators, and coordinators indicate strong positive outcomes in all five First Nations. The program has been very well-received, and strongly reinforces local cultural knowledge, identity, and both individual and collective self-esteem. The process of cultural adaptation and the delivery of the program by local partners is in itself a contributor to community empowerment, with indirect effects on youth well-being. Preliminary results suggest that wide latitude given in the adaptation process contributed to community interest, buy-in and engagement with the intervention. Despite the high degree of adaptation, with many creative innovations by communities, overall fidelity to program and session goals was maintained.

The intervention appears to have a positive impact at individual, family, and community levels. Recurrent themes in qualitative evaluation, include: increases in family bonding, communication skills, parenting skills, as well as increased enthusiasm for learning about their own cultures. There is some evidence for spillover effects to other children (who may or may not accompany a sibling in the program) and family members, positive interactions between participating families, and for wider community solidarity. Quantitative data confirm beneficial effects at the level of youth well-being, with reductions in feelings of distress, and increased feeling of connection to family and community. There is also evidence of positive effects of the program on adults in terms of knowledge of parenting and communication skills.

The *Listening to One Another* program illustrates the ways in which close community partnership and creative integration of culture can yield youth mental health promotion interventions that are consonant with local values. Challenges for future work include: further documenting effectiveness in terms of mental health outcomes; learning how to achieve the level of community engagement required for program delivery when there are not strong pre-existing partnerships with communities; and finding ways to modify and deliver the program for low resource settings, including through schools and the use of web-based training materials.

CONCLUSION

Indigenous peoples and communities have faced long histories of cultural oppression and dislocation. Recognition of this history and its impact across the generations is essential to develop ethically sound and culturally safe approaches to mental health services as population-level promotion of youth well-being and resilience. However, the challenges that youth face are not only related to historical events but reflect ongoing structural inequalities and dilemmas, involving political, economic, and bureaucratic structures that maintain negative stereotypes, racism, and discrimination; geographic isolation with limited educational and vocational opportunities; and collective marginalization and disempowerment. These structural problems point to the need for changes not only within Indigenous communities but also in the larger society among non-Indigenous people and institutions (Saul, 2014).

Indigenous youth increasingly participate in a wired world in which they are linked to a global youth culture that promotes values that may be at odds with local traditions and immediate opportunities. At the same time, the Internet holds the prospect of new educational, health, community and vocational opportunities that may make small, remote settlements viable places to advance a wider range of life projects and provides an opportunity to deliver mental health promotion interventions to remote communities (Kral, 2010).

Adults who are acutely aware of what they have lost and who want to reconnect with elders often drive cultural revitalization projects. However, evidence from our own and other studies indicates that many Indigenous youth are hungry for cultural knowledge. Indeed, the enthusiasm expressed by youth in our program served to engage parents in cultural learning projects. The need to valorize and reconnect with a devalued and suppressed collective history and identity is shared by many. Moreover, acknowledging and valuing one's roots need not conflict with being fully engaged in learning and benefitting from new technologies, knowledge, and ways of being. Youth today face the prospect of increasingly fluid and hybrid identities fed by multiple cultural streams and need space to find their own unique trajectories in relation to their histories, communities, and global society.

An ecosocial approach to mental health promotion is especially apposite for Indigenous youth and communities because it is consonant with core cultural values that emphasize interdependence with others and with the environment. This way of thinking is important not only in addressing the specific needs of Indigenous youth but in coming to grips with the major planetary challenges of climate change, urbanization, migration, and global mental health.

References

Adams, G., Fryberg, S. A., Garcia, D. M., & Delgado-Torres, E. U. (2006). The psychology of engagement with indigenous identities: a cultural perspective. *Cultural Diversity & Ethnic Minority Psychology, 12*(3), 493–508.

Adelson, N. (2000). Re-imagining aboriginality: an indigenous peoples' response to social suffering. *Transcultural Psychiatry, 37*(1), 11–34.

Alfred, T. (2005). *Wasáse: Indigenous pathways of action and freedom.* Peterborough: Broadview.

Allen, J., Hopper, K., Wexler, L., Kral, M., Rasmus, S., & Nystad, K. (2014). Mapping resilience pathways of Indigenous youth in five circumpolar communities. *Transcultural Psychiatry, 51*(5), 601–631.

Ames, M. E., Rawana, J. S., Gentile, P., & Morgan, A. S. (2013). The protective role of optimism and self-esteem on depressive symptom pathways among Canadian aboriginal youth. *Journal of Youth and Adolescence, 44*(1), 142–154.

Anderson, I., Baum, F., & Bentley, M. (Eds.). (2007). *Beyond bandaids: Exploring the underlying social determinants of aboriginal health.* Casuarina, Australia: Cooperative Research Centre for Aboriginal Health.

Barry, M. M., Clarke, A. M., Jenkins, R., & Patel, V. (2013). A systematic review of the effectiveness of mental health promotion interventions for young people in low and middle income countries. *BMC Public Health, 13*(1), 835.

Barry, M. M., & Jenkins, R. (2007). *Implementing mental health promotion.* Edinburgh: Churchill Livingston.

Bauer, G. R. (2014). Incorporating intersectionality theory into population health research methodology: challenges and the potential to advance health equity. *Social Science & Medicine, 110,* 10–17.

Bombay, A., Matheson, K., & Anisman, H. (2011). The impact of stressors on second generation Indian residential school survivors. *Transcultural Psychiatry, 48*(4), 367–391.

Bombay, A., Matheson, K., & Anisman, H. (2014). The intergenerational effects of Indian Residential Schools: implications for the concept of historical trauma. *Transcultural Psychiatry, 51*(3), 320–338.

Brady, M. (1995). Culture in treatment, culture as treatment. A critical appraisal of developments in addictions programs for indigenous North Americans and Australians. *Social Science & Medicine, 41*(11), 1487–1498.

Brascoupé, S., & Waters, C. (2009). Cultural safety: exploring the applicability of the concept of cultural safety to Aboriginal health and community wellness. *Journal of Aboriginal Health, 7*(1), 6–40.

Braveheart, M. Y. H., & DeBruyn, L. M. (1998). The American Indian holocaust: healing historical unresolved grief. *American Indian and Alaska Native Mental Health Research, 8*(2), 56–78.

Burack, J., Blidner, A., Flores, H., & Fitch, T. (2007). Constructions and deconstructions of risk, resilience and wellbeing: a model for understanding the development of Aboriginal adolescents. *Australasian Psychiatry, 15*(Suppl. 1), S18–S23.

Burack, J. A., Bombay, A., Flores, H., Stewart, J., & Ponizovsky, V. (2014). Developmental perspectives on the role of cultural identity in well-being: evidence from Aboriginal communities in Canada. In J. A. Burack, & L. A. Schmidt (Eds.), *Cultural and Contextual Perspectives on Developmental Risk and Well-being* (pp. 81–103). New York: Cambridge University Press.

Burack, J. A., D'Arrisso, A., Ponizovsky, V., Troop-Gordon, W., Mandour, T., Tootoosis, C., et al. (2013). 'Friends and grades': peer preference and attachment predict academic success among Naskapi youth. *School Psychology International, 34*(4), 371–386.

Burgess, C. P., Berry, H. L., Gunthorpe, W., & Bailie, R. S. (2008). Development and preliminary validation of the 'Caring for Country' questionnaire: measurement of an Indigenous Australian health determinant. *International Journal for Equity in Health, 7*, 26.

Cargo, M., & Mercer, S. L. (2008). The value and challenges of participatory research: strengthening its practice. *Annual Review of Public Health, 29*, 325–350.

Carson, B., Dunbar, T., Chenhall, R. D., & Bailie, R. S. (Eds.). (2007). *Social determinants of indigenous health*. Crows Nest, NSW: Allen & Unwin.

Carter, S. L., Straits, J. E., & Hall, M. (2007). *Project venture: Evaluation of a positive, culture-based approach to substance abuse prevention with American Indian youth* Technical Report Gallup, NM: The National Indian Youth Leadership Project. www.niylp.org.

Castellano, M. B., Archibald, L., & DeGagné, M. (Eds.). (2011). *From truth to reconciliation: Transforming the legacy of residential schools*. Ottawa: Aboriginal Healing Foundation.

Chandler, M. (2010). Social determinants of education outcomes in Indigenous learners. *Education Canada, 50*, 45–50.

Chandler, M., & Lalonde, C. (1998). Cultural continuity as a hedge against suicide in Canada's First Nations. *Transcultural Psychiatry, 35*(2), 191–219.

Chandler, M., & Lalonde, C. (2009). Cultural continuity as a moderator of suicide risk among Canada's First Nations. In L. J. Kirmayer, & G. G. Valaskakis (Eds.), *Healing traditions: The mental health of Aboriginal peoples in Canada* (pp. 221–248). Vancouver, BC: UBC Press.

Chino, M., & Debruyn, L. (2006). Building true capacity: indigenous models for indigenous communities. *American Journal of Public Health, 96*(4), 596–599.

Cicchetti, D. (2013). Resilient functioning in maltreated children–past, present, and future perspectives. *Journal of Child Psychology and Psychiatry, 54*(4), 402–422.

Clarke, A. M., Kuosmanen, T., & Barry, M. M. (2015). A systematic review of online youth mental health promotion and prevention interventions. *Journal of Youth and Adolescence, 44*(1), 90–113.

Clelland, N., Gould, T., & Parker, E. (2007). Searching for evidence: what works in indigenous mental health promotion? *Health Promotion Journal of Australia, 18*(3), 208–216.

Connors, E., & Maidman, F. (2001). A circle of healing: family wellness in aboriginal communities. In I. Prilletensky, G. Nelson, & L. Peirson (Eds.), *Promoting family wellness and preventing child maltreatment: Fundamentals for thinking and action* (pp. 349–416). Toronto, ON: University of Toronto Press.

Cotton, M.-E., Nadeau, L., & Kirmayer, L. J. (2014). Consultation to remote and Indigenous communities. In L. J. Kirmayer, J. Guzder, & C. Rousseau (Eds.), *Cultural consultation: Encountering the other in mental health care* (pp. 223–244). New York: Springer SBM.

Crooks, C. V. (2009). *Engaging and empowering Aboriginal youth: A toolkit for service providers.* Toronto: CAMH Centre for Prevention Science.

Crooks, C. V., Chiodo, D., Thomas, D., & Hughes, R. (2010). Strengths-based programming for First Nations youth in schools: building engagement through healthy relationships and leadership skills. *International Journal of Mental Health and Addiction, 8*(2), 160–173.

Currie, C. L., Wild, T. C., Schopflocher, D. P., Laing, L., & Veugelers, P. (2012). Racial discrimination experienced by Aboriginal university students in Canada. *Canadian Journal of Psychiatry, 57*(10), 617–625.

Dell, C. A., Seguin, M., Hopkins, C., Tempier, R., Mehl-Madrona, L., Dell, D., et al. (2011). From benzos to berries: treatment offered at an Aboriginal youth solvent abuse treatment centre relays the importance of culture. *Canadian Journal of Psychiatry, 56*(2), 75–83.

Duran, E. (2006). *Healing the soul wound: Counseling with American Indians and other Native People.* New York: Teachers College Press.

Duran, E., Duran, B., Heart, M. Y. H.B., & Horse-Davis, S. Y. (1998). Healing the American Indian soul wound. In Y. Danieli (Ed.), *International handbook of multigenerational legacies of trauma* (pp. 341–354). New York: Springer.

Durie, M. (2005). Indigenous health promotion. In H. Herrman, S. Saxena, & R. Moodie (Eds.), *Promoting mental Health: Concepts, emerging evidence, practice* (pp. 265–268). Geneva: World Health Organization.

Durie, M., Milroy, H., & Hunter, E. (2009). Mental health and the Indigenous peoples of Australia and New Zealand. In L. J. Kirmayer, & G. Valaskakis (Eds.), *Healing traditions: The mental health of aboriginal peoples in Canada* (pp. 36–55). Vancouver: University of British Columbia Press.

Elias, B., Mignone, J., Hall, M., Hong, S. P., Hart, L., & Sareen, J. (2012). Trauma and suicide behaviour histories among a Canadian Indigenous population: an empirical exploration of the potential role of Canada's residential school system. *Social Science & Medicine, 74*(10), 1560–1569.

Flanagan, T., Iarocci, G., D'Arrisso, A., Mandour, T., Tootoosis, C., Robinson, S., et al. (2011). Reduced ratings of physical and relational aggression for youths with a strong cultural identity: evidence from the Naskapi people. *Journal of Adolescent Health, 49*(2), 155–159.

Fleming, J. E., & Ledogar, R. (2008). Resilience, an evolving concept: a review of literature relevant to Aboriginal research. *Pimatisiwin: A Journal of Aboriginal and Indigenous Community Health, 6*(2), 7–23.

Fryberg, S. A., Troop-Gordon, W., D'Arrisso, A., Flores, H., Ponizovskiy, V., Ranney, J. D., et al. (2013). Cultural mismatch and the education of Aboriginal youths: the interplay of cultural identities and teacher ratings. *Developmental Psychology, 49*(1), 72–79.

Gone, J. P. (2013). Redressing First Nations historical trauma: theorizing mechanisms for Indigenous culture as mental health treatment. *Transcultural Psychiatry, 50*(5), 683–706.

Gone, J. P., & Trimble, J. E. (2012). American Indian and Alaska Native mental health: diverse perspectives on enduring disparities. *Annual Review of Clinical Psychology, 8*, 131–160.

Goodkind, J., LaNoue, M., Lee, C., Lance Freeland, C., & Freund, R. (2012). Feasibility, acceptability, and initial findings from a community-based cultural mental health intervention for American Indian youth and their families. *Journal of Community Psychology, 40*(4), 381–405.

Gracey, M., & King, M. (2009). Indigenous health part 1: determinants and disease patterns. *Lancet, 374*(9683), 65–75.

Guerin, B. (2010). A framework for decolonization interventions: broadening the focus for improving the health and wellbeing of Indigenous communities. *Pimatisiwin: A Journal of Aboriginal and Indigenous Community Health, 8*(3), 61–83.

Hallett, D., Chandler, M. J., & Lalonde, C. E. (2007). Aboriginal language knowledge and youth suicide. *Cognitive Development, 22*(3), 392–399.

Herrman, H., & Jané-Llopis, E. (2012). The status of mental health promotion. *Public Health Review, 34*, 1–21.

Hopkins, K. D., Zubrick, S. R., & Taylor, C. L. (2014). Resilience amongst Australian Aboriginal youth: an ecological analysis of factors associated with psychosocial functioning in high and low family risk contexts. *PLoS ONE, 9*(7), e102820. http://dx.doi.org/10.1371/journal.pone.0102820.

Hosman, C. M. H., & Jané-Llopis, E. (2005). The evidence of effective interventions for mental health promotion. In H. Herrman, S. Saxena, & R. Moodie (Eds.), *Promoting mental health: Concepts, emerging evidence, practice* (pp. 169–188). Geneva: World Health Organization.

Iarocci, G., Root, R., & Burack, J. A. (2009). Social competence and mental health among aboriginal youth: an integrative developmental perspective. In L. J. Kirmayer, & G. Valaskakis (Eds.), *Healing traditions: The mental health of Aboriginal peoples in Canada* (pp. 80–106). Vancouver: University of British Columbia Press.

Indigenous Physicians Association of Canada and the Royal College of Physicians and Surgeons of Canada. (2009). *Promoting improved mental health for Canada's Indigenous peoples: A curriculum for psychiatry residents and psychiatrists* (Winnipeg & Ottawa: IPAC-RCPSC Psychiatry Curriculum Development Working Group).

International Work Group for Indigenous Affairs. (2015). *The indigenous world: 2015.* Copenhagen: IWGIA.

Jacquez, F., Vaughn, L. M., & Wagner, E. (2013). Youth as partners, participants or passive recipients: a review of children and adolescents in community-based participatory research (CBPR). *American Journal of Community Psychology, 51*(1–2), 176–189.

Kant, S., Vertinsky, I., Zheng, B., & Smith, P. M. (2013). Social, cultural, and land use determinants of the health and well-being of Aboriginal peoples of Canada: a path analysis. *Journal of Public Health Policy, 34*(3), 462–476.

Kenyon, D. B., & Hanson, J. D. (2012). Incorporating traditional culture into positive youth development programs with American Indian/Alaska Native youth. *Child Development Perspectives, 6*(3), 272–279.

Keyes, C. L. (Ed.). (2012). *Mental well-being: International contributions to the study of positive mental health.* Springer Science & Business Media.

Kingsley, J., Townsend, M., Henderson-Wilson, C., & Bolam, B. (2013). Developing an exploratory framework linking Australian Aboriginal peoples' connection to country and concepts of wellbeing. *International Journal of Environmental Research and Public Health, 10*(2), 678–698.

King, M., Smith, A., & Gracey, M. (2009). Indigenous health part 2: the underlying causes of the health gap. *Lancet, 374*(9683), 76–85.

Kirmayer, L. J. (2007). Psychotherapy and the cultural concept of the person. *Transcultural Psychiatry, 44*(2), 232–257.

Kirmayer, L. J. (2012). Rethinking cultural competence. *Transcultural Psychiatry, 49*(2), 149.

Kirmayer, L. J. (2015). Re-visioning psychiatry: toward an ecology of mind in health and illness. In L. J. Kirmayer, R. Lemelson, & C. A. Cummings (Eds.), *Re-visioning psychiatry: Cultural phenomenology, critical neuroscience, and global mental health.* New York: Cambridge University Press.

Kirmayer, L. J., Bennegadi, R., & Kastrup, M. (2016). Cultural awareness and responsiveness in person-centered psychiatry. In J. Mezzich, M. Botbol, G. Christodoulou, C. R. Cloninger, & I. Salloum (Eds.), *Person-centered psychiatry.* Heidelberg: Springer Verlag.

Kirmayer, L. J., Brass, G. M., & Valaskakis, G. G. (2009). Conclusion: healing/invention/tradition. In L. J. Kirmayer, & G. G. Valaskakis (Eds.), *Healing traditions: The mental health of Aboriginal peoples in Canada* (pp. 440–472). Vancouver, BC: UBC Press.

Kirmayer, L. J., Dandeneau, S., Marshall, E., Phillips, M. K., & Williamson, K. J. (2011). Rethinking resilience from Indigenous perspectives. *Canadian Journal of Psychiatry, 56*(2), 84–91.

Kirmayer, L. J., Dandeneau, S., Marshall, E., Phillips, M. K., & Williamson, K. J. (2012). Toward an ecology of stories: Indigenous perspectives on resilience. In M. Ungar (Ed.), *The social ecology of resilience* (pp. 399–414). New York: Springer.

Kirmayer, L. J., Fletcher, C., & Watt, R. (2009). Locating the ecocentric self: Inuit concepts of mental health and illness. In L. J. Kirmayer, & G. G. Valaskakis (Eds.), *Healing traditions: The mental health of Aboriginal peoples in Canada* (pp. 289–314). Vancouver, BC: UBC Press.

Kirmayer, L. J., Fraser, S.-L., Fauras, V., Dandeneau, S., & Whitley, R. (2009a). *Current approaches to Aboriginal youth suicide prevention*. Ottawa: Health Canada, First Nations and Inuit Health Branch.

Kirmayer, L. J., Gone, J. P., & Moses, J. (2014). Rethinking historical trauma. *Transcultural Psychiatry, 51*(3), 299–319.

Kirmayer, L. J., Sedhev, M., Whitley, R., Dandeneau, S., & Isaac, C. (2009b). Community resilience: models, metaphors and measures. *Journal of Aboriginal Health, 7*(1), 62–117.

Kirmayer, L. J., Simpson, C., & Cargo, M. (2003). Healing traditions: culture, community and mental health promotion with Canadian Aboriginal peoples. *Australasian Psychiatry, 11*(Suppl.), 15–23.

Kolahdooz, F., Nader, F., Kyoung, J. Y., & Sharma, S. (2015). Understanding the social determinants of health among Indigenous Canadians: priorities for health promotion policies and actions. *Global Health Action, 8*. http://dx.doi.org/10.3402/gha.v8.27968.

Kral, I. (2010). *Plugged in: Remote Australian indigenous youth and digital culture*. Canberra, Australia: Australian National University (CAEPR Working Paper No. 69/2010).

Kral, M. J., & Idlout, L. (2012). It's all in the family: wellbeing among Inuit in Arctic Canada. In H. Selin, & G. Davey (Eds.), *Happiness across cultures* (pp. 387–398). New York: Springer.

Kral, M. J., Salusky, I., Inuksuk, P., Angutimarik, L., & Tulugardjuk, N. (2014). *Tunngajuq*: stress and resilience among Inuit youth in Nunavut, Canada. *Transcultural Psychiatry, 51*(5), 673–692.

Krieger, N. (2012). Methods for the scientific study of discrimination and health: an ecosocial approach. *American Journal of Public Health, 102*(5), 936–944.

LaFromboise, T. D., & Lewis, H. A. (2008). The Zuni life skills development program: a school/community-based suicide prevention intervention. *Suicide and Life-threatening Behavior, 38*(3), 343–353.

Langlois, S., & Turner, A. (2014). *Aboriginal languages and selected vitality indicators in 2011*. Ottawa: Statistics Canada.

Ledogar, R. J., & Fleming, J. (2008). Social capital and resilience: a review of concepts and selected literature relevant to Aboriginal youth resilience research. *Pimatisiwin, 6*(2), 25.

Liebenberg, L., Ikeda, J., & Wood, M. (2015). "It's just part of my culture": understanding language and land in the resilience processes of Aboriginal youth. In L. C. Theron, L. Liebenberg, & M. Ungar (Eds.), *Youth resilience and culture* (pp. 105–116). The Netherlands: Springer.

Liebenberg, L., Ungar, M., & Van de Vijver, F. (2012). Validation of the Child and Youth Resilience-28 (CYRM-28) among Canadian youth. *Research on Social Work Practice, 22*(2), 219–226.

Lippman, L., Moore, K. A., & McIntosh, H. (2009). *Positive indicators of child well-being: a conceptual framework, measures and methodological issues*. Florence: UNICEF Innocenti Research Centre.

MacDonald, J. P., Ford, J. D., Willox, A. C., & Ross, N. A. (2013). A review of protective factors and causal mechanisms that enhance the mental health of indigenous circumpolar youth. *International Journal of Circumpolar Health, 72*, 21775.

MacDonald, J. P., Willox, A. C., Ford, J. D., Shiwak, I., Wood, M., & IMHACC Team (2015). Protective factors for mental health and well-being in a changing climate: perspectives from Inuit youth in Nunatsiavut, Labrador. *Social Science & Medicine, 141,* 133–141.

Masten, A. S. (2014). Global perspectives on resilience in children and youth. *Child Development, 85*(1), 6–20.

McCormick, R. (2009). Aboriginal approaches to counselling. In L. J. Kirmayer, & G. Valaskakis (Eds.), *Healing traditions: The mental health of Aboriginal peoples in Canada* (pp. 337–355). Vancouver: University of British Columbia Press.

McMahon, T. R., Kenyon, D. B., & Carter, J. S. (2013). "My culture, my family, my school, me": identifying strengths and challenges in the lives and communities of American Indian youth. *Journal of Child and Family Studies, 22*(5), 694–706.

Mezzich, J. E., Salloum, I. M., Cloninger, C. R., Salvador-Carulla, L., Kirmayer, L. J., Banzato, C. E. M., et al. (2010). Person-centered integrative diagnosis: conceptual basis and structural model. *Canadian Journal of Psychiatry, 55*(11), 701–708.

Mohatt, N. V., Thompson, A. B., Thai, N. D., & Tebes, J. K. (2014). Historical trauma as public narrative: a conceptual review of how history impacts present-day health. *Social Science & Medicine, 106,* 128–136.

Molyneaux, H., O'Donnell, S., Kakekaspan, C., Walmark, B., Budka, P., & Gibson, K. (2014). Social media in remote First Nation communities. *Canadian Journal of Communication, 39*(2), 275–288.

Niezen, R. (2009). Suicide as a way of belonging: causes and consequences of cluster suicides in Aboriginal communities. In L. J. Kirmayer, & G. Valaskakis (Eds.), *Healing traditions: The mental health of Aboriginal peoples in Canada* (pp. 178–195). Vancouver: University of British Columbia Press.

Nystad, K., Spein, A. R., & Ingstad, B. (2014). Community resilience factors among indigenous Sámi adolescents: a qualitative study in Northern Norway. *Transcultural Psychiatry, 51*(5), 651–672.

Phinney, J. S., & Ong, A. D. (2007). Conceptualization and measurement of ethnic identity: current status and future directions. *Journal of Counseling Psychology, 54*(3), 271–281.

Reading, J. (2009). *The crisis of chronic disease among Aboriginal peoples: A challenge for public health, population health and social policy.* Victoria, BC: Centre for Aboriginal Health Research.

Richmond, C. A., Ross, N. A., & Egeland, G. M. (2007). Social support and thriving health: a new approach to understanding the health of Indigenous Canadians. *American Journal of Public Health, 97*(10), 1827–1833. http://dx.doi.org/10.2105/AJPH.2006.096917 AJPH.2006.096917 [pii].

Ritchie, S. D., Wabano, M. J., Russell, K., Enosse, L., & Young, N. L. (2014). Promoting resilience and well being through an outdoor intervention designed for Aboriginal adolescents. *Rural and Remote Health, 14,* 2523.

Ruiz-Casares, M., Guzder, J., Rousseau, C., & Kirmayer, L. J. (2014). Cultural roots of well-being and resilience in child mental health. In *Handbook of child well-being* (pp. 2379–2407). The Netherlands: Springer.

Sanders, M. R. (2012). Development, evaluation, and multinational dissemination of the Triple-P Positive Parenting Program. *Annual Review of Clinical Psychology, 8*(2012), 345–379.

Saul, J. R. (2014). *The comeback: How aboriginals are reclaiming power and influence.* Toronto: Penguin Canada.

Sinclair, R. (2007). Identity lost and found: lessons from the Sixties Scoop. *First Peoples Child & Family Review, 3*(1), 65–82.

Sissons, J. (2005). *First peoples: Indigenous cultures and their futures.* London: Reaktion Books.

Smith, L. T. (1999). *Decolonizing methodologies: Research and Indigenous peoples.* London: Zed Books.

Snowshoe, A., Crooks, C. V., Tremblay, P. F., Craig, W. M., & Hinson, R. E. (2015). Development of a cultural connectedness scale for First Nations youth. *Psychological Assessment, 27*(1), 249.

Spoth, R., Greenberg, M., Bierman, K., & Redmond, C. (2004). Prosper community-university partnership model for public education systems: capacity-building for evidence- based, competence-building prevention. *Prevention Science, 5*(1), 31–39.

Statistics Canada. (2013). *Aboriginal Peoples in Canada: First Nations People, Métis and Inuit. National household Survey, 2011.* Ottawa: Statistics Canada.

Stephens, C., Porter, J., Nettleton, C., & Willis, R. (2006). Disappearing, displaced, and under-valued: a call to action for Indigenous health worldwide. *Lancet, 367*(9527), 2019–2028.

Stewart, S. L. (2008). Promoting indigenous mental health: cultural perspectives on healing from native counsellors in Canada. *International Journal of Health Promotion and Education, 46*(2), 12–19.

Stuart, J., & Jose, P. E. (2014). The protective influence of family connectedness, ethnic iden-tity, and ethnic engagement for New Zealand Māori adolescents. *Developmental Psychol-ogy, 50*(6), 1817.

Taylor, J. (2008). Indigenous peoples and indicators of well-being: Australian perspectives on United Nations global frameworks. *Social Indicators Research, 87,* 111–126.

Thomas, A., Cairney, S., Gunthorpe, W., Paradies, Y., & Sayers, S. (2010). Strong souls: develop-ment and validation of a culturally appropriate tool for assessment of social and emotional well-being in indigenous youth. *Australian and New Zealand Journal of Psychiatry, 44*(1), 40–48.

Tiessen, M., Taylor, D. M., & Kirmayer, L. J. (2010). A key individual-to-community link: the impact of perceived collective control on Aboriginal youth well-being. *Pimatisiwin: A Journal of Indigenous and Aboriginal Community Health, 7*(2), 241–267.

Truth and Reconciliation Commission. (2015). *Honouring the truth, reconciling for the future: Summary of the final report of the Truth and Reconciliation Commission of Canada. Ottawa.*

Tsey, K., Wilson, A., Haswell-Elkins, M., Whiteside, M., McCalman, J., Cadet-James, Y., et al. (2007). Empowerment-based research methods: a 10-year approach to enhanc-ing Indigenous social and emotional wellbeing. *Australasian Psychiatry, 15*(Suppl. 1), S34–S38.

Turner, K., & Sanders, M. (2007). Family intervention in Indigenous communities: emergent issues in conducting outcome research. *Australasian Psychiatry, 15*(Suppl. 1), S39–S43.

Ulturgasheva, O., Rasmus, S., Wexler, L., Nystad, K., & Kral, M. (2014). Arctic indigenous youth resilience and vulnerability: Comparative analysis of adolescent experiences across five circumpolar communities. *Transcultural Psychiatry, 51*(5), 735–756.

Ungar, M. (2011a). The social ecology of resilience: addressing contextual and cultural ambi-guity of a nascent construct. *American Journal of Orthopsychiatry, 81*(1), 1–17.

Ungar, M. (2011b). Community resilience for youth and families: facilitative physical and social capital in contexts of adversity. *Children and Youth Services Review, 33*(9), 1742–1748.

Ungar, M. (2012). Researching and theorizing resilience across cultures and contexts. *Preven-tive Medicine, 55*(5), 387–389.

Ungar, M. (2015). Resilience and culture: the diversity of protective processes and positive adaptation. In L. Theron, L. Liebenberg, & M. Ungar (Eds.), *Youth resilience and culture* (pp. 37–48). The Netherlands: Springer.

Ungar, M., & Liebenberg, L. (2011). Assessing resilience across cultures using mixed meth-ods: construction of the child and youth resilience measure. *Journal of Mixed Methods Research, 5*(2), 126–149.

United Nations General Assembly. (2007). *United Nations declaration on the rights of Indigenous peoples.* Accessed 08.11.15. http://www.converge.org.nz/pma/decrips.htm.

Valeggia, C. R., & Snodgrass, J. J. (2015). Health of Indigenous peoples. *Annual Review of Anthropology, 44*(1), 117–135.

Wendt, D. C., & Gone, J. P. (2012). Rethinking cultural competence: insights from Indigenous community treatment settings. *Transcultural Psychiatry, 49*(2), 206–222.

Westerman, T. G. (2003). *The development of the Westerman Aboriginal Symptom Checklist for Youth: A measure to assess the moderating effects of cultural resilience with Aboriginal youth at risk of depression, anxiety and suicidal behaviours* (Unpublished doctoral thesis). Perth, Australia: Curtin University.

Wexler, L. (2014). Looking across three generations of Alaska Natives to explore how culture fosters indigenous resilience. *Transcultural Psychiatry*, *51*(1), 73–92.

Wexler, L., Chandler, M., Gone, J. P., Cwik, M., Kirmayer, L. J., LaFromboise, T., et al. (2015). Advancing suicide prevention research with rural American Indian and Alaska Native populations. *American Journal of Public Health*, *105*(5), 891–899.

Wexler, L., Joule, L., Garoutte, J., Mazziotti, J., & Hopper, K. (2014). "Being responsible, respectful, trying to keep the tradition alive": cultural resilience and growing up in an Alaska Native community. *Transcultural Psychiatry*, *51*(5), 693–712.

Whitbeck, L. B., Walls, M., & Hartshorn, K. (2014). *Indigenous adolescent development: Psychological, social and historical contexts*. New York: Routledge.

Whitbeck, L. B., Walls, M. L., & Welch, M. L. (2012). Substance abuse prevention in American Indian and Alaska Native communities. *American Journal of Drug and Alcohol Abuse*, *38*(5), 428–435.

Yasui, M., Dishion, T. J., Stormshak, E., & Ball, A. (2015). Socialization of culture and coping with discrimination among American Indian families: examining cultural correlates of youth outcomes. *Journal of the Society for Social Work and Research*, *6*(3), 317–341.

Yi, K. J., Landais, E., Kolahdooz, F., & Sharma, S. (2015). Factors influencing the health and wellness of urban Aboriginal youths in Canada: insights of in-service professionals, care providers, and stakeholders. *American Journal of Public Health*, *105*(5), 881–890.

Young, N. L., Wabano, M. J., Burke, T. A., Ritchie, S. D., Mishibinijima, D., & Corbiere, R. G. (2013). A process for creating the aboriginal children's health and well-being measure (ACHWM). *Canadian Journal of Public Health*, *104*(2), e136–e141.

Young, N. L., Wabano, M. J., Ritchie, S. D., Burke, T. A., Pangowish, B., & Corbiere, R. G. (2015a). Assessing children's interpretations of the Aboriginal Children's Health and Well-being Measure (ACHWM). *Health and Quality of Life Outcomes*, *13*(1), 1.

Young, N. L., Wabano, M. J., Usuba, K., Pangowish, B., Trottier, M., Jacko, D., et al. (2015b). Validity of the Aboriginal children's health and well-being measure: Aaniish Naa Gegii? *Health and Quality of Life Outcomes*, *13*(1), 148.

Zimmerman, M. A., Stoddard, S. A., Eisman, A. B., Caldwell, C. H., Aiyer, S. M., & Miller, A. (2013). Adolescent resilience: promotive factors that inform prevention. *Child development perspectives*, *7*(4), 215–220.

Psychological Consequences of Parental Migration for Left-Behind Children

Y. Zheng[1,2,3]

[1]Beijing Anding Hospital, Capital Medical University, Beijing, P.R. China; [2]The Chinese Society of Child and Adolescent Psychiatry; [3]The International Association for Child and Adolescent Psychiatry and Allied Professions (IACAPAP)

World population has increased by two billion people from 1990 to 2015. With increased globalization and population mobility, growing numbers of people are seeking better work opportunities outside their region of birth. In recent years, international migration has grown in scope and complexity. The number of international migrants, defined as persons living outside of their country of birth, rose by nearly five percent, from 221 million in 2010 to 232 million in 2013. According to the UN, in 2013, the number of international migrants worldwide reached 3.2 percent of the world population. If current trends continue, the next 15 years could see 30 million additional international migrants added worldwide (United Nations DoEaSA, 2013). To better account for the migrant worker phenomenon and the effect it may have on children, this chapter reviews current literature, explores the magnitude of the phenomenon, and highlights the multitude of mechanisms by which migration affects children's lives and psychological wellbeing in around the globe.

LEFT-BEHIND CHILDREN: THE ORIGIN AND SCOPE OF THE PHENOMENON

International Migration

The distribution of migrants has certain patterns around the world. Most migrants came from developing countries and migrated toward

Positive Mental Health, Fighting Stigma and Promoting Resiliency for Children and Adolescents
http://dx.doi.org/10.1016/B978-0-12-804394-3.00007-3

more developed regions. Almost one in every 10 persons living in more developed regions is a migrant compared to one of every 70 persons in developing regions. Latin American, Asia, Africa, and less developed parts of Europe are the major exporting countries of the world's migrant stock. For example, between 1990 and 2013, Northern America had the largest number of international migrants, and of the 25 million migrants added in this period, 57 percent were born in Latin America and the Caribbean, 35 percent originated from Asia, while 6 percent were born in Africa. The largest migration corridor in the world from 1985 to 2015 has been from Mexico to USA (United Nations DoEaSA, 2013). In addition, migration between countries in Southern Asia (eg, Bangladesh, India, Indonesia and Sri Lanka) and oil-producing countries in Western Asia (eg, Saudi Arabia and United Arab Emirates) are also major migration corridors. Approximately one-third of the most qualified African nationals have settled outside their country of origin. In the cases of Mozambique, Ghana, and Tanzania, almost half of the highly skilled workers in the population migrated to other countries (Sørensen, 2012).

Many migrants leave their hometowns in rural areas to seek employment in cities. All regions, with the exception of Europe, are projected to record increases in the sizes of their urban populations of at least 15 percent. Africa and Asia are projected to have the largest increases in the size of their urban populations (United Nations PDotDoEaSA, 2015).

Most international migrants are of working age. In 2013, 171 million international migrants, or 74 percent of global migrants, were between the ages of 20 and 64. In the developed regions persons of working age account for 77 percent of all international migrants (United Nations DoEaSA, 2013). During this timeframe, there has also been an increase in women migrants. In the early 2000s, a sharp increase in the proportion of women among the migrant workers from certain countries was observed, specifically emigrants from Sri Lanka, Indonesia, and the Philippines, as well as Latin American countries (Fund UNP, 2006). Between 1990 and 2013, the proportion of women among all international migrants increased in all major areas with the exception of Africa and Asia (Fund UNP, 2006).

Migration can contribute to sustainable development by expanding economic opportunities, reducing poverty, addressing labor market imbalances, and accelerating the diffusion of new ideas and technologies. But with most of the migrants being of working age with an increasing number of women migrants, the children of these migrants has become a population needing special attention. When mothers or primary caregivers migrate, they develop ways to care for their children, including paying childcare workers, and placing children with the extended family, such as grandmothers, aunts, or older sisters (Hondagneu-Sotelo & Avila, 1997). Child-shifting, or placing children with relatives or friends for a variety of reasons, is a relatively common practice in the Caribbean, Africa, the Philippines, and Peru (Lashley, 2000; Leinaweaver, 2010; Peterson, 1993).

The migrant mother usually pays the extended family for childcare with remittances and gifts, but the impact of these transformations on children is unknown (Isaksen, Devi, & Hochschild, 2008). There is substantial controversy around the impact of the outflow of the labor force on the welfare of children. Remittances reduce the depth and severity of poverty among those who receive them, which is often the children. On the other hand, international migration can lead to the absence of traditional cultural figures that frequently results in the breakdown of essential social norms and customs which can negatively affect the children left behind. Gender differences also play an important role in the psychological impacts of parents' migration on children left behind.

It should also be noted that migrant parents sometimes do not abandon parenting roles when they migrate. They may maintain close contact with their children and financially support them. These new parenting practices result in a new concept of transnational families (Cortés, 2007). This new form of family and the complexity of relationships that arise from transnational connections call for new insights into family bonds and relational stresses. It may also require that we as psychiatrists adopt new theory and treatment approaches.

Internal Migration

In 2013, the majority of all migration occurred within world regions rather than across regional boundaries (United Nations DoEaSA, 2013). During economic development, internal migration is inevitable. Like transnational migration, national (internal) migration plays an important role in poverty reduction and economic development. For some countries, internal migrants outnumber those who migrate internationally. The past three decades (from 1985 to 2015) witnessed what some called the largest human migration in history. This certainly applies to the internal migration of people seeking work in China. The result of this migration is a sharp rise in the Chinese urban population, from 191 million in 1980 to 665 million in 2010 (Chen, 2011). This increase is believed to be driven largely by internal rural-to-urban migration. From 2000 to 2010, 116 million people migrated from rural area to large cities (2010 National Census Data, 2013). This trend for urbanization in China is anticipated to continue in the coming years, and so the health consequences of such large-scale migration are important. There is also an increasing trend of internal migration in other Asian countries such as the Philippines and Vietnam (Anh, 1999). This is also true for many developing countries in sub-Saharan Africa and Latin America (Migration IOM, 2005). Overall, the evidence to date suggests that those with limited access to land and other assets are more likely to migrate (Liu and Zou, 2011).

Because the major goal of migration is to seek better employment and opportunities in cities, internal migrants tend to be young men and women in their 20s to 40s. Due to China's rigid household registration system (known as "Hukou"), workers who have migrated are not registered as "resident" in urban areas. This prevents them from getting access to public services such as health care, housing, and education in the cities. As a result, the children of migrant workers struggle to get education and health care if they go to cities with their parents. Furthermore, migrant workers often have low income, live in crowded living conditions, and cannot afford to bring children with them. Often the children are left behind to live in their rural hometowns. This creates the "Left-Behind Children" phenomenon.

According to the Chinese national 2010 census (National survey of left-behind children in rural areas and migrant children in urban and rural areas), the total number of left-behind children (defined as children under 17 years old living in their rural homes with one or both parents working outside their registered resident area) reached 61 million, making up 37.7 percent of the population of all rural children. About 50 percent of left-behind children are left by both parents, while single-father and single-mother migrations account for 36.4 percent and 16.9 percent, respectively. Of children left by both parents, the majority live with their grandparents, and about 20 percent live with other relatives. It should be noted that about 6 percent of left-behind children are left alone without a stable guardian. This translates to two million children living alone in the rural area. Their welfare should be of special concern. Some children are left behind at a fairly young age; 20 percent were separated from their parents before the age of one, which means breast feeding may not be possible for some infants who are left behind (Luo et al., 2008).

The early separation from parents and the absence of parental care during development could have widespread educational, psychological, and nutritional effects on children. The enormous scale of the "left-behind" children phenomenon makes it vitally important to policy makers and child mental health professionals to further investigate the living conditions and psychological wellbeing of these children across the world, and devise appropriate action plans.

EDUCATION OF LEFT-BEHIND CHILDREN

The overall effect of migration on educational attainment is mixed. Brown and Park found that school performance is strongly correlated with household income (Brown & Park, 2002). Migrants remit a large share of their income. With this income, families of migrants can invest more in their children's education, such as tutoring, computer-assisted learning, and other academic resources that may improve the children's academic performance (Amuedo-Dorantes & Pozo, 2010; Duan & Zhou, 2005; Edwards & Ureta, 2003). This is especially true in international migrant families with left-behind girls. For example, Antman (2012) found a statistically significant positive effect of parental US migration on educational attainment for girls. In this sense, remittances usually have a positive effect on education, but it is still unknown how remittances contribute to the quality of learning of left-behind children.

On the other hand, evidence regarding the positive impact of remittances on education must be weighed against the negative effect that parental absence has on the psychological development and overall school performance of children left behind (Castañeda & Buck, 2011; Funds UNCs, 2008). This is mostly problematic in rural areas with a shortage of labor. In these areas, parental migration could result in a lack of adult labor in the home, and the left-behind children have to perform household and farm work, which may lead the children to complete less schooling than children in non-migrant families (McKenzie & Rapoport, 2011). Adolescents are particularly affected due to the expectation to become the new caregiver after the migration of one or both of the parents (Mansuri, 2006). In China, most of the rural left-behind children have access to primary education. School enrollment of 6 to 14 years old is 96 percent, but some underdeveloped areas such as Sichuan and Yunan provinces have a lower school enrollment rate. Factor analysis shown that the mother working in another city is a risk factor for attaining, less education and the drop-out rate of adolescents is much higher, with only 88 percent of children 14 years old being enrolled in school (National survey of left-behind children in rural areas and migrant children in urban and rural areas). The absence of a parent results in the loss of parental attention and supervision over children, which leads to poorer school performance. Particularly, the absence of a parent may negatively affect the left-behind children's psychological wellbeing and, thus, lead to academic, behavioral, and emotional problems. A study done by Spera (2005) suggested that parental involvement and monitoring are robust predictors of children's academic achievement. Liang and Chen studied the school attendance of left-behind children in rural areas of Guangdong province, China, and found that parental migration was significantly associated with decreased school enrollment rate due to lack of parental oversight (Chen, Adams, Qu, Wang, & Chen, 2013). Furthermore, surrogate guardians such as grandparents may place a lower value on education than parents, or lack sufficient time or motivation to support the studies of the child. Children living in extended families were hindered in receiving education due to domestic problems and the limited space at home. At least in rural areas of China, grandparents are not satisfactory substitutes for parents, as they may not be well-educated and place less emphasis on education (Liang & Chen, 2007). Other studies carried out in China, corroborated Liang's findings, and found that children whose parents had migrated were worse off in terms of school enrollment and had fewer years of schooling than their counterparts whose parents stayed with them (Chen et al., 2013; Meyerhoefer & Chen, 2011).

II. RISK AND RESILIENCE

Zhao et al. analyzed survey data from more than 7600 4th and 5th grade students from 74 rural elementary schools in rural areas of the Ningxia Autonomous Region and the Qinghai province in northwest China, and found that having migrant parents can reduce a child's math score rank by 15.60 percent. Compared to children who have neither parent migrating, migration of the father reduces the rank of a child's math score by 8.37 percent, and migration of the mother reduces the rank by 23.30 percent. This suggests that academic performance is influenced mainly by the presence of the mother in the household (Zhao et al., 2014). This is also true for international migrants. Stirbu (2006) found that children whose mother is abroad tend to reject non-compulsory education. This implies that even though migration has short-term financial benefits for a family, it may have a negative impact on children's accumulation of human capital in the long term. To make economic growth sustainable and improve human rights, the government should take active measures to dismantle barriers of education for those who are left behind.

PSYCHOLOGICAL WELLBEING OF LEFT-BEHIND CHILDREN

Overall Wellbeing and Quality of Life

Migration can improve the welfare of children left behind when remittances are able to reduce the effects of poverty or abuse. Studies carried out in Moldova compared 75 left-behind children with 84 children without migrating parents, and found that the material situation of the former improved post-parental migration (Fund UNCs, 2008). But children left behind by migrating parents who are not able to financially support them over a long period of time experience particularly negative outcomes. It is prudent to conclude that the overall satisfaction and wellbeing of left-behind children are related to the financial situation of the family. For children whose parents migrate internationally and who send greater remittances, the quality of life is often better. However, for those who are forced to migrate, if the financial hardship persists, left-behind children usually experience a reduction in quality of life. Two studies carried out in different regions of China illustrated this pattern. One study was completed in the eastern, more developed area of China, and the other was completed in the midwest, underdeveloped area. Both studies showed that left-behind children have poorer health-related quality of life than children living with both parents. The study conducted in Shandong province in east China revealed that the left-behind children showed poorer health-related quality of life (HRQoL) than their counterparts only in psychosocial dysfunction, but the mean school performance of the left-behind children did not differ significantly from that of non-left-behind children. Particularly in households with high levels of remittances, as age increased, the average HRQoL scores of the left-behind children or adolescents were significantly improved (Jia, Shi, Cao, Delancey, & Tian, 2010). However the study carried out in Midwest China showed that left-behind children scored significantly lower in all aspects including total scores, physical functioning, emotional functioning, and social functioning compared with the non-left-behind children (Huang et al., 2015).

Separation and the Effects on Child Development

Overall, family separation appears to be the most negative consequence of parental migration. It results in children receiving less supervision, a loss of support and encouragement, and the loss of role models. Attachment theory is often used when trying to theorize the consequence of parental migration, especially in the case of a migrating mother. An attachment is a substantial, enduring, affective bond between individuals. The initial attachment a child forms is generally to his/her mother or other primary caregiver. In very young children, physical proximity tends to promote attachment to a primary caregiver. Migration of the caregiver can subsequently disrupt the physical proximity which is the basis of attachment. This may cause significant psychological distress among children and can lead to depression, anxiety, or anger (Bowlby, 1982). However, migration is different from other forms of separation because parents can supervise and care for children remotely and financially support them. Nobles compared the experiences of children of divorced and migrant fathers in Mexico (Nobles, 2011). Migrant fathers were found to communicate more consistently with their children and to invest more in their children than did divorced fathers.

Concerns also revolve around the way in which parental absence could increase the risk of neglect, reduce the quality of discipline and supervision, reduce parental support and guidance, and thus undermine parent–child bonding. Studies have shown that parent–child bonding is important for the psychological development of children. A study showed that the reaction of Jamaican children to their parents' migration was directly connected to long-term psychological difficulties and underperformance in school (Pottinger, 2005). Children under age 5, left behind by a migrant mother or both parents, face the highest risk of psychological trauma as a result of a lack of nurturing, which is crucial during the early stages of development. Virtually all such children were found having psychological problems after their parents migrated (Fund UNCs, 2008). Zhao et al. (2014) examined 1694 left-behind children and 1223 non-left-behind controls, aged 7 to 17 years, in Anhui province, China, using a structured survey. Left-behind children displayed higher social anxiety scores, more neglect, lower parental educational level, lower quality of life, and lower family function than controls. When children are left to the care of much older relatives, generational differences can become an obstacle to effective communication, further depriving migrant children of the emotional support that is so crucial to their healthy and prosperous development. Adolescents whose parents migrated often experienced difficulties in their social relations, isolating themselves into small groups of peers in a similar situation (Fund UNCs, 2008).

Children left behind are more prone to psychological and emotional stress, feelings of abandonment, and low self-esteem, all of which may ultimately cause damage to the child's overall development and patterns of socialization (Bryant, 2005; Graham & Jordan, 2011). Reactions to separation may vary by gender. Boys may be more prone to externalizing problems in an earlier age than girls. Studies done in Latin American found more behavioral issues in boys whose fathers had migrated, and a study of early adolescents in Mexico noted higher distress levels in boys (Aguilera-Guzman, de Snyder, Romero, & Medina-Mora, 2004). One Chinese study found that left-behind boys have higher rates of skipping breakfast, physical inactivity, and Internet addiction, while left-behind girls are more likely to drink excess amount of sweetened beverages and to watch more TV (Gao et al., 2010). Another Chinese study of children of migrant families found that girls whose parents left at younger ages had higher depression and anxiety scores than boys (Liu, Li, & Ge, 2009). The difference in gender predilection can be partly explained by local culture. In Latin American, depression and anxiety of boys may be related to the pressure of future migration. On the other hand, in China, the elderly often discriminate against girls.

Thus, being left behind can cause considerable psychological stress among children. This can have long-term repercussions for their development. Experience of the primary caregiver, who is often the mother, migrating and being left alone at a young age are risk factors for psychological problems. However, regular communication and long distance parenting can partly alleviate this problem. The study carried out in the Philippines showed that communication with parents helps lessen the negative impact of separation and makes it easier for children to come to terms with their parents' absence (Ehrenreich & Hochschild, 2004). A study from China also found that the children who reported a higher level of parent–child communication also demonstrated a higher level of life and school satisfaction and happiness (Su, Li, Lin, Xu, & Zhu, 2013). However, communication between distant parents and children may encounter emotional, as well as practical barriers. All studies documented parental strategies for connecting with their children, including making regular phone calls home and, more recently, e-mails, web chat, and social networking (Mitrani, Santisteban, & Muir, 2004; Schmalzbauer, 2004). Families with limited income and low socioeconomic level may not be able to afford regular international calls. Besides, in many underdeveloped rural areas, children may only have limited access to the Internet. Children reported that phone calls were difficult if they had no shared daily life experiences to discuss or if they had only dim memories of their parent.

Long-term effects may result from the experience of separation. Disruption of the parent–child bond may lead to the inability to establish stable adult relationships (Chase-Lansdale, Cherlin, & Kiernan, 1995; Peterson, 1993).

Specific Disorders

The results of the majority of existing studies show that left-behind children are prone to psychological stress and have greater mental health problems. A meta-analysis including six controlled studies compared 1465 left-behind children and 1401 children in a normal family environment in China. The findings from this and several other studies suggest that left-behind children have significantly higher scores in anxiety, loneliness, fear, and self-blame (Jia & Tian, 2010; Liu, Zhang, Song, & Shi, 2013; Zhao et al., 2014). Other studies found that although no significant differences in the overall mental outcomes between the left-behind children and other children existed, certain subgroups of left-behind children were at potential risk (Tao, Guan, Zhao, & Fan, 2014). Being raised by grandparents and going to boarding schools are two independent risk factors for mental disorders while higher education levels of mothers is a protective factor (Wu, Lu, & Kang, 2014).

Attention-Deficit Hyperactivity Disorder and Conduct Disorder

Higher prevalence of psychiatric disorders among left-behind children in China is seen with oppositional defiant disorder (ODD), attention-deficit hyperactivity disorder (ADHD), and poor social interaction being the most troubling problems in boys aged 12 to 16 years (Fan, Su, Gill, & Birmaher, 2010). Findings from this nationally representative study corroborates findings from smaller scale studies conducted in Sri Lanka that showed adverse behavioral outcomes, emotional, and conduct disorders in school-aged children of female migrant workers (Senaratne, Perera, & Fonseka, 2011). The burden of emotional problems and hyperactivity disorders is highest in children from migrant families than from children in comparison families. Two in every five left-behind children (43.3 percent) had clinically relevant child psychiatric disorders (Wickramage et al., 2015). Environmental factors are important influences on the prevalence of conduct disorder (CD). Studies have compared the prevalence of CD in Mexico migrants and indigenous children. The results suggest that there is a large difference in risk for CD between Mexicans in Mexico and children of Mexican descent in the US. While only 2 percent of people in families of migrants met DSM-IV criteria for CD, 11.5 percent of

US-born Mexican-Americans met these criteria (Breslau et al., 2011). The dramatic increase in CD symptoms across generations within this migrant population implicates environmental influences in the origin of this disorder. Unfortunately identification of the particular environmental factors remains elusive. The environmental changes experienced by migrating populations are wide-ranging, as are the factors involved in the life of left-behind children.

Affective Disorders: Depression and Anxiety

Early-onset depression is associated with low self-esteem and increased risk for suicidal behaviors (Hardt, Herke, & Schier, 2011; Renouf, Kovacs, & Mukerji, 1997). Adolescents with early-onset depression are at greater risk of substance abuse, recurring depression, and other emotional and mental health problems in adulthood (Wilcox & Anthony, 2004).

Some level of depression is expected in the initial phase of separation. Nevertheless, intense depression and feelings of abandonment have been observed as persisting well beyond initial stages of parental migration (Smith, Lalonde, Johnson, 2004). Smith et al. also found that children of Caribbean serial migrants often displayed low self-esteem and behavioral problems in the long term. Children in Sri Lanka and Romania with parents living abroad were also more likely to experience anxiety and depression as children without migrant parents (Siriwardhana et al., 2015; Tomşa & Jenaro, 2015). In their study of children who had been separated from their migrant parents prior to reunification in the United States, Suárez-Orozco, Todorova, and Louie (2002) found that separation and reunification corresponded to a higher incidence of anxiety and depression symptoms among children. An association between attachment and lower likelihood depression has been demonstrated in a number of empirical studies with evidence suggesting that secure attachment supports healthy development (Wu, Kao, Yen, & Lee, 2007). Decreased communication between left-behind children and their parents may account for some increase in depression risk (Wenbin, Wang, & Zhengkui, 2008).

A study found that the overall prevalence of emotional problems was 43.6 percent among left-behind children, and socioeconomic status was related to these problems among them (Zeng et al., 2009). Wang et al. (2015) found that in 4857 left-behind children and adolescents in Chongqing the total prevalence rate of depressive symptoms was 24.8 percent, which is much higher than the national average of Chinese children. The risk factors for depression were absence of parents, low frequency of parent–child communication, and communication by letter or about sensitive topics. The age group 16 to 17 years was at a higher risk of depression than other subgroups (Wang et al., 2015). This finding is consistent with previous studies in which the mean total CDI scores of left-behind children were higher than controls (Liu et al., 2009). Good social support in early adolescence can decrease mental problems (Rueger, Malecki, & Demaray, 2010). Children from lower socioeconomic background and who have less social support have to cope with more difficulties and psychosocial stressors when left behind. This will increase the risk for emotional and behavioral disturbances.

Special Issues: Injuries and Suicide, Juvenile Delinquency and Substance Abuse

A number of tragedies involving the neglect or assault of left-behind children in China have highlighted the fact that these children may be exposed to a range of developmental risks. A study focused on the left-behind adolescents revealed a higher level of Internet addiction, suicide ideation, and thoughts of running away from home along with other social behavioral issues such as smoking and binge drinking (Gao et al., 2010). When left behind at a young age, the surrogate caretakers often don't have the energy and resources to take good care of these children. A study in rural China found that the annual injury rate per 1000 among left-behind children was more than twice that of children living with both parents. Male left-behind children had the highest annual injury rate: 316.4 per 1000. The top three external causes of injury were similar for both groups of children: falls (33.8 percent), mechanical injuries (16.2 percent), and animal bites (14.5 percent). The left-behind group is more prone to accidents, which indicates that the left-behind children, especially the younger ones, receive a lower level of care and supervision (Shen et al., 2009).

Another crucial period of development that can be affected by migrating parents is the transition from primary to secondary school (Smith et al., 2004). During this period, there are increased demands and pressures faced by children who have to take over parental responsibilities. This often results in deterioration of academic performance. The trend in declining accomplishment in school is mainly associated with girls, since they are more likely to take over household tasks than their male siblings following the mother's migration. A heavier household workload and stresses from school can lead adolescents to resort to substance abuse as a coping mechanism. Various UNICEF country studies indicate that children left behind are more vulnerable to drug abuse, teenage pregnancy, psychosocial problems, and violent behavior (Cortes, 2008).

The psychological distress these adolescents experience often leads to the adoption of risky behavior. In Jamaica, a survey found that the absence of mothers was a key determinant of children's involvement with violence (Pottinger, 2005). This situation has raised concerns that the risk of juvenile crime is increased for left-behind children, particularly where they are in low-income families (Duan & Zhou, 2005). A cross-sectional study was conducted among adolescents in Fuyang, Guangdong, which found that "left-behind" boys were at higher risk of Internet addiction, tobacco smoking, and suicide ideation. Girls were more likely to smoke, binge drink, and even to consider leaving home (Gao et al., 2010). In addition, migration, especially of mothers, significantly increases risks for children to be physically and sexually abused or exploited. However comparison of children of migrants to children of non-migrants in the Philippines revealed no systemic differences in the psychological problems, reports of abuse, or experiences of delinquency (Bryant, 2005). By contrast, UNICEF found that the increase in juvenile crime rates in Moldova between 1993 and 2000 was positively correlated with the number of children left behind, who accounted for almost 60 percent of juvenile offenders during that period. More recently, a 2012 UNICEF study found that of all the juvenile offenders in Moldova in 2010, nearly 90 percent were unemployed and not attending school, and 20 percent had one or both parents living abroad. Adolescents left behind assume adult behavior in conjunction with adult responsibilities, and, as is evident in Moldova, are more likely than non-migrant children to partake in illegal and criminal activity (Fund UNCs, 2008).

IMPLICATIONS FOR FUTURE POLICY IMPROVEMENT AND RESEARCH DIRECTIONS

Socioeconomic development is inevitable, and unexpected problems often emerge as a result. Increased population and workforce mobility means that many children are left behind and not cared for in intact families involving both parents. At the root of this phenomenon is the inequality and imbalance of global development. This is too big a problem to be resolved quickly. As a result, the trend of population migration is expected to continue. In light of this global trend, we need to have a clear picture of the current status of left-behind children from international and internal migration. We also need future research to provide an evidence-based component to assessment of risks in order to resolve the problem.

In order to address the negative consequences of parents' migration on children left behind, measures should be taken to support the rights of development of all children. Current social protection policies frequently do not emphasize the specific needs of children left behind. This is partly due to the underestimation of the problem and partly because those countries most affected by migration often lack sufficient resources to implement policies that address the unique needs of these children.

It must be emphasized that more academic research and policy analysis is needed to fully understand how parents' migration affects children left behind. Current literature review indicates that although a number of negative consequences have been identified in past studies, we still do not know how many children actually experience them and how severely they are affected. Sound and up-to-date data regarding the demographics of the children of migrants as well as of their caregivers are needed, and the amount and type of remuneration caregivers receive are also pertinent to children's wellbeing. Efforts to generate such data should include multinational and state-specific representative surveys as well as coordinated rigorous qualitative analyses. International collaboration is vital to generate a global picture of left-behind children. In order to enhance children's rights in the context of the inevitable trend of migration and to formulate evidence-based policies, national level data across countries should be comparable in terms of definitions and methodologies. Data collection efforts should be sensitive to gender and age differences in order to take into account the potential modifying factors of the phenomenon.

As of 2016, most qualitative literature on this problem used cross-sectional data, and remained problem-focused, without enough exploration of factors related to the wellbeing and mental health status of left-behind children. More longitudinal studies are needed to address the long-term outcomes of these children, including their employment, social relationships, and achievement. Further research, which identifies resilience factors in left-behind children, will therefore be useful. Research is needed to examine the psychology and mental health of the new generations of children and adolescents who grow up to migrate and seek opportunities outside their region of origin.

Policy must be strengthened in order to secure children's basic social and economic rights. It is especially important that legislation to regulate child labor be introduced and increased. In many rural areas with a shortage of labor, parents' migration often forces children to drop out of school and work to help support their family. In addition, policies should be reinforced to better monitor and manage various forms of child abuse. This is particularly important for young girls, as they are vulnerable to sexual abuse. Remittances are not substitutes for government policies and institutional frameworks that need to address exclusion, inequalities, and the provision of social services. Poverty reduction strategies (including redistributive policies) need to address the issues of migration and development. Policy makers will need to develop coherent policies at national, regional, and local levels to address the ever-growing problem of international migrant children as well as children left behind. Policies can be made to mitigate the psychosocial impacts of migration on children by providing programs to caregivers on parenting skills, gender sensitivity, and management of peer relationships. These programs must be sensitive to migrant communities' own cultural values and mores, especially regarding gender roles, youth participation, and the mitigation of risky behaviors. Education officials should develop training programs that prepare staff to recognize traits associated with the psychosocial effects of parental migration.

Many studies in China found that school environment and national policy were significantly correlated with psychological and behavioral outcomes of left-behind children. These findings call our attention to the inequity in public education resource allocation between urban and rural areas, as well as the inequality in educational benefits that are tied to individual registered residency. In 2001, China's average financial education support from government was 4015 yuan for every student in urban areas, but only 900 yuan for those in rural areas. Government must make every effort to narrow the gap. In 2011, the Chinese central government announced its 12th Five-Year Plan, which stated its goal of granting more qualified migrant workers and their family members' urban residency during 2011 to 2015. The Plan also articulated the goal of ensuring migrant children receive equal access to compulsory education, with the support of local full-time public schools. Governments will also provide housing subsidy, healthcare, and other benefits to migrant workers who have a stable job in urban enterprises (National Health and Family Committee of PRC). These policies are expected to facilitate the interaction between local and migrant children, and help migrant children engage in the urban environment. More welfare benefits for migrant workers may also improve their family socioeconomic status and family relationship, both of which are protective factors for children's healthy development.

The phenomenon of left-behind children is global, and calls for international cooperation to resolve. Countries from which migrant workers originate should engage in dialogue with receiving countries to ensure bilateral agreements that allow migrant workers to take their children, in order to avoid the abandonment of children by parents working abroad (especially mothers). National governments should focus on designing and implementing co-development strategies between countries within a particular migration corridor. Policies and legal frameworks should focus primarily on reducing social, economic, educational, and health inequalities between countries. This should be the basis for incorporating migration, aiming at maximizing migration's developmental potentials, while reducing its negative consequences.

References

Aguilera-Guzman, R. M., de Snyder, V. N. S., Romero, M., & Medina-Mora, M. E. (2004). Paternal absence and international migration: stressors and compensators associated with the mental health of Mexican teenagers of rural origin. *Adolescence, 39*(156), 711–723.

Amuedo-Dorantes, C., & Pozo, S. (2010). Accounting for remittance and migration effects on children's schooling. *World Development, 38*(12), 1747–1759.

Anh, D. N. (1999). Market reforms and internal labor migration in Vietnam. *Asian and Pacific Migration Journal, 8*(3), 381–409.

Antman, F. (2012). Gender, educational attainment, and the impact of parental migration on children left behind. *Journal of Population Economics, 25*(4), 1187–1214.

Bowlby, J. (1982). Attachment and loss: retrospect and prospect. *American Journal of Orthopsychiatry, 52*(4), 664–678.

Breslau, J., Borges, G., Saito, N., Tancredi, D. J., Benjet, C., Hinton, L., … Aguilar-Gaxiola, S. (2011). Migration from Mexico to the US and conduct disorder: a cross-national study. *Archives of General Psychiatry, 68*(12), 1284–1293.

Brown, P. H., & Park, A. (2002). Education and poverty in rural China. *Economics of Education Review, 21*(6), 523–541.

Bryant, J. (2005). Children of international migrants in Indonesia, Thailand, and the Philippines: a review of evidence and policies. In *Innocenti working paper* (Vol. 5)UNICEF.

Castañeda, E., & Buck, L. (2011). Remittances, transnational parenting, and the children left behind: economic and psychological implications. *The Latin Americanist, 55*(4), 85–110.

Chase-Lansdale, P. L., Cherlin, A. J., & Kiernan, K. E. (1995). The long-term effects of parental divorce on the mental health of young adults: a developmental perspective. *Child Development, 66*(6), 1614–1634.

Chen, S., Adams, J., Qu, Z., Wang, X., & Chen, L. (2013). Parental migration and children's academic engagement: the case of China. *International Review of Education, 59*(6), 693–722.

Chen, J. (2011). Internal migration and health: re-examining the healthy migrant phenomenon in China. *Social Science & Medicine, 72*(8), 1294–1301.

Cortés, R. (2007). Children and women left behind in labor sending countries: an appraisal of social risk, global report on migration and children. In *UNICEF*. UNICEF.

Cortes, R. (2008). Children and women left behind in labour sending countries: an appraisal of social risks. In *UNICEF*. UNICEF.

Duan, C. R., & Zhou, F. L. (2005). Studies on "left behind" children in rural China. *Population Research, 29*(1), 29–36.

Edwards, A. C., & Ureta, M. (2003). International migration, remittances, and schooling: evidence from El Salvador. *Journal of Development Economics, 72*(2), 429–461.

Ehrenreich, B., & Hochschild, A. R. (2004). The care crisis in the Philippines: children and translational families in the new global economy. In *Global woman: Nannies, maids, and sex workers in the new economy* (pp. 39–54). New York: Holt Paperbacks.

Fan, F., Su, L., Gill, M., & Birmaher, B. (2010). Emotional and behavioral problems of Chinese left-behind children: a preliminary study. *Social Psychiatry and Psychiatric Epidemiology, 45*(6), 655–664.

Fund UNCs. (2008). The impacts of migration on children in Moldova. In M. A. Salah (Ed.), *United Nations children's fund*.

Fund UNP. (2006). *State of world population 2006, a passage to hope: Women and international migration*. United Nations Population Fund.

Gao, Y., Li, L. P., Kim, J. H., Congdon, N., Lau, J., & Griffiths, S. (2010). The impact of parental migration on health status and health behaviours among left behind adolescent school children in China. *BMC Public Health, 10*(1), 56.

Graham, E., & Jordan, L. P. (2011). Migrant parents and the psychological well-being of left-behind children in Southeast Asia. *Journal of Marriage and Family, 73*(4), 763–787.

Hardt, J., Herke, M., & Schier, K. (2011). Suicidal ideation, parent–child relationships, and adverse childhood experiences: a cross-validation study using a Graphical Markov Model. *Child Psychiatry and Human Development, 42*(2), 119–133.

Hondagneu-Sotelo, P., & Avila, E. (1997). "I'm here, but I'm there": the meanings of Latina transnational motherhood. *Gender and Society, 11*(5), 548–571.

Huang, Y., Zhong, X.-N., Li, Q.-Y., Xu, D., Zhang, X.-L., Feng, C., … Deng, B. (2015). Health-related quality of life of the rural-China left-behind children or adolescents and influential factors: a cross-sectional study. *Health and Quality of Life Outcomes, 13*(1), 29.

Isaksen, L. W., Devi, S. U., & Hochschild, A. R. (2008). Global care crisis: a problem of capital, care chain, or commons? *American Behavioral Scientist, 52*(3), 405–425.

II. RISK AND RESILIENCE

Jia, Z., & Tian, W. (2010). Loneliness of left-behind children: a cross-sectional survey in a sample of rural China. *Child: Care, Health and Development, 36*(6), 812–817.

Jia, Z., Shi, L., Cao, Y., Delancey, J., & Tian, W. (2010). Health-related quality of life of "left-behind children": a cross-sectional survey in rural China. *Quality of Life Research: An International Journal of Quality of Life Aspects of Treatment, Care and Rehabilitation, 19*(6), 775–780.

Lashley, M. (2000). The unrecognized social stressors of migration and reunification in Caribbean families. *Transcultural Psychiatry, 37*(2), 203–217.

Leinaweaver, J. B. (2010). Outsourcing care: how Peruvian migrants meet transnational family obligations. *Latin American Perspectives, 37*(5), 67–87.

Liang, Z., & Chen, Y. P. (2007). The educational consequences of migration for children in China. *Social Science Research, 36*(1), 28–47.

Liu, Y., & Zou, W. (2011). Rural-urban migration and dynamics of income distribution in China. *China & World Economy, 19*(6), 37–55.

Liu, Z., Li, X., & Ge, X. (2009). Left too early: the effects of age at separation from parents on Chinese rural children's symptoms of anxiety and depression. *American Journal of Public Health, 99*(11), 2049–2054.

Liu, Z., Zhang, Y. B., Song, A. Q., & Shi, J. Q. (2013). Meta analysis of mental health in left behind children. *Chinese Journal of Child Health Care, 21*(1), 68–70.

Luo, J., Peng, X., Zong, R., Yao, K., Hu, R., Du, Q., ... Zhu, M. (2008). The status of care and nutrition of 774 left-behind children in rural areas in China. *Public Health Reports, 123*(3), 382–389.

Mansuri, G. (2006). Migration, School attainment and child labor: evidence from rural Pakistan. In *World Bank policy research working paper.* World Bank.

McKenzie, D., & Rapoport, H. (2011). Can migration reduce educational attainment? Evidence from Mexico. *Journal of Population Economics, 24*(4), 1331–1358.

Meyerhoefer, C., & Chen, C. J. (2011). The effect of parental labor migration on children's educational progress in rural China. *Review of Economics of the Household, 9*(3), 379–396.

Migration IOM. (2005). In F. Laczko (Ed.), *Internal migration and development: A global perspective.* International Organization for Migration.

Mitrani, V. B., Santisteban, D. A., & Muir, J. A. (2004). Addressing immigration-related separations in hispanic families with a behavior-problem adolescent. *American Journal of Orthopsychiatry, 74*(3), 219–229.

2010 National Census Data. (April 23, 2013). National Bureau of Statistics of China.

National Health and Family Committee of the People's Republic of China, http://www.nhfpc.gov.cn/jkj/s5888/200805/81047a30f3c34141b12481de35930d78.shtml.

National survey of left-behind children in rural areas and migrant children in urban and rural areas, http://acwf.people.com.cn/n/2013/0510/c99013-21437965.html.

Nobles, J. (2011). Parenting from abroad: migration, nonresident father involvement, and children's education in Mexico. *Journal of Marriage and Family, 73*(4), 729–746.

Peterson, J. T. (1993). Generalized extended family exchange: a case from the Philippines. *Journal of Marriage and Family, 55*(3), 570–584.

Pottinger, A. M. (2005). Children's experience of loss by parental migration in inner-city Jamaica. *American Journal of Orthopsychiatry, 75*(4), 485–496.

Renouf, A. G., Kovacs, M., & Mukerji, P. (1997). Relationship of depressive, conduct, and Comorbid disorders and social functioning in childhood. *Journal of the American Academy of Child and Adolescent Psychiatry, 36*(7), 998–1004.

Rueger, S., Malecki, C., & Demaray, M. (2010). Relationship between multiple sources of perceived social support and psychological and academic adjustment in early adolescence: comparisons across gender. *Journal of Youth and Adolescence, 39*(1), 47–61.

Schmalzbauer, L. (2004). Searching for wages and mothering from Afar: the case of Honduran transnational families. *Journal of Marriage and Family, 66*(5), 1317–1331.

Senaratne, B., Perera, H., & Fonseka, P. (2011). Mental health status and risk factors for mental health problems in left-behind children of women migrant workers in Sri Lanka. *Ceylon Medical Journal, 56*, 153–158.

Shen, M., Yang, S., Han, J., Shi, J., Yang, R., Du, Y., ... Stallones, L. (2009). Non-fatal injury rates among the "left-behind children" of rural China. *Injury Prevention, 15*(4), 244–247.

Siriwardhana, C., Wickramage, K., Siribaddana, S., Vidanapathirana, P., Jayasekara, B., Weerawarna, S., ... Pieris, S. (2015). Common mental disorders among adult members of 'left-behind' international migrant worker families in Sri Lanka. *BMC Public Health, 15*, 299.

Smith, A., Lalonde, R. N., & Johnson, S. (2004). Serial migration and its implications for the parent-child relationship: a retrospective analysis of the experiences of the children of Caribbean immigrants. *Cultural Diversity & Ethnic Minority Psychology, 10*(2), 107–122.

Sørensen, N. N. (2012). Revisiting the migration–development Nexus: from social networks and remittances to markets for migration control. *International Migration, 50*(3), 61–76.

Spera, C. (2005). A review of the relationship among parenting practices, parenting styles, and adolescent school achievement. *Educational Psychology Review, 17*(2), 125–146.

Stirbu, M. (2006). Migration and impact on child welfare in Moldova: assessment of welfare policies against the rights of the child. In *Unicef social inclusion, policy and budgeting.* UNICEF.

Su, S., Li, X., Lin, D., Xu, X., & Zhu, M. (2013). Psychological adjustment among left-behind children in rural China: the role of parental migration and parent–child communication. *Child: Care, Health and Development, 39*(2), 162–170.

Suârez-Orozco, C., Todorova, I. L. G., & Louie, J. (2002). Making up for lost time: the experience of separation and reunification among immigrant families. *Family Process, 41*(4), 625–643.

Tao, X. W., Guan, H. Y., Zhao, Y. R., & Fan, Z. Y. (2014). Mental health among left-behind preschool-aged children: preliminary survey of its status and associated risk factors in rural China. *The Journal of International Medical Research, 42*(1), 120–129.

Tomşa, R., & Jenaro, C. (2015). Children left behind in Romania: anxiety and predictor variables. *Psychological Reports, 116*(2), 485–512.

United Nations DoEaSA. (2013). *Population division: international migration report.*

United Nations PDotDoEaSA. (2015). *Integrating population issues into sustainable development, including the post-2015 development agenda* A Concise Report.

Wang, L., Feng, Z., Yang, G., Yang, Y., Dai, Q., Hu, C., ... Xia, F. (2015). The epidemiological characteristics of depressive symptoms in the left-behind children and adolescents of Chongqing in China. *Journal of Affective Disorders, 177*, 36–41.

Wenbin, G., Wang, T., & Zhengkui, L. (2008). A study on depression characteristics and its influencing factors in children left in rural areas. *Chinese Journal of Behavioral Medical Science, 16*(3), 238–240.

Wickramage, K., Siriwardhana, C., Vidanapathirana, P., Weerawarna, S., Jayasekara, B., Pannala, G., ... Siribaddana, S. (2015). Risk of mental health and nutritional problems for left-behind children of international labor migrants. *BMC Psychiatry, 15*, 39.

Wilcox, H. C., & Anthony, J. C. (2004). Child and adolescent clinical features as forerunners of adult-onset major depressive disorder: retrospective evidence from an epidemiological sample. *Journal of Affective Disorders, 82*(1), 9–20.

Wu, W.-C., Kao, C.-H., Yen, L.-L., & Lee, T. S.-H. (2007). Comparison of children's self-reports of depressive symptoms among different family interaction types in northern Taiwan. *BMC Public Health, 7*, 116.

Wu, Q., Lu, D., & Kang, M. (2014). Social capital and the mental health of children in rural China with different experiences of parental migration. *Social Science & Medicine, 132*(C), 270–277.

Zeng, R., Zhang, L. L., Luo, J. Y., Gong, W. J., Du, Q. Y., & Wu, H. (2009). Study on emotional behavioral problems and related determinants among stranded children aged 4 to 7 years in the rural areas of China. *Chinese Journal of Epidemiology, 30*(7), 706–709.

Zhao, X., Chen, J., Chen, M. C., Lv, X. L., Jiang, Y. H., & Sun, Y. H. (2014). Left-behind children in rural China experience higher levels of anxiety and poorer living conditions. *Acta Paediatrica, 103*(6), 665–670.

PART III

INTERVENTIONS AND TREATMENTS

8

Mental Health Literacy for Students and Teachers: A "School Friendly" Approach

S. Kutcher, Y. Wei, M. Hashish

Dalhousie University and IWK Health Centre, Halifax, NS, Canada

HEALTH LITERACY AND MENTAL HEALTH LITERACY: AN INTRODUCTION

Mental health literacy (MHL) is the foundation for mental health promotion, effective acknowledgment of prevention of mental disorders, and provision of evidence-based mental health care (Jorm, 2012; Jorm, Korten, Jacomb et al., 1997; Kutcher, Bagnell, & Wei, 2015; Kutcher , Wei, & Coniglio, 2016; Kutcher, Wei, & Weist, 2015; Reavley & Jorm, 2011; McLuckie, Kutcher, Wei, & Weaver, 2014). Anchored in the larger concept of health literacy (HL), which has undergone substantial evolution over time (Nutbeam, 2008; World Health Organization (WHO), 2013), understanding of the nature and impact of MHL has similarly changed from its initial consideration as information about mental disorders to a more comprehensive construct considering MHL as an empowerment competency for people to participate in their own health care (Jorm et al., 1997; Kutcher et al., 2016). Most recently, mental health literacy has been defined to comprise four distinct but related components: understanding how to obtain and maintain good mental health, understanding mental disorders and their treatments, decreasing stigma, and enhancing help-seeking efficacy (knowing when and where to obtain evidence-based mental health care and having competencies to enhance self-care) (Kutcher et al., 2015, 2016).

Historically, HL was initially conceptualized as narrowly constructed within the health care delivery environment and focused primarily on the ability of people to be able to understand and apply medical information

Positive Mental Health, Fighting Stigma and Promoting Resiliency for Children and Adolescents
http://dx.doi.org/10.1016/B978-0-12-804394-3.00008-5

given to them by their health care providers, particularly with regards to improving adherence to treatment (American Medical Association Ad Hoc Committee on Health Literacy, 1992). Soon thereafter, however, this construct was expanded to include key components of health promotion and individual capacity for improvement of health-related behaviors: "the cognitive and social skills which determine the motivation and ability of individuals to gain access to, understand and use information in ways which promote and maintain good health" (Nutbeam, 1998).

More recently, understanding of HL has further evolved, now encompassing not only the individual's capacity to seek health improving and health maintaining interventions but also to include the ability for self-care and for participating in the development of health policy and related activities designed to enhance health outcomes (Kanj & Mitic, 2009; Institute of Medicine, 2012; Schillinger et al., 2003; WHO, 2013). This broader construct is now understood to be a key factor in improving both individual and population health outcomes and has been identified as an important intervention to be applied for the decrease of health inequalities in populations (Berkman et al., 2011; Kickbusch, 2001; WHO, 2013). Indeed, according to WHO (2013), HL is "a stronger predictor of an individual's health status than income, employment status, education and racial or ethnic group."

With the increasing application of patient-centered health care interventions (such as the Wagner Chronic Care Model), HL has become an essential competency for health care recipients (Coleman et al., 2009; Schillinger et al., 2005). Educational interventions designed to enhance HL are understood to be an important component of health care capacity-building (Nutbeam, 2008; IoM, 2012; WHO, 2013).

Currently, the construct of HL can be considered to comprise the following components: competencies required to help a person obtain and maintain good health and identify illnesses, understanding of how and where to access and evaluate health information and health care, understanding how to properly apply prescribed treatments, and understanding health-related human rights and how to advocate for health improvements (WHO, 2013). To achieve this, HL needs to be: developmentally appropriate, contextually applied, and widely available through existing institutional and social vehicles such as schools, the workplace, and media (Kanj & Mitic, 2009; Nutbeam, 2008; WHO, 2013).

A similar evolution in understanding of MHL is also underway. The initial important work of Jorm et al. (1997) on an individual's ability to recognize, manage, or prevent mental disorders, and early evaluations of educational interventions designed to address this focused primarily on one or two mental disorders (such as depression). This early construct was later broadened by Jorm and colleagues (Jorm, 2012; Reavley & Jorm, 2011) to additionally include: recognition of the development of mental disorders, knowledge of effective self-help strategies, and first-aid skills to assist others who have a mental disorder.

As the HL definition has evolved, so have others contributed to the evolving construct of MHL (Kutcher, Bagnell, et al., 2015; Kutcher et al., 2016). In step with the current conceptualization of HL, MHL is currently conceptualized to address the four constructs presented in the previous. section. This approach has integrated historically separate stigma interventions into the broader and more comprehensive construct of MHL. Such integration is supported both by the recognition that knowledge and stigma are not unique and separate constructs, but are related to each other and that knowledge enhancement does impact stigma reduction related to mental health and mental illness (eg, Chan, Mak, & Law, 2009; Corrigan, Morris, Michaels, Rafacz, & Rüsch, 2012; Pinfold et al., 2003; Thornicroft, 2006). This evolving understanding also parallels the WHO integration of human rights constructs into HL and other health care frameworks that have integrated health knowledge with stigma reduction strategies in other health conditions, such as HIV/AIDS and epilepsy (Birbeck, 2006; Brown, Macintyre & Trujillo, 2003; Heijnders & Van Der Meij, 2006; Sermrittirong, Van Brakel, & Bunbers-Aelen, 2014).

Global interest in school mental health is now becoming more evident (Kutcher, Wei, et al., 2015; Rowling & Weist, 2004). Foundational to all different school mental health approaches is the integration of MHL into the existing school curriculum structure because the school setting is contextually established to deliver interventions using a literacy approach (Jorm & Wright, 2007; Kutcher, Bagnell, et al., 2015). Furthermore, using educational strategies, including school curriculum and various knowledge-based interventions delivered in school settings may be more effective in addressing stigma in young people than other types of interventions (Corrigan et al., 2012; Kutcher et al., 2016; Pinfold et al., 2003). Finally, bringing mental health literacy into the school setting is not only consistent with a core activity of schools, but also fits well with the definition of literacy that is used by the United Nations Educational, Scientific and Cultural Organization (UNESCO, 2006), a construct also consistent with the WHO model for Health Promoting Schools (http://www.who.int/school_youth_health/gshi/hps/en/).

To date, a number of different types of interventions addressing some or all parts of the components of MHL have been reported in the school setting. Broadly speaking, these fall into one of two different strategies. First are strategies that introduce interventions to the school using external resources. For example, Skre et al.'s clinician-led intervention in a Norwegian sample (2013); Pino-Foltz et al.'s application of the In Our Own Voice intervention in two schools in the USA (2011); Stuart's evaluation of the Reaching Out program in a Canadian setting (2006); and Jorm's application of the very expensive corporate supplied Mental Health First

Aid program targeting teachers (eg, Kitchener & Jorm, 2002). Many more examples can be found in a recent systematic review on the effectiveness of school mental health literacy interventions (Wei et al., 2013). Taken as a group, these interventions are added to existing school activities, are usually not delivered by existing internal school resources, are episodic rather than continuous, require fidelity of delivery as a requirement of the intervention, do not usually strengthen existing school resources or communities, often focus primarily on one target group (such as students only), and are not likely to be sustainable, particularly in times of fiscal constraint, due to their costs and add-on nature.

Second, in contrast, are interventions that are substantially different from the above-described externally applied interventions. These are "School Friendly" interventions, designed to be delivered by existing school resources (primarily teachers) within existing school activities (primarily everyday classroom instruction) and have the following characteristics:

1. are designed to be a resource that can be easily integrated into existing school curriculum
2. are designed to be developmentally appropriate and educationally innovative
3. are designed to be learned by and then taught by usual classroom teachers within their usual classroom instruction periods
4. are designed to be pedagogically familiar in content and process
5. are designed to enhance and strengthen existing school systems
6. are designed to be able to fit into existing school mandated curriculum (such as health and physical education or life-skills management), and therefore become embedded and continuous rather than external and episodic interventions
7. are designed to build on the professional ability of teachers to teach, rather than requiring fidelity of implementation
8. are designed to improve MHL outcomes for both teachers and students simultaneously
9. are designed to be cost-effective and sustainable
10. have demonstrated significant and robust impacts on both teacher and student mental health literacy in two or more independent investigations conducted in different settings

As of 2016, these have been applied within a curriculum-based framework, where teachers can learn to apply a mental health literacy resource within the existing school curriculum that is consistent with established pedagogic procedures and existing school structures. For example, Perry et al. in their 2014 study of the *Headstrong* resource in Australia and McLuckie et al. (2014) in their study of the *Guide* resource in Canada illustrate this School Friendly approach.

CANADIAN APPROACHES TO SCHOOL FRIENDLY MENTAL HEALTH LITERACY

In Canada, there has been increasing recognition of the importance of school mental health. For example, a study by the School Based Mental Health and Substance Abuse Consortium, funded by the Mental Health Commission of Canada, recently reported on the substantial need to address the mental health of students in Canadian schools (Mental Health Commission of Canada, 2013). This work builds on earlier study by Santor, Short, and Ferguson (2009), which came to similar conclusions. Evergreen, the Canadian child and youth mental health framework, identified schools as a key site for the delivery of mental health-related interventions (Kutcher & McLuckie, 2010). The Canadian Teachers' Federation is a national organization supporting the importance of addressing child and youth mental health in the school setting, and recently, the faculty of education at the University of Western Ontario established a center for school-based mental health to encourage the development of research into various components of this topic (http://www.edu.uwo.ca/).

To respond to the national considerations referenced in the previous section, a collaboration between the Canadian Mental Health Association (the leading national mental health Non-Government Organization in Canada) and Dr. Stan Kutcher, the Sun Life Financial Chair in Adolescent Mental Health at Dalhousie University, resulted in the development, field testing, and subsequent delivery and evaluation of a "School Friendly" mental health literacy approach (Kutcher & Wei, 2013; Kutcher, Wei, McLuckie, & Bullock, 2013; McLuckie et al., 2014), Mental Health & High School Curriculum Guide (the Guide) (Kutcher & Canadian Mental Health Association, 2009). The Guide consists of six web-based modules addressing knowledge, attitudes, and help-seeking efficacy. This includes: stigma of mental illness, understanding mental health and mental illness, information about specific mental illness, experiences of mental illness, seeking help and finding support, and the importance of positive mental health. Further information about this freely available resource can be found at www.teenmentalhealth.org.

This intervention takes the form of a classroom-ready resource (the Guide) designed to be delivered by usual classroom teachers to students in Canadian schools enrolled in grades 9 or 10 (ages 13 to 15 years). These grade levels were chosen because at this point most young people would still be attending school, they would all tend to be exposed to the same standard curriculum (few, if any, individualized curriculum options), and this period in the life span is the point of departure for the rapid increase in psychiatric diagnoses that occurs prior to age 25 years (Costello, Mustillo, Erkanli, Keeler, & Angold, 2004; Kessler et al., 2005), making the development of mental health literacy at this point an important foundational component for potentially improving mental health outcomes. The Guide was certified by the Curriculum Services Canada, a national curriculum standards and evaluation agency and was initially field-tested in various provinces across the country (www.curriculum.org). On the basis of that evaluation, curriculum materials were revised, input from students and parents was sought, a new section designed for teacher self-study, a teachers' self-evaluation test was added, and a teacher training program on how to apply the Guide in the classroom was developed by Kutcher and members of his team. Recently the Guide has been updated by Kutcher and Wei in response to teacher suggestions for improvement and to ensure compatibility with new diagnostic nomenclature. Further development of a train-the-trainer model that can be embedded in schools and school boards maintains the sustainability of the intervention. As a result, teachers and trainers received the Guide in concert with web-based access to all the components of the Guide intervention (teacher self-study, teacher self-evaluation, student evaluation resource, six classroom-ready modules consisting of prepared lesson plans, and in-class teaching resources such as powerpoint slides, animated videos, and print-ready materials).

The initial application of this approach was conducted and evaluated in the Province of Nova Scotia where it was subsequently embedded in the 2012 Provincial education policy framework—Kids and Learning First (Nova Scotia Department of Education and Early Childhood Development, 2012; Wei et al., 2015). Two cross-sectional studies assessing the impact of this intervention specifically on teachers were conducted with educators from the Halifax Regional School Board and from the larger Province of Nova Scotia (Kutcher et al., 2013; Wei, Kutcher, Heather, & Mackay, 2014). Additionally, two cross-sectional cohort studies assessing the impact of this intervention on students were conducted in a number of school boards in the province of Ontario including the largest school board in Canada, the Toronto District School Board (Kutcher et al., 2016; McLuckie et al., 2014), as well as a randomized-controlled trial in the Ottawa District School Board in Canada (Milin, Kutcher, Lewis, Walker, & Ferrill, 2013).

In all of the research and evaluations of the Guide, classroom teachers who were identified as having the responsibility for applying the Guide in their classrooms were provided with a one-day training program designed to be able to fit into existing teacher professional development day sessions. Evaluation of the impact of this simple intervention demonstrated significant and substantial improvements in teachers' knowledge (Cohen's effect size: $d = 1.48$–2.03) and substantial decreases in teachers stigma as a result of the intervention (Cohen's effect size: $d = 0.21$–1.26) (see Table 8.1) (Wei et al., 2014; Kutcher et al., 2016).

With regards to the impact of this intervention on students' mental health literacy, research conducted in the three different Canadian school districts at different times all demonstrated similar results. Teachers who

TABLE 8.1 Research Summary of the Guide Impact

Province	Study Type	Year	Participants	Increased Knowledge	Improved Attitudes		Improved Help-Seeking	
Nova Scotia	Program evaluation	2012–2013	218 educators	Yes	$p < 0.0001, d = 1.85$	Yes	$p < 0.0001, d = 0.51$	
Ontario	RCT	2011–2012	362 students	Yes	$p = 0.0001, d = 0.46$	Yes	$p = 0.0001, d = 0.30$	Yes	$p = 0.01; d = 0.18$
	Cross-sectional study	2012	409 students	Yes	$p < 0.001, d = 0.9;$ $p < 0.001^a, d = 0.73^a$	Yes	$p < 0.001, d = 0.25; p < 0.007^a, d = 0.18^a$	
	Program evaluation	2013	74 educators	Yes	$p < 0.001, d = 1.48$	Yes	$p < 0.03, d = 1.26$	
	Cross-sectional study	2013	175 students	Yes	$p < 0.0001, d = 1.11; p < 0.001^a, d = 0.91^a$	Yes	$p < 0.001, d = 0.66; p < 0.001^a, d = 0.52^a$	
Alberta	Program evaluation	2013	25 educators	Yes	$p < 0.0001, d = 2.03$	Yes	NS, $d = 0.21$	

[a] Results from three-month follow-up.

III. INTERVENTIONS AND TREATMENTS

taught the Guide had all received a one-day training session for the classroom use of the Guide resource as part of a professional development program provided by either the Ontario Shores Mental Health Center or the Royal Ottawa Hospital. In all cases, student outcomes demonstrated significant and substantial improvements in knowledge (Cohen's effect size: $d = 0.46–1.11$) and significant decreases in stigma as a result of the intervention (Cohen's effect size: $d = 0.18–0.66$) (Kutcher et al., 2016; McLuckie et al., 2014; Milin et al., 2013). These impacts were sustained over a three-month follow-up. The Ottawa study also investigated student self-reported help-seeking efficacy, which also showed significant impact with a more modest effect size (see Table 8.1).

Feedback from teachers using the Guide indicated that it was easy to apply in the classroom, that it did not entail the use of additional resources, and that the students thought that the topic was timely and important, found the material engaging, and enjoyed the various classroom and learning activities supported by the modules.

DISCUSSIONS AND CONCLUSIONS

This series of interventions all used the "School Friendly" approach to address MHL. The Guide resource was available at no cost, easily accessible via the web, and teacher friendly. Teachers were able to simply download the various modules and supporting materials and immediately apply them in their classrooms once they had received training on the use of the resource. A simple one-time training opportunity, compatible with existing professional development activities, provided them with the information they required for classroom application and concurrently demonstrated significant and substantial impact on improving their knowledge and decreasing their stigma. This approach used well-understood and historically comfortable pedagogic approaches, which enabled teachers to apply the resource in their own classroom using their own professional skills. This did not require fidelity of delivery (just as no other school curriculum resource—be it mathematics textbooks or geography curriculum—requires fidelity of delivery) and was able to be modified by teachers to fit each of their own teaching styles. Teaching of the resource embedded into usual classroom curriculum demonstrated the positive impact on students' knowledge, attitudes, and help-seeking efficacy. Additionally, this impact was sustained over time.

Finally, unlike the traditional costly, stand-alone school mental health programs that are added to existing school activities, "School Friendly" mental health literacy intervention is tied into a larger education and health system integrated model that promotes a horizontal and seamless pathway through mental health care for young people who may require

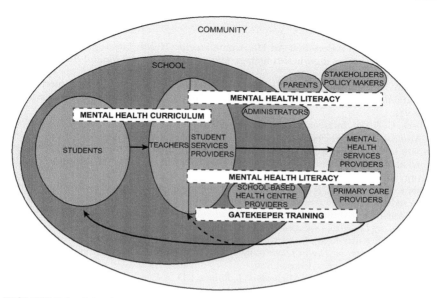

FIGURE 8.1 School-Based Integrated Pathway to Care Model. *From Wei, Y., Kutcher, S., & Szumilas, M. (2011). Comprehensive school mental health: an integrated "School-Based pathway to care" model for Canadian secondary schools. McGill Journal of Education, 46(2), 213–229. doi:10.7202/1006436ar. Copyright by McGill Journal of Education. Reprinted with permission.*

various types and levels of intervention (see Fig. 8.1). Mental health literacy, delivered by a single classroom intervention that enhances both teacher and student knowledge and decreases both teacher and student stigma, may be the first impactful stepping-stone along this pathway to better youth mental health (Wei, Kutcher, & Szumilas, 2011).

Thus, the "School Friendly" mental health literacy approach has the impact of not only effectively addressing the various components of mental health literacy, but it also has the role of enhancing the opportunity for young people to be able to access appropriate mental health care if they need it. In this way, the "School Friendly" mental health literacy approach provides an opportunity to bridge the long-standing gap between public health/population health interventions and clinical interventions, perhaps beginning a new care delivery framework, applicable wherever schools and health providers co-exist in the same community. Additional work by the authors on other components of this framework such as the "Go To Educators" program (Wei & Kutcher, 2014) and child and youth mental health care competency building in primary health care (Garcia-Ortega et al., 2003, 2013) suggests that such an integrated approach, beginning with "School Friendly" mental health literacy may be adapted, modified, and considered for global application (Kutcher, Wei, et al., 2015).

References

American Medical Association Ad Hoc Committee on Health Literacy. (1992). Report of the scientific council on health literacy. *Journal of the American Medical Association, 281,* 552–557.

Berkman, N. D., Sheridan, S. L., Donahue, K. E., et al. (2011). Health literacy interventions and outcomes: an updated systematic review. *Evidence Report/Technology Assessment, 199,* 1–941.

Birbeck, G. (2006). Interventions to reduce epilepsy associated stigma. *Psychology, Health & Medicine, 11*(3), 364–366. http://dx.doi.org/10.1080/13548500600595343.

Brown, L., Macintyre, K., & Trujillo, L. (2003). Interventions to reduce HIV/AIDS stigma: what have we learned? *AIDS Education and Prevention, 15*(1), 49–69. http://dx.doi.org/10.1521/aeap.15.1.49.23844.

Chan, J. Y., Mak, W. W., & Law, L. S. (2009). Combining education and video-based contact to reduce stigma of mental illness: "The Same or Not the Same" anti-stigma program for secondary schools in Hong Kong. *Social Science & Medicine, 68*(8), 1521–1526. http://dx.doi.org/10.1016/j.socscimed.2009.02.016.

Coleman, C., Kurtz-Rossi, S., McKinney, J., Pleasant, A., Rootman, I., & Shohet, L. (2009). *Calgary Charter on Health Literacy.* Retrieved from http://www.centreforliteracy.qc.ca/Healthlitinst/Calgary_Charter.htm.

Corrigan, P. W., Morris, S. B., Michaels, P. J., Rafacz, J. D., & Rüsch, N. (2012). Challenging the public stigma of mental illness: a meta-analysis of outcome studies. *Psychiatric Services, 63*(10), 963–973. http://dx.doi.org/10.1176/appi.ps.201100529.

Costello, E. J., Mustillo, E., Erkanli, A., Keeler, G., & Angold, A. (2004). Prevalence and development of psychiatric disorders in childhood and adolescence. *Archives of General Psychiatry, 60*(8), 837–844. http://dx.doi.org/10.1001/archpsyc.60.8.837.

Garcia-Ortega, I., Kadlec, H., Kutcher, S., Hollander, M., Kallstorm, L., & Mazowita, G. (2003). Program evaluation of a child and youth mental health training program for family physicians in British Columbia. *Journal of Canadian Child Adolescent Psychiatry, 22*(4), 296–302.

Garcia-Ortega, I., Rodrigues, J., Escobar-Martinez, A., & Kutcher, S. (2013). Implementing an educational program to enhance identification, diagnosis and treatment of adolescent depression into primary care in Guatemala. *Family Medicine & Medical Science Research, 2*(1). http://dx.doi.org/10.4172/2327-4972.1000104.

Heijnders, M., & Van Der Meij, S. (2006). The fight against stigma: an overview of stigma-reduction strategies and interventions. *Psychology, Health & Medicine, 11*(3), 353–363. http://dx.doi.org/10.1080/13548500600595327.

Institute of Medicine. (2012). *Facilitating state health exchange communication through the use of health literate practices.* Washington, DC: The National Academies Press.

Jorm, A. (2012). Mental health literacy: empowering the community to take action for better mental health. *The American Psychologist, 67*(3), 231–243. http://dx.doi.org/10.1037/a0025957.

Jorm, A. F., Korten, A. E., Jacomb, P. A., Christensen, H., Rodgers, B., & Pollitt, P. (1997). "Mental health literacy": a survey of the public's ability to recognise mental disorders and their beliefs about the effectiveness of treatment. *The Medical Journal of Australia, 166*(4), 182–186.

Jorm, A. F., & Wright, A. (2007). Beliefs of young people and their parents about the effectiveness of interventions for mental disorders. *The Australian and New Zealand Journal of Psychiatry, 41*(8), 656–666. http://dx.doi.org/10.1080/00048670701449179.

Kanj, M., & Mitic, W. (2009). *Promoting health and development: Closing the implementation gap.* World Health Organization. Available at: http://www.who.int/healthpromotion/conferences/7gchp/Track1_Inner.pdf. Accessed July 16, 2014.

Kessler, R. C., Berglund, P., Demler, O., Jin, R., Merikangas, K. R., & Walter, E. E. (2005). Lifetime prevalence and age-of-onset distributions of DSM-IV disorders in the national comorbidity survey replication. *Archives of General Psychiatry, 62*(6), 593–602. http://dx.doi.org/10.1001/archpsyc.62.6.593.

Kickbusch, I. S. (2001). Health literacy: addressing the health and education divide. *Health Promotion International, 16*(2), 289–297.

Kitchener, B. A., & Jorm, A. F. (2002). Mental health first aid training for the public: evaluation of effects on knowledge, attitudes and helping behavior. *BMC Psychiatry, 2*, 10. http://dx.doi.org/10.1186/1471-244X-2-10.

Kutcher, S., Bagnell, A., & Wei, Y. (2015). Mental health literacy in secondary schools: a Canadian approach. *Child and Adolescent Psychiatric Clinics of North America, 24*(2), 233–244. http://dx.doi.org/10.1016/j.chc.2014.11.007.

Kutcher, S., & Canadian Mental Health Association National Office (2009). *Mental health & high school curriculum guide.* Halifax, NS and Ottawa, on: Sun life financial Chair in adolescent mental health and Canadian mental health association national office.

Kutcher, S., McLuckie, A., & Child for Youth Advisory Committee, Mental Health Commission of Canada (2010). *Evergreen: A child and youth mental health framework for Canada.* Calgary, AB: Mental Health Commission of Canada.

Kutcher, S., & Wei, Y. (2013). Challenges and solutions in the implementation of the school-based pathway to care model: the lessons from Nova Scotia and beyond. *Canadian Journal of School Psychology, 28*(1), 90–102. http://dx.doi.org/10.1177/0829573512468859.

Kutcher, S., Wei, Y., & Coniglio, C. (2016). Mental health literacy: past, present, and future. *Canadian Journal of Psychiatry, 61*(3), 154–158.

Kutcher, S., Wei, Y., McLuckie, A., & Bullock, L. (2013). Educator mental health literacy: a program evaluation of the teacher training education on the Mental Health & High School Curriculum Guide. *Advances in School Mental Health Promotion, 6*(2), 83–93. http://dx.doi.org/10.1080/1754730X.2013.784615.

Kutcher, S., Wei, Y., & Weist, M. (2015). Global school mental health: considerations and future directions. In S. Kutcher, Y. Wei, & M. Weist (Eds.), *International school mental health for adolescents: Global opportunities and challenges* (pp. 299–310). UK: Cambridge University Press.

McLuckie, A., Kutcher, S., Wei, Y., & Weaver, C. (2014). Sustained improvements of students' mental health literacy with use of a mental health curriculum in Canadian schools. *BMC Psychiatry, 14*, 379. http://dx.doi.org/10.1186/s12888-014-0379-4.

Mental Health Commission of Canada. (2013). *School based mental health in Canada* a final report. Retrieved from http://www.mentalhealthcommission.ca/English/system/files/private/document/ChildYouth_School_Based_Mental_Health_Canada_Final_Report_ENG.pdf.

Milin, R., Kutcher, S., Lewis, S., Walker, S., & Ferrill, N. (2013). Randomized controlled trial of a school-based mental health literacy intervention for youth: impact on knowledge, attitudes, and help-seeking efficacy. In *Poster presentation at the 60th AACAP Annual Meeting, Orlando, USA.*

Nova Scotia Department of Education. (2012). *Kids & learning first: A plan to help every student succeed.* Halifax: Nova Scotia Department of Education, NS.

Nutbeam, D. (1998). Health promotion glossary. *Health Promotion International, 13*, 349–364.

Nutbeam, D. (2008). The evolving concept of health literacy. *Social Science & Medicine, 67*(12), 2072–2078. http://dx.doi.org/10.1016/j.socscimed.2008.09.050.

Pinfold, V., Toulmin, H., Thornicroft, G., Huxley, P., Farmer, P., & Graham, T. (2003). Reducing psychiatric stigma and discrimination: evaluation of educational interventions in UK secondary schools. *The British Journal of Psychiatry, 182*(4), 342–346. http://dx.doi.org/10.1192/bjp.182.4.342.

Pino-Foltz, M. D., Logsdon, M. C., & Myers, J. A. (2011). Feasibility, acceptability, and initial efficacy of a knowledge-contact program to reduce mental illness stigma and improve mental health literacy in adolescents. *Social Science & Medicine, 72*(12), 2011–2019. http://dx.doi.org/10.1016/j.socscimed.2011.04.006.

Reavley, N. J., & Jorm, A. F. (2011). *National survey of mental health literacy and stigma.* Canberra: Department of health and ageing. http://dx.doi.org/10.3109/00048674.2011.621060.

III. INTERVENTIONS AND TREATMENTS

Rowling, L., & Weist, M. D. (2004). Promoting the growth, improvement and sustainability of school mental health programs worldwide. *International Journal of Mental Health Promotion, 6*(2), 3–11. http://dx.doi.org/10.1080/14623730.2004.9721925.

Santor, D., Short, K., & Ferguson, B. (2009). *Taking mental health to school: A policy- oriented paper on school-based mental health for Ontario.* Ottawa, ON: The Provincial Centre of Excellence for Child and Youth Mental Health at CHEO.

Schillinger, D., Piette, J., Grumbach, K., Wang, F., Wilson, C., Daher, C., et al. (2003). Closing the loop: Physician communication with diabetic patients who have low health literacy. *Archives of Internal Medicine, 163,* 83–90.

Schillinger, D., Machtinger, E. L., Wang, F., Chen, L., Win, K., Palacios, J., et al. (2005). Language, Literacy, and Communication Regarding Medication in an Anticoagulation Clinic: Are Pictures Better Than Words? In K. Henriksen, J. B. Battles, E. S. Marks, & D. I. Lewin (Eds.), *Advances in Patient Safety: From Research to Implementation* (Vol. 2). Rockville, MD: Agency for Healthcare Research and Quality.

Sermrittirong, S., Van Brakel, W. H., & Bunbers-Aelen, J. F. (2014). How to reduce stigma in leprosy – a systematic literature review. *Leprosy Review, 85*(3), 149–157. Retrieved from: http://www.ncbi.nlm.nih.gov/pubmed/25509715.

Skre, I., Friborg, O., Breivik, C., Johnsen, L. I., Arnesen, Y., & Wang, C. E. (2013). A school intervention for mental health literacy in adolescents: effects of a non-randomized cluster controlled trial. *BMC Public Health, 13,* 873. http://dx.doi.org/10.1186/1471-2458-13-873.

Stuart, H. (2006). Reaching out to high school youth: the effectiveness of a video-based anti-stigma program. *Canadian Journal of Psychiatry, 51*(10), 647–653. Retrieved from http://www.ncbi.nlm.nih.gov/pubmed/17052032.

Thornicroft, G. (2006). *Shunned: Discrimination against people with mental illness.* Oxford: Oxford University Press.

UNESCO. (2006). *Education for all: A global monitoring report.* UNESCO.

Wei, Y., Hayden, J. A., Kutcher, S., & McGrath, P. J. (2013). The effectiveness of school mental health literacy programs to address knowledge, attitudes and help seeking among youth. *Early Intervention in Psychiatry, 7*(2), 109–121. http://dx.doi.org/10.1111/eip.12010.

Wei, Y., & Kutcher, S. (2014). Innovations in Practice: 'Go-to' Educator Training on the mental health competencies of educators in the secondary school setting: a program evaluation. *Child and Adolescent Mental Health, 19*(3), 219–222. http://dx.doi.org/10.1111/camh.12056.

Wei, Y., Kutcher, S., Blackwood, A., Glover, D., Weaver, C., MacKay, A., et al. (2015). A collaborative and sustainable approach to address mental health promotion and early identification in schools in the Canadian province of Nova Scotia and beyond. In S. Kutcher, Y. Wei, & M. Weist (Eds.), *International school mental health for adolescents: Global opportunities and challenges* (pp. 30–45). UK: Cambridge University Press.

Wei, Y., Kutcher, S., Heather, H., & Mackay, A. (2014). Successfully embedding mental health literacy into Canadian classroom curriculum by building on existing educator competencies and school structures: the Mental Health and High School Curriculum Guide for secondary schools in Nova Scotia. *Literacy Information and Computer Education Journal, 5*(3), 1158–1163.

Wei, Y., Kutcher, S., & Szumilas, M. (2011). Comprehensive school mental health: an integrated "School-Based pathway to care" model for Canadian secondary schools. *McGill Journal of Education, 46*(2), 213–229. http://dx.doi.org/10.7202/1006436ar.

World Health Organization. (2013). *The solid facts: Health literacy.* Geneva: World Health Organization. Retrieved from http://www.euro.who.int/__data/assets/pdf_file/0008/190655/e96854.pdf.

Transforming Cultures for the Mental Health Care of Young People: The Service Reform Imperative

P. McGorry, S. Goldstone

Orygen, The National Centre of Excellence in Youth Mental Health, Parkville, VIC, Australia

INTRODUCTION

Although mental health issues are the key health concern for young people today, contributing 45 percent of the total burden of disease for those aged 10 to 24 years (Gore et al., 2011), young people have the poorest access to mental health care of all ages across the lifespan. Despite the disproportionate impact that mental ill-health has on young people, they are the age group the least likely of all across the lifespan to receive professional care. The vast majority of young people from low- and middle-income countries are unable to access mental health care, simply because it is rarely available to them, while less than a third of young people in high-income countries who experience mental health issues access professional help (McGorry, Goldstone, Parker, Rickwood, & Hickie, 2014; World Health Organization, 2014).

A number of reasons contribute to this state of affairs. Young people may not recognize or acknowledge a need for mental health care, and often feel that they should manage their emotional difficulties themselves. Poor mental health literacy and unhelpful beliefs around strength and autonomy are major factors that prevent help-seeking in this age group (Rickwood, Deane, & Wilson, 2007). In the developed world at least, another crucial factor is the current structure of our health care system.

Positive Mental Health, Fighting Stigma and Promoting Resiliency for Children and Adolescents
http://dx.doi.org/10.1016/B978-0-12-804394-3.00009-7

Primary health care services, the first port of call for most people, are geared to catering for physical ill-health and are largely designed for young children or older adults, and can be highly alienating to young people. Moreover, because young people are usually in good physical health, they may not routinely visit a general practitioner, and when they do, they often do not feel comfortable enough to discuss emotional concerns (Rickwood et al., 2007). Other service-level factors such as accessibility, confidentiality, and cost are particularly concerning for young people, and even the location, milieu, and décor of the service can also be critical barriers (Ambresin, Bennett, Patton, Sanci, & Sawyer, 2013; Roberts, Sanci, & Haller, 2012).

The situation is even more difficult for young people and their families who seek help from the specialist mental health system. Young people tend to present with complex and evolving symptom profiles that often do not meet the stringent diagnostic criteria required for acceptance, particularly into an adult service, despite the significant distress and functional impairment they are obviously enduring. All too often, they are also ineligible for child and adolescent services, particularly from mid-adolescence, as they approach the age cut-off for these services.

This state of affairs is largely driven by poor resourcing and design. Our current child and adolescent services focus on the needs of younger children within their family, educational, and social contexts. In an effort to accommodate older adolescents, many have reached upwards and imposed an age cut-off of 18, or even 16 years that is tied to the end of formal secondary schooling and the legal age of adulthood (Patel, Flisher, Hetrick, & McGorry, 2007). However, the largely pediatric focus of these services is inappropriate for many older adolescents, especially those with more severe disorders, who frequently find that their only access to care is via older adult services. The adult services, which are largely designed around the needs of middle-aged adults with established disorders, have also attempted to reach down to young people, but with limited success. This artificially imposed division of health services at age 18 presents serious problems for certain physical health conditions; however, for mental health it is a fatal design flaw, because the discontinuity between them falls right within the age range where the incidence of new onsets peaks, rendering the system weakest where it should be strongest (McGorry, 2007).

Accessing mental health services can be difficult for young people; but for those with existing mental health issues who must transition between the child and adolescent stream and the adult stream for ongoing care, the situation is even more complex. Although the majority of these young people are referred on to adult services, around one-third are not, and of those that are accepted by adult services, a quarter are discharged without having been seen (Paul et al., 2013; Singh et al., 2010). In part, this is because most adult services do not cater for those who have received help in childhood for developmental disorders; for example, young people with intellectual disabilities or neurodevelopmental disorders such as autism or attention-deficit/hyperactivity disorder. For those who are referred on, while some transfer does occur, optimal transition is rare. This is largely due to differences in the service cultures and work practices between the child and adolescent and adult services, poor communication and collaboration between services, poor transfer protocols, and the rigid structure and culture of the adult services , which young people can find alienating and intimidating (McLaren et al., 2013; Paul, Street, Wheeler, & Singh, 2015).

A NEW APPROACH TO MENTAL HEALTH CARE FOR YOUNG PEOPLE

Clearly, a new approach is required to improve young people's access to mental health care, as well as the quality and continuity of that care. There are strong arguments to support the need for a specific youth mental health stream that is able to recognize the unique biopsychosocial needs of this age group. The first is clinical, in that young people in the early stages of a mental illness tend to present with heterogeneous blends of comorbidities of variable intensity, particularly substance abuse and challenging personality traits, which usually do not meet strict diagnostic thresholds and require an integrated model of care. Thus, services that acknowledge the particularly complex and evolving pattern of symptoms and morbidity seen in this age group are needed. Second, developmentally and culturally appropriate approaches are essential for the management of emerging disorders; young people's individual and group identity and their help-seeking needs and behaviors need to be central to any service model (McGorry et al., 2014). Ideally, this means creating a service model with its own discrete culture and expertise, but with seamless linkages to systems for younger children and older adults (McGorry, Tanti, et al., 2007). This will overcome many of the issues contributing to young people's poor access to care and difficulties in transition between the current service streams (Singh et al., 2010).

Addressing the barriers to access to mental health care for young people requires a multifaceted approach. First and foremost, young people need to be able to recognize when, how, and where to seek help. Awareness-raising and education is key to this, and the media, education, and health care sectors all play an important role. At the system level, accessible, affordable, and acceptable care that is developmentally appropriate for the young person and their stage of illness should be available. However, the sheer scale of the incidence and prevalence of mental ill-health among young people demands a new and comprehensive approach to service provision that has the capacity to deal with the scale of this need, as well as the ability to manage its complexity and diversity. Service levels that cover the full spectrum of illness severity are required, ranging from e-health and primary care services or enhanced primary care services for those with mild to moderate mental health issues, through to specialized services for those with complex presentations or more severe illness (McGorry, Tanti, et al., 2007). The key principles for such services are outlined in Box 9.1.

PROMOTING ACCESSIBLE, APPROPRIATE, AND ACCEPTABLE CARE

Although up to 80 percent of young people will experience mental health issues at some point during adolescence, much of this mental ill-health is mild to moderate in nature (Copeland, Shanahan, Costello, & Angold, 2011; Gibb, Fergusson, & Horwood, 2010; McGorry, 2007; Patton et al., 2014). Typically, young people present with complex and fluctuating blends of symptoms, most commonly depression, anxiety, and other

---

BOX 9.1

KEY PRINCIPLES FOR YOUTH MENTAL HEALTH SERVICES

Youth mental health services should:

- welcome youth participation at all levels, to ensure the service offers an accessible, welcoming, stigma-free environment that provides the care that young people and their families need
- adopt a preventive and optimistic framework that emphasizes early intervention and offers holistic, evidence-informed, stepped care that is governed by risk-benefit considerations and shared decision-making, with social and vocational outcomes as key targets
- operate as a "one-stop shop," where care providers are organized around the young person, his/her family, and his/her unique needs, in which a dedicated team of clinical and non-clinical personnel provides the full cycle of care for the young person and his/her family
- offer flexible tenure of care (including entry, exit, and re-entry) as needed throughout this critical developmental period
- eliminate discontinuities at peak periods of need for care during developmental transitions by providing positive and seamless linkages with services for younger children and older adults

---

more non-specific symptoms, including withdrawal, apathy, and sleep and appetite disturbance. Self-harm and substance abuse are also prevalent in this age group. While it is true that there is a tendency for many of these issues to resolve by the late 20s, if left untreated, this neglect too often comes at a significant cost to the young person in terms of underachievement or even educational/vocational failure and poor social functioning, as well as to the wider community in terms of non-participation and lost productivity (Patton et al., 2014). Furthermore, current evidence strongly suggests that persistent mental health problems in adolescence significantly increases the risk of mental illness in adulthood (Copeland et al., 2011; Gibb et al., 2010; McGorry, Purcell, Hickie, & Jorm, 2007; Patton et al., 2014).

The complexity and relative non-specificity of these symptom profiles mean that different treatment approaches are required than those that are employed for full-threshold illness, with the emphasis being on offering care that is appropriate to the very early stages of illness, pre-emptive in nature, and with a strong preventive focus. This sits best with a clinical staging approach, which differentiates earlier and milder clinical phenomena from those that accompany illness extension and progression. This enables an agnostic, rather than a diagnostic, approach to treatment, at least in the early stages of illness, where the persistence of symptoms, distress, and impairment indicate a need for care both on immediate clinical grounds as well as to mitigate the risk of progression of illness (McGorry, Purcell, et al., 2007). An explicit acknowledgment of the early stages of illness provides a more clinically useful framework, in that it is sensitive to risk/benefit considerations and favors the selection of earlier and safer interventions, and prioritizes a preventive, or at least pre-emptive, approach to treatment. This is particularly relevant for young people, who are the most likely to experience the onset of illness, and thus have the most to gain from early and pre-emptive intervention (McGorry, 2007).

DEVELOPING NEW SERVICE MODELS FOR YOUNG PEOPLE

The available evidence indicates that for the majority of young people, mental health care is best provided in the context of stigma-free, youth-friendly primary or enhanced primary care structures based in their local communities. These services must be backed up by specialized services for those with more severe or complex presentations, also in community-based settings, but with additional outreach services and the ability to provide step-up/step-down inpatient care when necessary. These face-to-face services can be both supported and extended by online services that offer instant information, monitoring, or support across a range of mobile or fixed platforms, so that young people can choose to access help whenever they choose, in whatever way they wish.

Over the last few years, reform in the delivery of youth mental health services has been gaining ground, particularly in Australia, the United Kingdom, Canada, Denmark, and Asia, and more recently in the United States (Birchwood & Singh, 2013; Illback & Bates, 2011; McGorry, 2007; McGorry, Bates, & Birchwood, 2013; Rao et al., 2013; Verma, Poon, Lee, Rao, & Chong, 2012). The most fully evolved of these service reforms is Australia's new youth mental health stream, **headspace**, which was established in 2006 by the Federal Government and tasked with devising and building a national youth mental health service stream designed to provide highly accessible, youth-friendly centers to promote and support early intervention for mental and substance use disorders in young people. This came about as the result of a targeted awareness-raising campaign and intense lobbying by academic, clinical, and community group leaders, as well as the increasing demand for investment in youth mental health by the Australian community. The first 10 headspace centers opened in 2007, and since then headspace has been successfully scaled up to reach over 70 Australian communities, and many more via **eheadspace**, its online support service (www.headspace.org.au). By 2017, 100 sites will be in operation, allowing coverage for 50 percent of Australia's young people in a face-to-face setting.

Headspace operates on an enhanced primary care model, providing a multidisciplinary care structure with close links to local specialist services, schools, and other community-based organizations. Each site is an independent local consortium, overseen by the headspace National Office, and offers evidence-based care within a clinical staging framework (McGorry, Tanti, et al., 2007). headspace caters to the broader health needs of young people, offering four core streams: mental health care, drug and alcohol services, physical and sexual health care, and vocational and educational consulting. Access is open to all young people, regardless of their presenting symptoms, and as of 2016, headspace has offered support to over 100,000 young Australians.

A stepped model of care is employed in all headspace centers, with simple brief psychosocial approaches offered as first-line therapy and medication only being used as an additive therapy if the young person does not respond to initial psychosocial interventions, or presents at the outset with more severe symptoms or risk. This links the care offered to the stage of illness and allows a preventive and proactive stance to therapeutic intervention, with the aim being to prevent the development of sustained illness. As well as the four core service streams, each headspace center also delivers local community awareness campaigns to enhance young peoples' help-seeking behavior, the ability of families and local service providers to identify emerging mental health concerns in young people early, and to strengthen the referral pathways into the service.

In addition to these face-to-face services, headspace also runs a nationwide online support service (eheadspace; www.eheadspace.org.au) where young people can "chat'" with a mental health professional either online or by telephone, and access assessment and therapeutic care. This has greatly expanded access to expert mental health care for young Australians, who can now access care when, where, and how they choose to. In recognition of the issue of youth suicide in Australia, headspace also provides a support service for schools affected by student suicide (headspace school support), which offers a range of services, including assistance with managing the immediate response following a student suicide or suicide attempt; staff and parent information sessions; education and training related to suicide and evidence-based resources; a postvention toolkit; secondary and tertiary consultation; assistance with critical incident review; and media liaison and advice.

The majority of the young people using headspace services, even when highly distressed, are experiencing mild to moderate levels of mental ill-health and are in the early stages of illness; however, at most headspace sites there is also a substantial subset of young people with more complex, severe, and enduring problems who currently are unable to gain access to the traditional CAMHS/adult system (Rickwood et al., 2014). To begin to address this need, in 2011 the Australian Government funded the creation of up to nine "enhanced headspace" services, which are now beginning to deliver evidence-based early psychosis services, offering early detection, acute care during an initial psychotic episode, and recovery-focused continuing care featuring multimodal interventions to support the young person (and his/her family) to maintain or regain their social, academic, and/or career trajectory during the critical first two to five years following the onset of a psychotic illness (Hughes et al., 2014). The first of these enhanced services (known as hYEPPs or headspace Youth Early Psychosis Programs) commenced operation in 2013, embedded with clusters of headspace centers at a regional level, and drawing on their links with locally available services. It is hoped that ultimately they will be expanded to cover not only all headspace communities, but also the full diagnostic spectrum in young people with any severe mental illness.

A comprehensive sample of 22,000 young people assessed by headspace nationally revealed that headspace appears to be successfully addressing the issues of access and engagement, a conclusion supported by the heavy demand for eheadspace services from across the nation (Rickwood et al., 2014). Moreover, very recent census data from 33,038 young people attending the 55 fully operational headspace centers between 2013 and 2014 has shown that 85 percent presented with mental health issues, including behavioral and situational issues (bullying, difficulty with relationships, grief). Physical or sexual health issues were the next most common, at 7.1 percent of presentations. Very few young people presented primarily for alcohol or drug issues (3.1 percent) or for vocational consultations (1.8 percent). The average wait time for a first appointment was two weeks, and the mean number of sessions attended varied depending on the presenting problem, with those who presented for mental health issues attending a mean of 4.4 sessions, though a sizable proportion of this group attended more than five sessions (approximately 30 percent). Interestingly, many of the clients who presented for reasons other than mental health issues also received mental health care. Most consultations (approximately 80 percent) were with either a psychologist or another allied mental health staff member, with only 10 percent provided by general practitioners (GPs) and 1.2 percent by psychiatrists. Alcohol and drug services were usually provided by specialist workers, with contributions from other allied mental health workers (Rickwood, Telford, et al., 2015).

Among the 24,034 young people from this cohort who had first presented to headspace centers with mental health concerns, depression and anxiety accounted for over two-thirds of all first visits for both young women and young men. Clients' level of psychological distress (measured by the K10 scale) and psychosocial functioning (measured with the SOFAs scale) were assessed at their first visit, and then at Visits 3, 6, 10, and 15 as appropriate, and then by a follow-up survey at 90 days after their final visit. Cognitive-behavioral therapy (CBT) was the most common treatment for all primary presenting concerns, with the second-most common treatment being supportive counseling, followed by psychoeducation, interpersonal therapy, and acceptance and commitment therapy. Approximately one-third of clients showed a significant improvement in their levels of distress, with one-quarter showing reliable improvement, and 20 percent showing a clinically significant improvement. Similar results were seen for psychosocial functioning, and for those clients for whom data on both measures was available, 60 percent showed a significant improvement on one or both scales, while 50 percent showed a reliable improvement, and 40 percent showed clinically significant improvement on one or both scales (Rickwood, Mazzer, et al., 2015).

Together, these data provide important evidence to show that headspace has been successful in meeting its goals of improving access and outcomes for young people: headspace is clearly seen as accessible and acceptable to young people, who present primarily for mental health concerns. Interestingly, for those who present with physical or sexual health issues, a significant proportion also accessed mental health care, and thus headspace provides both direct and indirect pathways to care. While it is difficult to compare the outcomes of headspace clients with those from clients of a comparable service, within the limits of currently available data, it seems that headspace compares favorably, and is able to reduce distress and improve psychosocial functioning for the majority of clients.

However, headspace is still a work in progress. Important gaps remain, notably the fact that more than half of the Australian community is not yet covered, as the current level of funding does not yet allow full national coverage. Furthermore, access rates for young men, indigenous young people, and certain ethnic populations, while improved, are still too low, and the program does not yet adequately cover those with serious mental illness. The long-term aim of these reforms is to develop a nationwide youth mental health stream of care that fully integrates care for young people with other service systems; notably education, employment, housing, and justice, in order to provide a seamless coverage of mental health care from puberty to mature adulthood at around 25 years of age, with soft transitions with child and adult mental health care, and strong links with other mainstream services. This system acknowledges biopsychosocial development and recognizes the complexity and challenges faced by young people as they become independent adults, as well the burden of disease imposed on this age group by poor mental health. By taking this multidisciplinary approach it also deliberately seeks to blur the distinctions between the traditionally separate tiers of primary and specialist care, including some aspects of acute care. This recognizes the complexity of much of the mental ill-health apparent in young people and allows a more flexible and appropriate response for each individual, depending on his/her own unique needs.

Clearly, the success of this reform will only be able to be assessed after careful evaluation, and evidently more health services research is necessary to develop, refine, adapt, and evaluate this new model of care. An independent evaluation of headspace is currently being finalized and will no doubt inform the evolution of this model. However, the indications to date are that the model is justified, if only purely on the grounds of the significant improvement it offers in terms of access to care, which has been acknowledged by policymakers both nationally and internationally. However, on purely pragmatic terms, we believe that offering evidence-informed care within a system that is accessible and acceptable to young people, as headspace clearly is, should continue as a "best bet," while we continue to accumulate the research evidence that will allow the development of a truly evidence-based care stream for this uniquely vulnerable group.

Another key reason for the need for services such as headspace is their role in driving genuine reform in mental health care. Real-world clinical laboratories such as headspace, that have been developed by clinician researchers and include an integrated research capacity, are crucial for the accumulation of new evidence, as well as the development of the new skills and professional workforces to support these reforms (McGorry et al., 2014). All the available evidence—the epidemiological data, our new knowledge of the developmental changes that occur during transition to adulthood, and perhaps decisively, the economic imperatives—indicates that this transformational reform should be based on the principles of early intervention and a priority focus on the developmental period of greatest need and capacity to benefit from investment: emerging adulthood. Psychiatry needs to move away from our historically largely palliative approach to care, and toward the more pre-emptive and personalized approach that is used in today's physical medicine if we are to achieve the greatest possible public health gains. Another advantage of this 21st century clinical infrastructure is that it will greatly facilitate the population-based and universal programs that link with mental health awareness and promotion activities, as well as with the new Internet-based technologies that are already dramatically changing the face of mental health awareness and care.

We already have proof of concept of the value of early and pre-emptive intervention from the early psychosis movement that has developed and evolved over the last two decades and is now widespread; this has largely driven the growing interest in youth mental health worldwide (Chan et al., 2014; Hegelstad et al., 2012; Nordentoft, Rasmussen, Melau, Hjorthøj, & Thorup, 2014; Norman et al., 2011). This by no means argues against investments earlier or later in life, which are also essential, both in terms of preventive/pre-emptive interventions, as well as for ongoing care. However, the current widespread neglect of young people's mental health concerns has a double effect of downgrading the value of existing early-life investments, as well as contributing to the ongoing pressure on our already overstretched adult services. Appropriate, accessible, and acceptable youth mental health services are the missing link here. Examples of such modern stigma-free cultures of care that have been designed and are operated with young people themselves, such as headspace, already exist (Birchwood & Singh, 2013; Illback & Bates, 2011; McGorry, 2007; McGorry et al., 2013; Rao et al., 2013; Verma et al., 2012). These transformational reforms are highly valued in their communities, and the arguments for them are increasingly being accepted by policymakers worldwide. Perhaps most importantly, they represent our best available bet to reduce the lifelong impact of mental ill-health on the individual, his/her family, and society more broadly.

References

Ambresin, A. E., Bennett, K., Patton, G. C., Sanci, L. A., & Sawyer, S. M. (2013). Assessment of youth-friendly health care: a systematic review of indicators drawn from young people's perspectives. *The Journal of Adolescent Health: Official Publication of the Society for Adolescent Medicine, 52*, 670–681.

Birchwood, M., & Singh, S. P. (2013). Mental health services for young people: matching the service to the need. *The British Journal of psychiatry*, (Suppl. 54), s1–s2.

Chan, S. K., So, H. C., Hui, C. L., Chang, W. C., Lee, E. H., Chung, D. W., ... Chen, E. Y. (2014). 10-year outcome study of an early intervention program for psychosis compared with standard care service. *Psychological Medicine*, 1–13.

Copeland, W., Shanahan, L., Costello, E. J., & Angold, A. (2011). Cumulative prevalence of psychiatric disorders by young adulthood: a prospective cohort analysis from the Great Smoky Mountains Study. *Journal of the American Academy of Child and Adolescent Psychiatry, 50*, 252–261.

Gibb, S. J., Fergusson, D. M., & Horwood, L. J. (2010). Burden of psychiatric disorder in young adulthood and life outcomes at age 30. *The British Journal of Psychiatry: the Journal of Mental Science, 197*, 122–127.

Gore, F. M., Bloem, P. J., Patton, G. C., Ferguson, J., Joseph, V., Coffey, C., … Mathers, C. D. (2011). Global burden of disease in young people aged 10–24 years: a systematic analysis. *Lancet, 377*, 2093–2102.

Hegelstad, W. T., Larsen, T. K., Auestad, B., Evensen, J., Haahr, U., Joa, I., … McGlashan, T. (2012). Long-term follow-up of the TIPS early detection in psychosis study: effects on 10-year outcome. *The American Journal of Psychiatry, 169*, 374–380.

Hughes, F., Stavely, H., Simpson, R., Goldstone, S., Pennell, K., & McGorry, P. (2014). At the heart of an early psychosis centre: the core components of the 2014 Early Psychosis Prevention and Intervention Centre model for Australian communities. *Australasian Psychiatry: Bulletin of Royal Australian and New Zealand College of Psychiatrists, 22*, 228–234.

Illback, R. J., & Bates, T. (2011). Transforming youth mental health services and supports in Ireland. *Early Intervention in Psychiatry, 5*(Suppl. 1), 22–27.

McGorry, P. D. (2007). The specialist youth mental health model: strengthening the weakest link in the public mental health system. *The Medical Journal of Australia, 187*, S53–S56.

McGorry, P. D., Bates, T., & Birchwood, M. (2013). Designing youth mental health services for the 21st century: examples from Australia, Ireland and the UK. *The British Journal of Psychiatry: the Journal of Mental Science, 202*, s30–s40.

McGorry, P. D., Goldstone, S. D., Parker, A. G., Rickwood, D. J., & Hickie, I. B. (2014). Cultures for mental health care of young people: an Australian blueprint for reform. *Lancet Psychiatry, 1*, 559–568.

McGorry, P. D., Purcell, R., Hickie, I. B., & Jorm, A. F. (2007). Investing in youth mental health is a best buy. *The Medical Journal of Australia, 187*, S5–S7.

McGorry, P. D., Tanti, C., Stokes, R., Hickie, I. B., Carnell, K., Littlefield, L. K., & Moran, J. (2007). Headspace: Australia's National Youth Mental Health Foundation–where young minds come first. *The Medical Journal of Australia, 187*, S68–S70.

McLaren, S., Belling, R., Paul, M., Ford, T., Kramer, T., Weaver, T., … Singh, S. P. (2013). 'Talking a different language': an exploration of the influence of organizational cultures and working practices on transition from child to adult mental health services. *BMC Health Services Research, 13*, 254.

Nordentoft, M., Rasmussen, J. O., Melau, M., Hjorthøj, C. R., & Thorup, A. A. (2014). How successful are first episode programs? A review of the evidence for specialized assertive early intervention. *Current Opinion in Psychiatry, 27*, 167–172.

Norman, R. M., Manchanda, R., Malla, A. K., Windell, D., Harricharan, R., & Northcott, S. (2011). Symptom and functional outcomes for a 5 year early intervention program for psychoses. *Schizophrenia Research, 129*, 111–115.

World Health Organization. (2014). *Health for the world's adolescents: A second chance in the second decade.* Geneva: World Health Organization.

Patel, V., Flisher, A. J., Hetrick, S., & McGorry, P. (2007). Mental health of young people: a global public health challenge. *Lancet, 369*, 1302–1313.

Patton, G. C., Coffey, C., Romaniuk, H., Mackinnon, A., Carlin, J. B., Degenhardt, L., … Moran, P. (2014). The prognosis of common mental disorders in adolescents: a 14-year prospective cohort study. *Lancet, 383*, 1401–1411.

Paul, M., Ford, T., Kramer, T., Islam, Z., Harley, K., & Singh, S. P. (2013). Transfers and transitions between child and adult mental health services. *The British Journal of psychiatry. Supplement, 54*, s36–s40.

III. INTERVENTIONS AND TREATMENTS

Paul, M., Street, C., Wheeler, N., & Singh, S. P. (2015). Transition to adult services for young people with mental health needs: a systematic review. *Clinical Child Psychology and Psychiatry, 20*, 436–457.

Rao, S., Pariyasami, S., Tay, S. A., Lim, L. K., Yuen, S., Poon, L. Y., … Verma, S. (2013). Support for Wellness Achievement Programme (SWAP): a service for individuals with at-risk mental state in Singapore. *Annals of the Academy of Medicine, Singapore, 42*, 552–555.

Rickwood, D. J., Deane, F. P., & Wilson, C. J. (2007). When and how do young people seek professional help for mental health problems? *The Medical Journal of Australia, 187*, S35–S39.

Rickwood, D. J., Mazzer, K. R., Telford, N. R., Parker, A. G., Tanti, C. J., & McGorry, P. D. (2015). Changes in psychological distress and psychosocial functioning in young people visiting headspace centres for mental health problems. *The Medical Journal of Australia, 202*, 537–542.

Rickwood, D. J., Telford, N. R., Mazzer, K. R., Parker, A. G., Tanti, C. J., & McGorry, P. D. (2015). The services provided to young people through the headspace centres across Australia. *The Medical Journal of Australia, 202*, 533–536.

Rickwood, D. J., Telford, N. R., Parker, A. G., Parker, A. G., Tanti, C. J., & McGorry, P. D. (2014). Headspace – Australia's innovation in youth mental health: who are the clients and why are they presenting? *The Medical Journal of Australia, 200*, 108–111.

Roberts, J., Sanci, L., & Haller, D. (2012). Global adolescent health: is there a role for general practice? *The British Journal of General Practice: the Journal of the Royal College of General Practitioners, 62*, 608–610.

Singh, S. P., Paul, M., Ford, T., Kramer, T., Weaver, T., McLaren, S., … White, S. (2010). Process, outcome and experience of transition from child to adult mental healthcare: multiperspective study. *The British Journal of Psychiatry: the Journal of Mental Science, 197*, 305–312.

Verma, S., Poon, L. Y., Lee, H., Rao, S., & Chong, S. A. (2012). Evolution of early psychosis intervention services in Singapore. *East Asian Archives of Psychiatry: Official Journal of the Hong Kong College, 22*, 114–117.

Evidence-Based Parenting Interventions: Current Perspectives and Clinical Strategies

D.J. Hawes[1], J. Allen[2]

[1]The University of Sydney, NSW, Australia; [2]University College
London, London, United Kingdom

INTRODUCTION

The effective treatment of child psychopathology is often determined by the effectiveness with which a clinician is able to facilitate targeted and sustained change in parenting. The literature is now replete with evidence-based parenting programs for a range of problems, in which parents are cast as the primary agents of therapeutic change. In addition to these programs, parenting processes are often core to formulation-driven treatment plans in which they may be conceptualized and targeted alongside any number of other child and family risk processes. The benefits of targeting quality of parenting have been demonstrated dramatically in recent decades, as evidence has grown regarding mechanisms of change and long-term outcomes among children with various disorders. At the same time, such interventions present clinicians with a range of unique challenges that call for unique theoretical perspectives and process strategies.

THEORETICAL PERSPECTIVES ON PARENTING AND CHILD PSYCHOPATHOLOGY

It is now well recognized that competencies related to the self-regulation of emotion, cognition, and goal-directed behavior, are shaped through

Positive Mental Health, Fighting Stigma and Promoting Resiliency for Children and Adolescents
http://dx.doi.org/10.1016/B978-0-12-804394-3.00010-3

repeated transactions between children's biologically based characteristics and the social contexts in which they develop (Rothbart & Posner, 2006). The earliest and most profound such context is the parent–child relationship. Parenting practices often not only control variables for child behavior patterns but may also serve to potentiate the expression of biological vulnerabilities, and in doing so enhance risk that is carried forward across the life span (Dadds, Moul, Hawes, Mendoza Diaz, & Brennan, 2015; Hawes, Dadds, Frost, & Russell, 2013). At the same time, the very parenting processes that operate on child outcomes may themselves arise from child-driven effects associated with child characteristics (eg, temperament) and behavior.

In contrast to the notion that parenting risk factors are unique to specific disorders, research has emphasized considerable overlap among the parenting processes that are common to trajectories of both externalizing and internalizing dysfunction (Levy, Hawes, & Johns, 2015). Indeed, there is now strong evidence that parenting plays a significant role in shaping the self-regulatory capacities, or executive functions, that are associated with disorders of both types, as well as a range of broader developmental and academic outcomes (Fay-Stammbach, Hawes, & Meredith, 2014). However, as outlined in the next section, the family-based risk models that have received the strongest empirical support, and have been translated into the most established parenting interventions, have been those related to disruptive behavior disorders or conduct problems (ie, oppositional defiant disorder and conduct disorder) and childhood anxiety disorders.

Parenting and Externalizing Problems

The models that have received the strongest empirical support in explaining the emergence and maintenance of childhood conduct problems are those in which family risk mechanisms are conceptualized based on social learning (operant) theory (Hawes & Dadds, 2005a; Patterson & Fisher, 2002). These conceptualizations attribute the maintenance and amplification of child conduct problems to escalating cycles of parent–child coercion that function as interlocking "reinforcement traps". These coercive cycles are maintained by escape-avoidance mechanisms through which aversive control tactics (eg, whining, nagging, shouting, hitting) are rewarded, and positive/warm family interactions are extinguished (Dishion & Patterson, 2006). The contingencies supplied by parents in terms of relative rates of reinforcement for socially competent versus deviant behavior are seen to represent the most proximal influences on child outcomes. Likewise, the same reinforcement mechanisms that operate on child behavior are assumed to encompass the alteration and shaping of parenting behavior.

In addition to specifying the risk processes through which parent–child contingencies play out on a moment-to-moment timescale, coercion theory also emphasizes the longer term, developmental timescale across which cascading risk processes are set in train. Often first initiated by 2 years of age, the longer that coercive cycles persist over time, the more rapidly they are likely to escalate, and the higher they are likely to push the upper amplitudes of family aggression. As children become increasingly skilled in their use of coercion, discipline becomes increasingly challenging for parents. Deficits in social competencies expand to other domains of development, and soon generalize to contexts outside of the home (Dishion & Patterson, 2006). Parenting processes continue to shape antisocial trajectories across later childhood and adolescence; however, the precise parenting processes of proximal importance in this period shift from those related to setting limits on behavior in the home, to those related to the regulation of children's peer activities in external settings. As such, evidence-based interventions for adolescent conduct problems often provide youth with skills training related to self-regulation, while also targeting parenting practices related to monitoring and supervision (Dishion & Kavanagh, 2003; Henggeler & Sheidow, 2012).

Parenting and Internalizing Problems

The critical/rejecting parenting associated with coercion in the families of children with conduct problems has also been associated with risk for internalizing problems—in particular child and adolescent depression (McLeod, Weisz, & Wood, 2007). Alternatively, risk for anxiety disorders has been associated most strongly with overprotective/overcontrolling parenting, wherein parents excessively restrict children's engagement with situations or behaviors based on anticipation of potential threat (Rapee, Schniering, & Hudson, 2009). This may extend to psychological control expressed through intrusive or passive–aggressive parenting behaviors that inhibit autonomy-granting. Such parents may withdraw affection or induce guilt as means of discipline, creating a family environment in which acceptance is contingent on a child's behavior (Barber, 1996). These parenting behaviors have been proposed to confer risk through a number of mechanisms, potentially functioning to (1) model anxious responding to innocuous events, (2) enhance children's threat interpretations, (3) prevent the habituation of anxious arousal by limiting children's exposure to fear-provoking events, and (4) interfere with the adaptive development of children's emotion regulation skills (Ollendick, Costa, & Benoit, 2010).

Guided by the conceptualization of transactional parent–child dynamics emphasized in models of conduct problems, research has likewise supported the occurrence of transactional parent–child dynamics in accounts of internalizing problems (LaFrenière & Dumas, 1992). In line with this, Dadds and Roth (2001) proposed an "anxious–coercive cycle", in which fearful children solicit attention, comfort, and protection from their parents during novel situations, which in turn functions to reinforce children's avoidance and dependence on parents. There has since been considerable support for the notion that child anxiety is maintained by parenting responses that are in part a product of maladaptive child behavior (Williams, Kertz, Schrock, & Woodruff-Borden, 2012). Such evidence suggests that interventions for anxiety that ignore parent–child interactions may place children at risk of reinstating relationship dynamics that contribute to the amplification of anxiety in the family. At present, evidence-based treatments for internalizing problems place considerably less emphasis on parenting targets than those for externalizing problems; however, growing treatment outcome research has emphasized the therapeutic value of training parents in strategies that emphasize calm and consistent responding, and teaching parents to respond to child anxiety using cognitive-behavioral strategies such as graded exposure, structured problem-solving, and behavioral experiments (Cartwright-Hatton et al., 2011).

KEY ISSUES IN THE PLANNING AND DELIVERING OF PARENTING INTERVENTIONS

The clinical assessment of parents and parenting serves a number of key functions. First, such assessment is essential to formulation-driven clinical practice, informing functional hypotheses about the controlling variables (eg, patterns of social rewards and punishment) that can be targeted to produce child behavior change. This formulation often benefits from comprehensive measurement strategies that incorporate parent interviews, self-report inventories, and structured observational procedures that allow for the assessment of family process variables that may not otherwise be accessible (Hawes & Dadds, 2013). Evidence-based models of childhood disorders such as those already presented provide a means to map out the domains of parenting that are likely to be of most proximal importance to children and adolescents characterized by various diagnostic and developmental features. These models specify the optimal starting points from which to plan the assessment of parenting and family variables, and guide the interpretation of the resulting data in relation to data on a child's behavior and development. Second, a range of parent and family factors represent potential barriers to treatment, with data on those factors often needed to guide the effective implementation of parenting interventions. Such factors include a parent's resources for change (eg, self-regulatory capacities, social support), as well as parents' readiness for change and motivation for treatment (Geffken, Keeley, Kellison, Storch, & Rodrigue, 2006). Third, data on parents' capacities to meet children's current and future developmental needs, and the appropriateness of the demands being made by the child's environment, are crucial to making clinical judgments about a child's prognostic status—potentially within the context of high-risk scenarios involving neglect or maltreatment. Finally, the collection of data on parenting throughout an intervention may provide information of key importance to the evaluation of treatment progress and outcomes. Such data may allow a therapist faced with poor treatment adherence to understand and address barriers to change (eg, parents' self-defeating cognitions, interference from other family members), and inform important revisions to problem formulation across therapy.

Although the collection of reliable data on family functioning is essential to planning effective parenting interventions, such data alone offers no guarantee that an intervention will act on those dynamics effectively. We assume that the process of therapeutic change is also driven by the process of consultation, the most important of which concerns the early contacts between a therapist and family. The effective management of this process is particularly crucial when working with distressed, multiproblem families (Scott & Dadds, 2009). It is important from the outset to recognize that the planning and delivery of interventions that address issues related to parenting and the family is often complicated by the very nature of these domains. By the time many children and adolescents are referred to clinical services, their parents have suffered a long history of defeats in their attempts to manage the presenting problem. In addition to the distress associated with this, many of the family factors implicated in parenting problems (eg, parent psychopathology, negative parental attributions and feelings toward the child, marital conflict, lack of social support) are distressing in their own right. Such factors are likewise associated with poor engagement in child and adolescent mental health services.

Promoting Engagement in Parenting Interventions

The most valuable strategies for assessing parenting and family domains are those that support the dual aim of eliciting reliable data while at the same time promoting a strong therapeutic relationship with parents. Our approach to managing this process (Dadds & Hawes, 2006) draws on a structural model of the family system. According to Minuchin (1974), a healthy family is characterized by overlapping but independent parent, child, and extended family subsystems, that are organized hierarchically. Most importantly, parents act as an executive subsystem, wherein they maintain a positive relationship independent of the parenting role and can function cooperatively to solve family problems. While the data to show that problematic structural dynamics are a direct causal variable for child psychopathology is complex for methodological reasons, evidence suggests that these dynamics may confer broad risk for childhood problems. In the families of children with conduct problems, for example, it has been found that the boundaries between parent and child subsystems often become unclear; the parents' relationship becomes conflicted; and extended family get drawn into failed attempts to manage the child's behavior (Green, Loeber, & Lahey, 1992; Shaw Criss, Schonberg, & Beck, 2004). We assume that the first critical process of therapy is to join with the parental subsystem of the family to form a therapeutic team, and that it is through this parent-centered partnership that a therapist is best placed to impact on the broader family system.

In our work we have found that many of the process difficulties encountered by therapists in engaging parents in family-based interventions stem from a failure to structure initial contacts that are compatible with this aim (Dadds & Hawes, 2006). The effective management of the consultation process begins with the first telephone contact, at which point it is important to clarify who is involved in the parenting of the child, and to take the necessary steps to ensure that the relevant members of the parenting subsystem attend the initial assessment session whenever possible. Many therapists trained in family-systems approaches believe that the first session should involve all family members so that the system as a whole can be observed. This opportunity for observation can, however, come at a significant cost. A therapist's attempts to explore issues beyond those directly associated with the child are in many cases rejected by parents whose experience and perception of the problem has not first been sufficiently validated. This relies on parents being free to express and explore their experiences in the family, no matter how distressing or controversial. Complaints about the effect of the child's behavior on the parents' lives and marriage, catastrophic fears about the child's future, and hostile feelings toward the child, are common themes. Parents may withhold such disclosures in the presence of children, while therapists may be forced to similarly restrict the scope of the interview when such expressions intensify. We therefore recommend scheduling the initial assessment interview with parents alone, in order to allow for the full expression and exploration of the issues impacting on the family, and the planning of future contacts as an adult team. There can be important benefits to including older children and adolescents in the initial assessment session; however, this is generally most advantageous within a session structure that permits the therapist to build relationships with the adolescent and his/her parents separately (eg, dividing the session to accommodate one-on-one time with respective subsystems). We recommend not proceeding to more formal assessments of parenting and family dynamics until open and trusting relationships have been established with relevant parents and caregivers.

Establishing Shared Therapeutic Goals with Parents

Parents who feel forced into a particular intervention, or disagree with the goals upon which it is focused, will be unlikely to comply with therapist recommendations. Likewise, parents who do not understand how the goals and components of an intervention relate to the causes of a child problem will often lack the motivation to work on them. Rather, the therapeutic goals that are most likely to be achieved in parenting interventions are those that are shared by therapists and parents, and emerge from a shared perception and conceptualization of the problem. The building of such a perception represents a central aim of the consultation models that is recommended here, and can be facilitated using a number of strategies (Dadds & Hawes, 2006; Sanders & Dadds, 1993).

Clinicians often first explore issues related to parenting and family functioning in the course of an initial interview that also addresses a range of topics more directly related to the referred child (eg, dimensions of the presenting problem, developmental and treatment history, social and academic functioning). The successful investigation of parent-focused issues in this interview often relies on effective strategies for managing these respective child and parent foci in relation to one another. The strategies that are most likely to facilitate a shared perception of the child problem at this stage are those that shift parents away from definitions of the presenting problem as simply a child issue, toward a perspective that allows this problem to be considered alongside other issues in the family and their own lives. This is reflected by the structure of the initial interview recommended by Dadds and Hawes (2006), within which an initial focus on the child's presenting problem gradually expands to encompass issues of importance to the broader family system. As such, careful attention is paid to the order in which topics are raised, and the management of transitions between these topics.

The various issues that may be adversely impacting on a family system represent an essential, yet challenging focus within the parent interview. Included here are issues related to parents' mental health and substance use, social support, feelings and attributions about the parent–child relationship, family history of mental health problems, and distress or violence in the marital relationship. These issues may be sensitive, highly emotional, or frightening—both to parents and therapists alike. They can also be the issues that carry the most critical implications for the planning and delivery of family-based interventions with complex cases. The likelihood that parents will be receptive to the assessment of these issues can be maximized by a number of steps taken prior to, and during, this component of the interview. First and foremost, we advise that inquiries about other problems or stressors in the family are initiated only after parents' presenting concerns about the child have been adequately addressed. Doing so reflects a basic respect for those concerns, while at the same time allowing elementary rapport to be established before more sensitive issues are broached. In our assessment model the focus on these issues is therefore reserved for the final topic of the interview.

III. INTERVENTIONS AND TREATMENTS

Second, the manner in which this component of the interview is introduced to parents can be an important factor in their willingness to shift the focus of discussion from the referred child to their own lives. Parents are often not expecting to be faced with personal questions of this kind when seeking help for their child, and may react adversely when caught off guard. The smooth transition to this focus can be facilitated by first summarizing the child-focused information gathered up to this point, and providing a plain-language rationale for turning to issues in the broader family system (eg, "With my questions today I've been trying to build a complete picture about Nicholas' difficulties and his life in general, which is what will allow me to work out the best way that I can help. As part of this I was also hoping to also ask some standard questions about yourselves and family life more generally, so I can really understand the big picture of what's important. Is that alright with you?"). We make it a rule to explicitly ask parents' permission to proceed at this point—a gesture that should not be underestimated.

Third, by structuring the order in which these issues are raised, it is possible to confront those more sensitive issues most gradually. Although the specific parent and family issues addressed in such an interview may vary depending on the nature of the referral and the clinical setting, we recommend always proceeding from the least to most potentially threatening. The flow of this discussion can also be facilitated by organizing these issues around related domains. We typically begin with parents' physical health (eg, any recent or current illnesses or medical conditions), which follows naturally onto parent's mental health (eg, stress, mood problems, coping strategies) and in turn social support and quality of life (eg, availability of social networks, pleasant events outside of the parenting role). This is typically followed by questions pertaining to parents' relationships in the family, beginning with the parent–child relationship. This can commence with inquiries into how the parent's time with the child is spent, and the parent's role in relation to various caregiver duties, before moving onto the parents' feelings and attributions about the child and the presenting problem. Broader relationships in the family may then be explored, in particular the parents' own relationship, and the child's relationships with significant others. It is important to also invite parents to identify any additional issues that may qualify as stressors in the family, such as financial strain, problematic work schedules, or difficulties related to broader social contexts (eg, interference from relatives, neighborhood safety).

Fourth, when exploring these issues in an interview attended by multiple parents or caregivers, it is important that each is able to respond to these questions without interruption. Given the nature of these issues, the comments provided by one parent can at times evoke strong responses from the other. While the discussion of such responses can be important to the aim of forming a shared perception of the problem, it is not generally compatible with eliciting necessary details about these issues. Our strategy for facilitating this questioning is to set up a process, whereby the respective sequence of issues is addressed with each parent in turn. This can be introduced with a simple rationale and invitation (eg, "To help me keep track of the things that may be important for me to know, I would like to ask these next questions first to one of you and then the other. Who would like to go first?"). Any interruptions from the other parent can then be dealt with through reminders that they will soon have their chance to comment, and while appealing for their patience as firmly as necessary.

Unique sensitivities related to the parent–child relationship warrant distinct interviewing strategies. From a clinical perspective, parents' cognitive attributions about their child and the meaning of the presenting problem represent a critical aspect of the parent–child relationship; one that is associated with risk for both externalizing and internalizing disorders (Chen, Johnston, Sheeber, & Leve, 2009; Dadds, Mullins, McAllister, & Atkinson, 2003). These attributions may include ideas that a child's behavior/emotion is intentional and under the child's control, is designed to deliberately upset the parent, is a sign of serious mental problems, is inherited from other (disliked) family members (eg, an abusive ex-spouse) or is in some way a punishment that the parent deserves. Parent attributions may be directly incompatible with the assumptions of the respective treatment model (eg, expectations that exposure to anxiety-provoking stimuli will cause the child harm). These attributions may also be associated with intense emotion, including explosive anger in reaction to provocative child behavior, and intense guilt following impulses of rejection and resentment toward the child. The intensity of such emotion can easily "flood" a parents' capacity to manage child behavior and emotion effectively, and overwhelm their attempts to initiate and maintain change (Mence et al., 2014; Snyder, Edwards, McGraw, Kilgore, & Holton, 1994).

Therapy may later target such attributions through various means; however, the critical process at the initial assessment stage is often to help parents to make these thoughts explicit. This can usually be done using a line of questioning that begins with direct, open-ended, inquiries (eg, "How would you describe your feelings toward Oscar at the moment?"), and progresses to close-ended questions oriented toward the parents' distress (eg, "How did you feel the last time he really tried to hurt you?", "In those moments when you are really struggling with Oscar's behavior, how bad does it get?", "What is the worst thought that you have had at that time?", "What is your greatest fear about Oscar's behavior?", "In your darkest moments, what do you think is happening with Oscar?"). The rationale for actively eliciting parent cognitions in this way does not simply concern the collection of important parenting data but also the therapeutic gains associated with expressing these largely unspoken ideas. We advise against attempts to challenge the irrational cognitions of parents at this point, which may be counter-therapeutic. It is usually more appropriate that the fears and concerns presented by parents are simply responded to empathically, normalized, and explored openly. As suggested by Scott and Dadds (2009), the most appropriate way to conclude a discussion of these attributions may be with a simple acknowledgment of their importance (eg, "OK, so let's keep an eye on how you are doing with these thoughts and feelings).

Collaborative Formulation and Treatment Planning

Many issues of resistance and poor engagement in parenting interventions can be traced back to a breakdown in the clinical processes that mark the transition from the assessment phase to the formal commencement of treatment. It is now well-recognized that parenting interventions are most effective when they emphasize therapist–parent collaboration; however, this collaboration can easily be undermined by failure to empower parents to make their own decisions about treatment. When clinical recommendations are presented to parents during the course of initial assessment, or therapists drift from assessment to treatment without distinguishing between these distinct stages, parents may be denied the opportunity to make an explicit decision to participate in that treatment. The active and cooperative participation of parents in the therapeutic process often relies on parents first having a sufficient opportunity to make such a decision, and doing so based on a clear understanding of assessment findings and their implications for treatment.

Sanders and Dadds (1993) outlined a guided participation model for communicating assessment results that is well-suited to parenting interventions. The therapist begins by outlining the specific types of data (eg, interview, questionnaire, observation) that were gathered from the various informants involved in the assessment (eg, mother, father, teacher, child). Each source of data is then shared, with the therapist checking for the parent's understanding and reactions before moving on to the next. Care is taken to avoid jargon and technical terms, and to encourage parents to ask questions and express any concerns about the meaning or integrity of the results. It is important that adequate attention is also given to the emotional impact of assessment results that may be distressing for parents to hear. Parents may be most receptive to receiving such results when they are presented in a sequence that prioritizes the information that they themselves have provided, and addresses the results that are likely to be least unexpected before progressing to those that may be more confronting or controversial. The therapist then presents a concise summary that integrates the overall assessment results, and checks for parent agreement with the conclusions suggested therein. These simple steps are often highly effective in promoting a shared conceptualization of a presenting problem, and facilitating collaborative treatment planning when implemented following the completion of initial assessment.

PARENTING PROGRAMS AND EXTERNALIZING PROBLEMS

Parenting interventions are recommended as a first-line intervention for conduct problems in children aged 3 to 11 years, and numerous programs meet the criteria by which "well-established" interventions are typically defined (NICE, 2013). These parent training programs typically commence with skills-training to increase positive reinforcement of desirable child behavior, followed by discipline-focused components in which parents are trained to use consistent, nonforceful consequences (eg, time-out) to set limits on negative behavior. Research examining the mechanisms through which such interventions operate has found child outcomes to be accounted for both by reductions in harsh/inconsistent parenting, and increases in positive parenting practices (Beauchaine, Webster-Stratton, & Reid, 2005; Brotman et al., 2009; Hawes & Dadds, 2006). Three of the most widely disseminated of these are the Triple P: Positive Parenting Program (Triple P) (Sanders, 2012), Incredible Years (Webster-Stratton & Reid, 2003), and Parent–Child Interaction Therapy (PCIT) (Brinkmeyer & Eyberg, 2003; McNeil & Hembree-Kigin, 2010).

Triple P (Sanders, 2012) is a multilevel treatment system comprising five levels of intensity that correspond to the severity of a child's conduct problems and the complexity of family's needs. Standard Triple P (Level 4), is a parent training program delivered in group, individual, and self-directed formats, in up to 12 sessions by mental health practitioners. Parents are trained in the use of 17 parenting skills (eg, talking with children, physical affection, attention, setting limits, planned ignoring) designed to increase positive child behaviors and decrease negative child behaviors, as well as strategies (planned activities training) to increase generalization of treatment effects to a broad range of settings. Enhanced Triple P (Level 5) builds on this by incorporating additional components that target systemic stressors such as parent depression and marital problems, and may include home visits to enhance skill implementation. A major review of treatment outcome data demonstrating durable and generalized gains resulting from Triple-P was recently reported by Sanders (2012).

The Incredible Years (IY) group format intervention (see Bywater, 2012; Webster-Stratton & Reid, 2003) utilizes a collaborative model of parental engagement to enhance positive parent–child relationships through the modeling and rehearsal of reward/praise and discipline techniques (eg, effective commands, logical consequences, time-out). Parents are also taught how to teach problem-solving skills to their children. IY comprises three linked programs for children, parents, and teachers, with the parent program's structured curriculum delivered to small groups of parents/caregivers (of children aged 0 to 12 years) by two facilitators over

4 to 18 weeks (2 h/week). Brief videotape vignettes demonstrating social learning and child development principles are used extensively throughout skills training. Significant long-term reductions in child conduct problems have been reported in multiagency randomized-controlled trials of the intervention (Bywater et al., 2009; McGilloway et al., 2012).

PCIT (Brinkmeyer & Eyberg, 2003; McNeil & Hembree-Kigin, 2010) is another widely disseminated parent training program for young children (aged 2 to 7 years) with conduct problems. Therapists coach the parents via an ear-piece—usually from behind a one-way mirror—as they interact with their child during the treatment sessions, teaching them to apply skills in the clinic until they achieve competency and are deemed ready to implement them on their own. Families meet for weekly 1-hour sessions for an average of 12 to 16 weeks, during which they are trained in two basic interaction patterns. These comprise an initial "child-directed interaction" phase in which parents learn specific positive attention skills (eg, labeled praises), and a subsequent "parent-directed interaction" phase in which parents learn and practice giving clear instructions and implementing time-out during in vivo discipline situations. The effectiveness of PCIT in reducing childhood conduct problems has been characterized by large effect sizes in *meta*-analytic research (Thomas & Zimmer-Gembeck, 2007). A number of other evidence-based programs for use with this younger age-group have been widely disseminated and form the basis for ongoing research into treatment innovations, including the Parent Management Training Oregon Model (PMTO) (Patterson, Reid, Jones, & Conger, 1975), Helping the Noncompliant Child (McMahon & Forehand, 2003), and Integrated Family Intervention (Dadds & Hawes, 2006).

The most effective interventions for conduct problems in late childhood and adolescence are those that combine parent training components with child-focused skills training targeting social-cognitive deficits related to emotion regulation and social problem-solving (eg, Multisystemic Therapy). The effects of such interventions are likewise mediated in part by changes in parenting practices, thereby emphasizing the importance of parenting mechanisms to child adjustment across both childhood and adolescence (Dekovic et al., 2012). Three such treatments that can be considered well-established are Multisystemic Therapy (Henggeler & Lee, 2003), Functional Family Therapy (Sexton & Alexander, 1999), and Multidimensional Treatment Foster Care (Chamberlain & Smith, 2003).

Improving Interventions for Externalizing Problems

Parenting interventions based on coercion theory have been shown to benefit the majority of children with conduct problems; however, the effect sizes associated with these interventions are often small. For example, meta-analytic research has indicated that parent training interventions are associated with a mean effect size of only 0.47 (range from 1.68 to −0.06) (McCart, Priester, Davies, & Azen, 2006). Efforts to enhance these benefits have taken various forms, based on the recognition that multiple theoretical perspectives are needed to account for the synergistic processes that shape child outcomes within the family. For examples, the unique dynamics that characterize the attachment system help to explain some child behavior that social learning principles cannot, such as why some children seem driven to elicit potentially harmful attention from parents, and why parent attention is so powerful a reinforcer at particular ages (Greenberg, Speltz, & DeKlyen, 1993). This perspective has informed parent training programs such as that created by Dadds and Hawes (2006), which aims not simply to improve attachment security, but to act on operant mechanisms in the family using strategies that are compatible with concurrent attachment dynamics. This includes maximizing parents' use of contingent reinforcement strategies that emphasize caregiver emotion and proximity, and training them to implement limit-setting strategies (eg, time-out) in ways that do not inadvertently threaten attachment security.

Poor response to parenting interventions for conduct problems has been associated with a range of social adversity factors that may interfere with families' implementation of treatment strategies and engagement with clinical services. These include socioeconomic disadvantage, minority group status, younger maternal age, and parental psychopathology (Beauchaine et al., 2005; Gardner, Hutchings, Bywater, & Whitaker, 2010; Lundahl, Risser, & Lovejoy, 2006; Reyno & McGrath, 2006). More recently, however, the notion that child characteristics may contribute to individual differences in treatment response has received growing attention. Most notably, there is now considerable evidence that poor response to such interventions is more likely to be seen among children with callous-unemotional (CU) traits (eg, lack of guilt and empathy), compared to those without such traits (eg, Hawes & Dadds, 2005b).

The development of parenting interventions that target the unique needs of children with conduct problems and CU traits has become a significant focus of emerging research. This work has been informed by models of the neurocognitive deficits that characterize these children, with evidence indicating that children with CU traits show deficits in the allocation of attention to emotional cues including the eyes of attachment figures (Dadds et al., 2012, 2014). As outlined by Hawes, Price, and Dadds (2014), a multisite program of clinical research is currently underway to develop and evaluate adjunctive treatment components that target precise aspects of parent–child emotional engagement (eg, eye contact) in the families of these children, and can be delivered alongside core components of social learning–based parenting interventions.

PARENTING INTERVENTIONS FOR INTERNALIZING PROBLEMS

The most established family-based interventions for childhood internalizing problems are for anxiety, and among these, the strongest evidence base can be seen for cognitive behavioral therapy (CBT) interventions (Connolly & Bernstein, 2007). Current CBT interventions are derived largely from Kendall's (1994) "Coping Cat" program, and have been informed by current evidence regarding the role of parent factors and family process in the development and maintenance of anxiety. The balance of parent and child-focused content differs from protocol to protocol, with child-focused, parent-focused, and family-based CBT programs available. The nature and extent of parental involvement generally reflects the child's developmental level, with parent-focused programs directed at young children (2 to 8 years), and child-focused programs featuring no or minimal parent involvement directed at older children and adolescents. The content of CBT programs for child anxiety varies, but typically includes psychoeducation covering the nature of anxiety, the framework and rationale for CBT, and familial processes implicated in the etiology and maintenance of child anxiety. Parents give their child support when learning skills (eg, cognitive restructuring) and concepts (eg, the link between thoughts, feelings, physical/somatic symptoms and behavior), the implementation of strategies (eg, graded exposure), completion of homework activities, and relapse prevention.

Family-based CBT also includes components that specifically target family factors (Wei & Kendall, 2014). Parent training involves the identification of unhelpful parenting practices such as overinvolvement, rejection, and overprotection. Parents are encouraged to replace these practices with problem-solving, graded exposure, and cognitive restructuring to support their child to develop these same coping skills. Parent modeling of coping emphasizes the importance of modeling effective coping strategies when faced with anxiety-provoking situations themselves. Contingency management involves explanation of behavioral/learning theories, emphasizing the removal of parent responses that reinforce anxious behaviors, instead instructing parents to encourage their children to face their fears, often through the use of praise and rewards. Collaborative problem-solving aims to help parents and children deal with challenging situations by learning a shared step-by-step process (ie, defining the problem, brainstorming solutions, evaluating proposed solutions, and selecting the one with the greatest likelihood of success). Communication skills training involves replacing unhelpful parent behaviors such as interrupting and criticizing with active listening, praise, and expression of positive emotions. Finally, parental anxiety management aims to reduce parent anxiety using CBT strategies (eg, cognitive restructuring, graded exposure).

The role of the parent may differ somewhat across these programs. Some view the therapist and parents as forming an expert collaborative team (Barrett, Dadds, & Rapee, 1996), while others view parents as "co-clients", with parental difficulties such as parent anxiety addressed within treatment (Breinholst, Esbjørn, Reinholdt-Dunne, & Stallard, 2012). Some family-based programs place an emphasis on "transfer of control" (Ginsburg et al., 1995), a process that involves the gradual transfer of knowledge and skills from therapist to parent, and then from parent to child (Thirlwall et al., 2013). This is a major benefit of family CBT, as parents can support their child to successfully implement strategies following the completion of therapy. Indeed, family-based CBT that aims to change child behavior via contingency management or transfer of control appears to offer superior long-term gains (Manassis et al., 2014).

Improving Interventions for Internalizing Problems

CBT interventions can be regarded as an effective treatment for childhood anxiety disorders, with an average of 60 percent of children anxiety diagnosis-free following treatment (James, James, Cowdrey, Soler, & Choke, 2013). Treatment gains appear to be achieved and maintained irrespective of the presence of comorbid mood or externalizing disorders (Benjamin, Harrison, Settipani, Brodman, & Kendall, 2013). Importantly, however, the parenting processes that contribute to child anxiety are exacerbated when parents are anxious themselves (Murray, Creswell, & Cooper, 2009), and can be problematic for parents' implementation of CBT strategies. For example, anxious parents may find it challenging to watch their children face feared situations and thus avoid planning and implementing exposure tasks. They may display anxiety during exposure, reinforcing their child's belief that the situation is unsafe and he or she is unable to cope. Not surprisingly, parental anxiety is associated with poor treatment response in anxious children (Hudson et al., 2014). Interestingly, however, Creswell, Willetts, Murray, Singhal and Cooper (2008) found that the effective treatment of parent anxiety did not modify parenting behaviors known to increase the risk for anxiety in children. This suggests that even when parent anxiety is successfully treated, parent anxiety management and CBT programs need to specifically target parenting practices characteristic of anxious parents that serve to maintain child anxiety (eg, parent overinvolvement).

Furthermore, despite a clear rationale for parental involvement, meta-analyses indicate that studies have failed to demonstrate an advantage of family/parent CBT for child anxiety compared to child-focused CBT (Reynolds, Wilson, Austin, & Hooper, 2012). However, concluding that parental involvement does not produce an added benefit would be pre-emptive given that programs vary considerably in the nature and extent of parental involvement, program content, and delivery format. When and how to include parents may depend on additional factors, including child (age, gender, presenting problem) and family/parent factors (parent psychopathology, parent–child conflict). Parent factors are rarely assessed in trials, making it difficult to determine if treatment was successful in changing parenting practices, and if so, how these changes relate to treatment outcomes (Breinholst et al., 2012). Wei and Kendall (2014) proposed a targeted approach that provides guidance on when, how, and under what circumstances to involve parents in treatment. In this implementation model, parent involvement is indicated when parent anxiety, maladaptive parenting, and/or parent–child conflict is present. This model serves as a guideline for much needed future research to answer the question of "what works best for whom" with regard to parent involvement in interventions for child anxiety.

CONCLUSIONS

Child development and psychopathology are highly embedded in the dynamics that play out in the parent–child relationship. The interventions that are most likely to produce durable improvements for children and their families are therefore those that impact on these dynamics, particularly when delivered early in childhood. Much progress has been made in the evaluation and dissemination of evidence-based parenting programs in recent years, most notably for conduct problems and anxiety disorders. However, the effective care of clinic-referred families often calls for professional capacities that extend well beyond the immediate contents of manualized programs, especially when dealing with highly distressed and multiproblem families. Indeed, many clinicians working in community settings find that the outcomes achieved in their own practice fall short of those promised in the literature. In our view, optimal outcomes often rely not only on access to evidence-based programs but also on a clinician's capacity to formulate child problems according to valid family-based models of psychopathology, and to apply effective consultation strategies to engage parents in the earliest stages of assessment and treatment planning (Hawes & Dadds, 2013). We would argue that the integration of these aspects of clinical practice should be regarded as a key priority for such therapists, and for the systems through which these therapists receive professional training and support.

References

Barber, B. K. (1996). Parental psychological control: revisiting a neglected construct. *Child Development*, *67*, 3296–3319. http://dx.doi.org/10.1111/j.1467-8624.1996.tb01915.x.
Barrett, P., Dadds, M., & Rapee, R. (1996). Family treatment of childhood anxiety: a controlled trial. *Journal of Consulting and Clinical Psychology*, *64*(2), 333–342.

Beauchaine, T. P., Webster-Stratton, C., & Reid, M. J. (2005). Mediators, moderators, and predictors of 1-year outcomes among children treated for early-onset conduct problems: a latent growth curve analysis. *Journal of Consulting and Clinical Psychology, 73,* 371–388. http://dx.doi.org/10.1037/0022-006X.73.3.371.

Benjamin, C. L., Harrison, J. P., Settipani, C. A., Brodman, D. M., & Kendall, P. C. (2013). Anxiety and related outcomes in young adults 7 to 19 years after receiving treatment for child anxiety. *Journal of Consulting and Clinical Psychology, 81*(5), 865–876.

Breinholst, S., Esbjørn, B. H., Reinholdt-Dunne, M. L., & Stallard, P. (2012). CBT for the treatment of child anxiety disorders: a review of why parental involvement has not enhanced outcomes. *Journal of Anxiety Disorders, 26*(3), 416–424.

Brinkmeyer, M., & Eyberg, S. M. (2003). Parent-child interaction therapy for oppositional children. In A. E. Kazdin, & J. R. Weisz (Eds.), *Evidence-based psychotherapies for children and adolescents* (pp. 204–223). New York: Guildford.

Brotman, L. M., O'Neal, C. R., Huang, K. Y., Gouley, K. K., Rosenfelt, A., & Shrout, P. E. (2009). An experimental test of parenting practices as a mediator of early childhood physical aggression. *Journal of Child Psychology and Psychiatry, 50,* 235–245. http://dx.doi.org/10.1111/j.1469-7610.2008.01929.x.

Bywater, T. J. (2012). Perspectives on the incredible years programme psychological management of conduct disorder. *British Journal of Psychiatry, 201,* 85–87. http://dx.doi.org/10.1192/bjp.bp.111.107920.

Bywater, T. J., Hutchings, J., Daley, D., Whitaker, C., Yeo, S. T., Jones, K., … Edwards, R. T. (2009). Long-term effectiveness of parenting intervention for children at risk of developing conduct disorder. *British Journal of Psychiatry, 195,* 318–324. http://dx.doi.org/10.1192/bjp.bp.108.056531.

Cartwright-Hatton, S., McNally, D., Field, A. P., Rust, S., Laskey, B., Dixon, C., … Woodham, A. (2011). A new parenting-based group intervention for young anxious children: results of a randomised controlled trial. *Journal of the American Academy of Child and Adolescent Psychiatry, 50,* 242–251. http://dx.doi.org/10.1016/j.jaac.2010.12.015.

Chamberlain, P., & Smith, D. K. (2003). Antisocial behavior in children and adolescents: the Oregon Multidimensional Treatment Foster Care model. In A. E. Kazdin, & J. R. Weisz (Eds.), *Evidence-based psychotherapies for children and adolescents* (pp. 282–300). New York: Guildford Press.

Chen, M., Johnston, C., Sheeber, L., & Leve, C. (2009). Parent and adolescent depression: the role of parental attributions. *Journal of Abnormal Child Psychology, 37,* 119–130. http://dx.doi.org/10.1007/s10802-008-9264-2.

Connolly, S. D., & Bernstein, G. A. (2007). Practice parameter for the assessment and treatment of children and adolescents with anxiety disorders. *Journal of the American Academy of Child and Adolescent Psychiatry, 46*(2), 267–283.

Creswell, C., Willetts, L., Murray, L., Singhal, M., & Cooper, P. (2008). Treatment of child anxiety: an exploratory study of the role of maternal anxiety and behaviours in treatment outcome. *Clinical Psychology and Psychotherapy, 15,* 38–44.

Dadds, M., Allen, J., McGregor, K., Woolgar, M., Viding, E., & Scott, S. (2014). Callous-unemotional traits in children and mechanisms of impaired eye contact during expressions of love: a treatment target? *Journal of Child Psychology and Psychiatry, 55*(7), 771–780.

Dadds, M. R., Allen, J. L., Oliver, B. R., Faulkner, N., Legge, K., Moul, C., … Scott, S. (2012). Love, eye contact, and the developmental origins of empathy versus psychopathy. *British Journal of Psychiatry, 200,* 191–196.

Dadds, M. R., & Hawes, D. J. (2006). *Integrated family intervention for child conduct problems.* Brisbane, Queensland: Australian Academic Press.

Dadds, M. R., Moul, C., Hawes, D. J., Mendoza Diaz, A., & Brennan, J. (2015). Individual differences in childhood behavior disorders associated with epigenetic modulation of the cortisol receptor gene. *Child Development, 86*(5), 1311–1320.

Dadds, M. R., Mullins, M. J., McAllister, R. A., & Atkinson, E. (2003). Attributions, affect, and behavior in abuse-risk mothers: a laboratory study. *Child Abuse and Neglect, 27,* 21–45.

Dadds, M. R., & Roth, J. H. (2001). Family processes in the development of anxiety problems. In M. W. Vasey, & M. R. Dadds (Eds.), *The developmental psychopathology of anxiety* (pp. 75–81). London: Oxford University Press.

Deković, M., Asscher, J. J., Manders, W. A., Prins, P. J. M., & van der Laan, P. (2012). Within-intervention change: mediators of intervention effects during multisystemic therapy. *Journal of Consulting and Clinical Psychology, 80,* 574–587. http://dx.doi.org/10.1037/a0028482.

Dishion, T. J., & Kavanagh, K. (2003). *Intervening in adolescent problem behaviour: A family centered approach.* New York: Guildford.

Dishion, T. J., & Patterson, G. R. (2006). The development and ecology of antisocial behavior. In D. Cicchetti, & D. J. Cohen (Eds.), *Developmental psychopathology: Vol. 3. Risk, disorder, and adaptation* (2nd ed., pp. 503–541). Hoboken, NJ: Wiley.

Fay-Stammbach, T., Hawes, D. J., & Meredith, P. (2014). Parenting influences on executive function in early childhood: a review. *Child Development Perspectives, 8,* 258–264. http://dx.doi.org/10.1111/cdep.12095.

Gardner, F., Hutchings, J., Bywater, T., & Whitaker, C. (2010). Who benefits and how does it work? Moderators and mediators of outcome in an effectiveness trial of a parenting intervention. *Journal of Clinical Child and Adolescent Psychology, 39*(4), 568–580.

Geffken, G. R., Keeley, M., Kellison, I., Storch, E. A., & Rodrigue, J. R. (2006). Parental adherence to child psychologists' recommendations from psychological testing. *Professional Psychology: Research and Practice, 37,* 499–505. http://dx.doi.org/10.1037/0735-7028.37.5.499.

Ginsburg, G. S., Silverman, W. K., & Kurtines, W. K. (1995). Family involvement in treating children with phobic and anxiety disorders: a look ahead. *Clinical Psychology Review, 15,* 457–473.

Greenberg, M. T., Speltz, M. L., & DeKlyen, M. (1993). The role of attachment in the early development of disruptive behavior problems. *Development and Psychopathology, 5,* 191–213.

Green, S. M., Loeber, R., & Lahey, B. B. (1992). Child psychopathology and deviant family hierarchies. *Journal of Child and Family Studies, 1,* 341–349.

Hawes, D. J., & Dadds, M. R. (2005a). Oppositional and conduct problems. In J. Hudson, & R. Rapee (Eds.), *Current thinking on psychopathology and the family* (pp. 73–91). New York: Elsevier.

Hawes, D. J., & Dadds, M. R. (2005b). The treatment of conduct problems in children with callous-unemotional traits. *Journal of Consulting and Clinical Psychology, 73*(4), 737–741.

Hawes, D. J., & Dadds, M. R. (2006). Assessing parenting practices through parent-report and direct observation during parent-training. *Journal of Child and Family Studies, 15,* 554–567. http://dx.doi.org/10.1007/s10826-006-9029-x.

Hawes, D. J., & Dadds, M. R. (2013). Parent and family assessment strategies. In B. D. McLeod, A. Jensen-Doss, & T. Ollendick (Eds.), *Handbook of child and adolescent diagnostic and behavioral assessment* (pp. 316–347). New York: Guilford Press.

Hawes, D. J., Dadds, M. R., Frost, A. D. J., & Russell, A. (2013). Parenting practices and prospective levels of hyperactivity/inattention across early- and middle-childhood. *Journal of Psychopathology and Behavioral Assessment, 35*(3), 273–282.

Hawes, D. J., Price, M. J., & Dadds, M. R. (2014). Callous-unemotional traits and the treatment of conduct problems in childhood and adolescence: a comprehensive review. *Clinical Child and Family Psychology Review, 17*(3), 248–267.

Henggeler, S. W., & Lee, T. (2003). Multisystemic treatment of serious clinical problems. In A. E. Kazdin, & J. R. Weisz (Eds.), *Evidence-based psychotherapies for children and adolescents* (pp. 301–322). New York: Guilford Press.

Henggeler, S. W., & Sheidow, A. J. (2012). Empirically supported family-based treatments for conduct disorder and delinquency in adolescents. *Journal of Marital and Family Therapy, 38*(1), 30–58.

Hudson, J. L., Newall, C., Rapee, R. M., Lyneham, H. J., Schniering, C. C., Wuthrich, V. M., … Gar, N. S. (2014). The impact of brief parental anxiety management on child anxiety treatment outcomes: a controlled trial. *Journal of Clinical Child and Adolescent Psychology, 43*(3), 370–380.

James, A. C., James, G., Cowdrey, F. A., Soler, A., & Choke, A. (2013). Cognitive behavioural therapy for anxiety disorders in children and adolescents. *Cochrane Database of Systematic Reviews* (6):CD004690. http://dx.doi.org/10.1002/14651858.CD004690.pub3.

Kendall, P. C. (1994). Treating anxiety disorders in children: results of a randomised clinical trial. *Journal of Consulting and Clinical Psychology, 65*(3), 724–730.

LaFrenière, P. J., & Dumas, J. E. (1992). A transactional analysis of early childhood anxiety and social withdrawal. *Development and Psychopathology, 4*, 385–402. http://dx.doi.org/10.1017/S0954579400000857.

Levy, F., Hawes, D. J., & Johns, A. (2015). Externalizing and internalizing comorbidity. In T. P. Beauchaine, & S. P. Hinshaw (Eds.), *The Oxford handbook of externalizing spectrum disorders* (pp. 443–460). New York, NY: Oxford University Press.

Lundahl, B., Risser, H., & Lovejoy, M. C. (2006). A meta-analysis of parent training: moderator and follow up effects. *Clinical Psychology Review, 26*, 86–104.

Manassis, K., Lee, T. C., Bennett, K., Zhao, X. Y., Mendlowitz, S., Duda, S., … Wood, J. J. (2014). Types of parental involvement in CBT with anxious youth: a preliminary meta-analysis. *Journal of Consulting and Clinical Psychology, 82*(6), 1163–1172.

McCart, M. R., Priester, P. E., Davies, W. H., & Azen, R. (2006). Differential effectiveness of behavioral parent-training and cognitive-behavioral therapy for antisocial youth: a meta-analysis. *Journal of Abnormal Child Psychology, 34*(4), 527–543. http://dx.doi.org/10.1007/s10802-006-9031-1.

McGilloway, S., Ni Mhaille, G., Bywater, T., Furlong, M., Leckey, Y., Kelly, P., … Donnelly, M. (2012). A parenting intervention for childhood behavioral problems: a randomised controlled trial in disadvantaged community based settings. *Journal of Consulting and Clinical Psychology, 80*, 116–127. http://dx.doi.org/10.1037/a0026304.

McLeod, B. D., Weisz, J. R., & Wood, J. J. (2007). Examining the association between parenting and childhood depression: a meta-analysis. *Clinical Psychology Review, 27*, 986–1003. http://dx.doi.org/10.1016/j.cpr.2007.03.001.

McMahon, R. J., & Forehand, R. (2003). *Helping the noncompliant child: A clinician's guide to effective parent training* (2nd ed.). New York: Guildford.

McNeil, C., & Hembree-Kigin, T. (2010). *Parent-child interaction therapy* (2nd ed.). New York: Springer.

Mence, M., Hawes, D. J., Wedgwood, L., Morgan, S., Barnett, B., Kohlhoff, J., & Hunt, C. (2014). Emotional flooding and hostile discipline in the families of toddlers with disruptive behaviour problems. *Journal of Family Psychology.* http://dx.doi.org/10.1037/a0035352.

Minuchin, S. (1974). *Families and family therapy.* Cambridge, MA: Harvard University Press.

Murray, L., Creswell, C., & Cooper, P. J. (2009). The development of anxiety disorders in childhood: an integrative review. *Psychological Medicine, 39*, 1413–1423.

National Institute for Clinical Excellence. (2013). *Antisocial behavior and conduct disorders in children and young people: Recognition, intervention and management.* Retrieved 1/5/13 from http://nice.org.uk/cg158.

Ollendick, T. H., Costa, N. M., & Benoit, K. E. (2010). Interpersonal processes and the anxiety disorders of childhood. In G. Beck (Ed.), *Interpersonal processes in the anxiety disorders: Implications for understanding psychopathology and treatment* (pp. 71–95). Washington, DC: APA Books.

Patterson, G. R., & Fisher, P. A. (2002). Recent developments in our understanding of parenting: birdirectional effects, causal models, and the search for parsimony. In M. H. Bornstein (Ed.), *Handbook of parenting: Vol. 5. Practical issues in parenting* (pp. 59–88). Mahwah, NJ: Erlbaum.

Patterson, G. R., Reid, J. B., Jones, R. R., & Conger, R. E. (1975). *A social learning approach to family intervention*. Eugene, OR: Castalia Publishing.

Rapee, R. M., Schniering, C. A., & Hudson, J. L. (2009). Anxiety disorders during childhood and adolescence: origins and treatment. *Annual Review of Clinical Psychology, 5*, 335–365. http://dx.doi.org/10.1146/annurev.clinpsy.032408.153628.

Reyno, S., & McGrath, P. (2006). Predictors of parent training efficacy for child externalizing behaviour problems: a meta-analytic review. *Journal of Child Psychology and Psychiatry, 47*, 99–111.

Reynolds, S., Wilson, C., Austin, J., & Hooper, L. (2012). Effects of psychotherapy for anxiety in children and adolescents: a meta-analytic review. *Clinical Psychology Review, 32*, 251–262.

Rothbart, M. K., & Posner, M. I. (2006). Temperament, attention, and developmental psychopathology. In D. Cicchetti, & D. J. Cohen (Eds.), *Handbook of developmental psychopathology, revised* (pp. 167–188). New York: Wiley.

Sanders, M. R. (2012). Development, evaluation, and multinational dissemination of the triple P positive parenting program. *Annual Review of Clinical Psychology, 8*, 345–379. http://dx.doi.org/10.1146/annurev-clinpsy-032511-143104.

Sanders, M. R., & Dadds, M. R. (1993). *Behavioral family intervention*. Needham Heights, MA: Allyn & Bacon.

Scott, S., & Dadds, M. R. (2009). Practitioner review: when parent training doesn't work:theory driven clinical strategies. *Journal of Child Psychology and Psychiatry and Allied Disciplines, 50*, 1441–1450. http://dx.doi.org/10.1111/j.1469-7610.2009.02161.x.

Sexton, T. L., & Alexander, J. F. (1999). *Functional family therapy: Principles of clinical intervention, assessment, and implementation*. Henderson, NV: RCH Enterprises.

Shaw, D. S., Criss, M., Schonberg, M., & Beck, J. (2004). Hierarchies and pathways leading to school age conduct problems. *Development and Psychopathology, 16*, 483–500. http://dx.doi.org/10.1017/S0954579404004638.

Snyder, J., Edwards, P., McGraw, K., Kilgore, K., & Holton, A. (1994). Escalation and reinforcement in mother-child conflict: social processes associated with the development of physical aggression. *Development and Psychopathology, 6*, 305–321. http://dx.doi.org/10.1017/S0954579400004600.

Thirlwall, K., Copper, P. J., Karalus, J., Voysey, M., Willetts, L., & Creswell, C. (2013). Treatment of child anxiety disorders via guided parent-delivered cognitive-behavioural therapy: randomised controlled trial. *British Journal of Psychiatry, 203*(6), 436–444. http://dx.doi.org/10.1192/bjp.bp.113.126698.

Thomas, R., & Zimmer-Gembeck, M. J. (2007). Behavioral outcomes of parent-child interaction therapy and triple P—Positive parenting program: a review and meta analysis. *Journal of Abnormal Child Psychology, 35*, 475–495. http://dx.doi.org/10.1007/s10802-007-9104-9.

Webster-Stratton, W., & Reid, M. J. (2003). Treating conduct problems and strengthening social and emotional competence in young children: the dina dinosaur treatment program. *Journal of Emotional and Behavioral Disorders, 11*, 130–146. http://dx.doi.org/10.1177/10634266030110030101.

Wei, C., & Kendall, P. C. (2014). Parental involvement: contribution to childhood anxiety and its treatment. *Clinical Child and Family Psychology Review, 17*(4), 319–339.

Williams, S. R., Kertz, S. J., Schrock, M. D., & Woodruff-Borden, J. (2012). A sequential analysis of parent–child interactions in anxious and nonanxious families. *Journal of Clinical Child and Adolescent Psychology, 41*, 64–74. http://dx.doi.org/10.1080/15374416.2012.632347.

Psychopharmacological Treatment for Depression in Children and Adolescents: Promoting Recovery and Resilience

M.R. Chapman, J.L. Hughes, B.D. Kennard,
T.L. Mayes, G.J. Emslie

UT Southwestern Medical Center, Dallas, TX, United States

INTRODUCTION

Depression is prevalent in youth, with estimates ranging from around 2 percent in childhood to 4 to 8 percent of adolescents (Avenevoli, Swendsen, He, Burstein, & Merikangas, 2015; Birmaher et al., 2007). In fact, large population surveys estimate between 11 and 18 percent of youth will experience a depressive disorder by age 18 (Avenevoli et al., 2015). Rates of depression are similar across gender during childhood; however, subsequent to puberty, females are twice as likely to suffer from depression than males (Birmaher et al., 2007). Clinically, major depressive disorder (MDD) in youth is similar to the adult presentation with a few exceptions; children may experience more irritability, impulsivity, and somatic complaints compared to adolescents and adults, who may present with more suicide attempts and symptoms of melancholy. Adolescents with depression are also at risk for a number of negative outcomes, including suicide attempts and death by suicide, future depressive episodes, substance abuse, early pregnancy, legal problems, and diminished academic and occupational success (Birmaher et al., 2007).

Positive Mental Health, Fighting Stigma and Promoting Resiliency for Children and Adolescents
http://dx.doi.org/10.1016/B978-0-12-804394-3.00011-5

Efficacious evidence-based psychosocial and psychopharmacological treatments are available for depressed youth, but many youth do not receive sufficient treatment. There is often a significant delay, sometimes years, between the onset of mental health symptoms and appropriate care (Wang, Berglund, Olfson, & Kessler, 2004). Few studies in children and adolescents have considered barriers to depression treatment. Wisdom and colleagues found that adolescent report of primary care providers attending to the developmental desires to feel normal, connected, and autonomous was related to more acceptance of treatment and reported success (Walker, Coleman, Lee, Squire, & Friesen, 2008; Wisdom, Clarke, & Green, 2006). For adolescents in the process of developing a mature identity, obtaining a diagnosis of depression or a "mental illness identity" can be quite problematic (Charmaz, 1993). Other potential barriers include: treatment cost, lack of awareness in families or health care providers, and effectiveness of available treatments.

Stigma is one ubiquitously recognized factor that acts as a barrier to receipt, continuity, and good outcomes of mental health care (Link & Phelan, 2001; Link, Phelan, Bresnahan, Stueve, & Pescosolido, 1999; Markowitz, 1998). Peers, family, or society at large may hold public stigma or negative attitudes about mental illness. Internalized stigma or self-stigma occurs when the individual comes to hold these same attitudes that may take the form of fear, avoidance, distrust, and/or bias. Children with depression may in fact be perceived more negatively by their peers than adults with depression, leading to peer exclusion and low social status (Connolly, Geller, Marton, & Kutcher, 1992). Even with appropriate treatment and newly learned behaviors, peers may be slow to change these negative perceptions (Walker et al., 2008). A vicious cycle may begin, such that youth become depressed, experience and internalize stigma, experience avoidance and increased social isolation, and depressive symptoms worsen. Ultimately, the consequence may be avoidance of seeking helpful treatments (Kanter, Rusch, & Brondino, 2008). Teen perceived barriers to care, including stigma and uncertainty about family's response, have been associated with decreased use of treatment, particularly antidepressants (Meredith et al., 2009).

Historically, the focus on treating depression has been on reducing depressive symptoms and promoting remission (or absence of symptoms), however, promoting health and well-being cannot be overlooked as the focus ideally of treatment is to not only achieve the absence of illness but also promote the presence of wellness. This chapter will provide a framework for fighting stigma, enhancing wellness, and promoting resiliency in depressed youth by (1) summarizing the foundation necessary to assess depression and partner with youth and their families, (2) reviewing systematic psychopharmacological treatment strategies, and (3) focusing on achieving wellness, not simply symptom reduction.

SETTING THE STAGE

Depressive disorders in youth have been noted to often be more contextual in nature than in their adult counterparts. As a result, conducting a rigorous assessment and providing thorough education about the illness and treatment alternatives to both the patient and his/her caregiver is a critical component.

Assessment

The diagnostic criteria for youth depression are the same as adult depression; however, the assessment process and presentation in youth differ from adults. Children and adolescents are often brought to treatment by a worried caregiver or at the recommendation of a teacher or other concerned adult, so addressing the youth's understanding of the assessment process, as well as what to expect with regard to recommendations, is vital. Clinicians use multiple informants (including the youth, parents, caregivers, and teachers) to understand the duration and nature of depressive symptoms. Generally, youths more accurately report internalizing symptoms, while caregivers often more accurately report behavioral symptoms. Additionally, younger children also demonstrate difficulty in reporting frequency and duration of symptoms, thus caregiver reports are needed to establish onset dates and course of illness (Herjanic & Reich, 1997; Hope et al., 1999; Jensen et al., 1999). Teachers may also provide useful information about internalizing symptoms, even more so than primary caregivers (Mesman & Koot, 2000).

Depressive disorders are categorized the same across the lifespan. The Diagnostic and Statistical Manual of Mental Disorders—5th edition (DSM-5) includes several diagnoses which fall in the depressive disorders category: major depressive disorder (MDD), persistent depressive disorder (dysthymia), substance/medication-induced depressive disorder, depression due to another medical condition, other specified depressive disorder, unspecified depressive disorder, and two newer diagnoses, disruptive mood dysregulation disorder (DMDD) and premenstrual dysphoric disorder. Both pediatric and adult MDD involve essentially the same symptoms for diagnosis including depressed or irritable mood, anhedonia, sleep and appetite disturbance, worthlessness, guilt, psychomotor disturbance, decreased concentration, decreased energy, and suicidal ideation. One possible exception is the symptom of irritability, as children may present with irritable mood without explicit sadness.

Evaluation of children and adolescents with affective disorders includes a detailed biological family history, including first-, second-, and third-degree relatives. Also, the current mental state of the caregiver is significant, as the child's treatment outcome may be impacted by parental disorders. For example, maternal depression has been shown to impact treatment outcomes in children with depression. In addition to the symptoms detailed in the DSM-5 criteria, depression presents with a variety of other common features. Depressed children have been shown to have negative cognitive functioning, including increased cognitive distortions, negative attributions, hopelessness, and low self-esteem, which is a frequent treatment target and affects treatment outcome (Asarnow & Bates, 1988; Beevers, Keitner, Ryan, & Miller, 2003; Garber & Hilsman, 1992; Garber, Weiss, & Shanley, 1993; Lewinsohn & Clarke, 1999; Marton & Kutcher, 1995). Certain psychosocial difficulties are also common features of depression, including increased school problems (behavior problems, poor academic achievement), social impairment, and poorer family relationships (Hamilton, Asarnow, & Tompson, 1997; Hops, Lewinsohn, Andrews, & Roberts, 1990; Kashani, Burbach, & Rosenberg, 1988; Puig-Antich et al., 1993; Puig-Antich et al., 1985a, 1985b; Strober, Lampert, Schmidt-Lackner, & Morrell, 1993). Additionally, it is important to assess for comorbid psychiatric and general medical conditions, as there are several areas of overlap worth consideration. Various physical health diagnoses are associated with high rates of pediatric depression, including diabetes mellitus, asthma, and neurological conditions. Other disorders can present primarily with depressive symptoms that mimic a primary psychiatric etiology (eg, hypothyroidism and systemic lupus erythematous). Various studies have identified high rates of psychiatric disorders in children and adolescents with neurological conditions (Cantwell, Baker, & Mattison, 1980; Rutter, 1970), including brain injury (Robinson, Boston, Starkstein, & Price, 1988; Robinson & Starkstein, 1990; Starkstein et al., 1990), epilepsy (Barraclough, 1981; Ring & Trimble, 1993; Robertson, 1989; Rutter, Tizard, Yule, Graham, & Whitmore, 1976), migraine headache (Ling, Oftedal, & Weinberg, 1970), and learning disabilities (Brumback & Weinberg, 1990; Emslie, Kennard, & Kowatch, 1995; Livingston, 1985; Weinberg & Rehmet, 1983; Weinberg, Rutman, Sullivan, Penick, & Dietz, 1973). Concurrent psychiatric disorders, including anxiety, disruptive disorders, attention-deficit/hyperactivity disorder, and substance use disorders, occur frequently with depression. Up to half of youth have two or more comorbid diagnoses. In addition to causing increased impairment, comorbid psychiatric disorders can affect treatment outcomes in children and adolescents.

Cultural Considerations

Limited research is available on cultural differences in depression presentation, both across international cultures and in specific ethnic minority groups within cultures. Stewart et al. (2002) found symptomatology similarities and differences between Hong Kong and United States adolescents, with both groups reporting similar prevalence rates of depression. More United States youth reported irritability, whereas Hong Kong youth reported more fatigue (Stewart et al., 2002). Little is known about the difference in the pharmacodynamics and pharmacokinetics of depression across ethnic groups (Stewart, Simmons, & Habibpour, 2012). Ethnic differences in attribution and treatment expectancies in families with depressed adolescents have been examined in a United States sample, with European American parents being more likely to attribute depression to physical causes than African American parents, and African American parents reporting more beliefs that cognitive-behavioral therapy would be helpful than other parents (Jacobs et al., 2008). The underrepresentation of cross-cultural and ethnic minority populations in depression research make it difficult to speak to specific evidence-based diagnostic and treatment guidelines for these youth; however, it is important for clinicians to assess the youth and caregivers' understanding of symptoms and depression, particularly in the context of cultural factors such as ethnicity, level of acculturation into mainstream culture, spiritual beliefs, and values (Stewart et al., 2012). Future research is needed to investigate cultural differences in presentation and understanding of depression, particularly given that perceptions of depression can differ across groups which can lead to additional stigma in some populations.

Screening Instruments

Both diagnostic and severity measures are available for the pediatric age group. Measures vary in length, ranging from semi-structured interviews designed to assess a variety of diagnoses to short, unstructured, and semi-structured interviews specific to depressive symptoms. Self-report screening measures, such as the Patient Health Questionnaire 9—Adolescent (PHQ-9-A) or the Quick Inventory of Depressive Symptomatology—Self-Report-16 (QIDS-SR-16) are useful in identifying youths in need of further evaluation. Ideally, a blend of clinician-rated, and parent- and self-report rating scales are used to diagnose the presence and severity of depression in the pediatric age group. Table 11.1 lists validated measures of depression for children and adolescents.

In sum, the assessment process for identifying depression in children and adolescents often requires considerable clinical acumen to determine (1) present symptoms and course of illness, (2) attribution of symptoms, (3) psychosocial difficulties (both prior to the depressive episode and as a consequence of the depressive episode), (4) primary disorder requiring treatment, (5) secondary or comorbid disorders, and (6) the best course of treatment.

Assessment Feedback and Treatment Planning

Once a depression diagnosis has been made, there are several important factors to address before moving forward in care, such as educating

TABLE 11.1   Rating Scales for Assessing Depression in Youth

Rating scales	Completed by	References
Beck Depression Inventory (BDI)	Child	Beck, Epstein, Brown, and Steer (1988)
Center for Epidemiologic Studies Depression Scale (CESD) and CESD-R	Child	Eaton, Muntaner, Smith, Tien, and Ybarra (2004), Radloff (1977)
Children's Depression Inventory (CDI)	Child	Kovacs (1985)
Children's Depression Rating Scale—Revised (CDRS-R)	Provider	Poznanski and Mokros (1996)
Mood and Feelings Questionnaire (MFQ)	Child, Parent	Daviss et al. (2006)
Patient Health Questionnaire—9 (PHQ-9)	Child	Richardson et al. (2010)
Patient Health Questionnaire—9 Adolescent (PHQ-A)	Child	Johnson, Harris, Spitzer and Williams (2002)
Quick Inventory of Depressive Symptomatology—Adolescent (QIDS-A)	Child, Parent, provider	Moore et al. (2007)
Reynolds Adolescent Depression Scale (RADS) and RADS-2	Child	Osman, Gutierrez, Bagge, Fang, and Emmerich (2010)

the youth and caregivers about depression, discussing treatment options, and addressing child and family concerns. The clinician should provide feedback on the assessment to the youth and caregiver, providing the opportunity for both to ask questions.

Motivational Interviewing

Studies have shown that a motivational interviewing style approach to providing feedback about depression and treatment options is beneficial in linking children to care and even reduced symptoms months later (Hoek et al., 2011; Van Voorhees et al., 2009). While a full presentation of motivational interviewing techniques is out of the scope of this chapter, interested readers are referred to the texts by Miller and Rollnick (2002; 2012) and to the motivational interviewing website (http://www.motivationalinterviewing.org/) for information about trainings. The four key principles of motivational interviewing include: expressing empathy, developing discrepancy, rolling with resistance, and supporting self-efficacy (Miller & Rollnick, 2002). With depressed youth, this style of interaction would be applied by the clinician in order to better understand the youth and caregiver's perspectives about depression and their readiness to address the illness, as well as to foster a collaborative discussion including psycho-education about depression and treatment options.

Motivational interviewing may be particularly useful with depressed youth, given its focus on enhancing motivation, which is often low in youth as a result of the depressive illness and the treatment being sought out by caretakers (Arkowitz & Burke, 2008). Motivational interviewing emphasizes reducing resistance to treatment with the non-directive presentation of suggestions (versus "recommendations"), and the emphasis on the development of a genuine, empathic, and warm therapeutic relationship between the clinician and youth (which has been shown to be particularly important in treating depression). The motivational interviewing style also allows the clinician flexibility to address the youth and families' understanding and attribution of depression while integrating useful education about depression and treatment options, working to help the family tailor an evidence-based treatment plan to their treatment preferences (Brody, 2009).

Psycho-education

Psycho-education is no doubt a vital component of depression treatment, and should include educating the patient and family that depression is an illness, with biological and genetic underpinnings, and that it is treatable. Depression has been called the "common cold" of mental illness, due to high prevalence rates. However, depression is still poorly understood by the general public. One recent campaign in the United States, called the Campaign to Change Direction, which partnered with several important mental health agencies and entities, has called attention to five common signs of mental illness: personality changes, agitation, withdrawal, poor self-care, and hopelessness. Several of the signs are symptoms of depression, and it is the hope of those involved in the campaign that increased knowledge of these symptoms will result in increased recognition and treatment, as well as decreased stigma. Table 11.2 lists useful components to include in psycho-education about depression in children and adolescents.

Additional psycho-education about the course of illness is also helpful. Duration of major depressive episodes varies significantly. In clinically referred youth, the duration of a major depressive episode averages 8 months, while community samples suggest approximately 1- to 2-month episodes (Birmaher et al., 2007). While most youth recover from their first episode of depression, recurrence rates are high. Within 1 to 2 years of remission, 20 to 60 percent experience recurrence, and by 5 years recurrence rates increase to up to 70 percent (Birmaher et al., 2007; Emslie, 2008; Kennard et al., 2009, 2014). Depression impacts every facet of a youth's life, including emotional, social, and cognitive domains, and family relationships. If untreated, significant sequelae include suicide attempts and death by suicide, as well as future depressive episodes in adulthood.

TABLE 11.2   Psycho-education Components

1. Information about the diagnosis, including common signs and symptoms, etiology, pathophysiology, and prognosis. Efforts should be made to individualize this feedback to the youth and family.
2. Information about suicide risk, including youth's current reported suicidal ideation and/or behavior, common warning signs, safety precautions such as increased supervision and lethal means restriction, crisis procedures, and relation to primary diagnosis. It can be helpful to provide the National Suicide Prevention Lifeline (800-273-TALK) to the youth and family.
3. Information about treatment, including general treatment options (including pharmacological, psychotherapeutic, and other psychosocial options), relative benefits and risks of treatment options, including specific medication side effects, drug–drug interactions, and medication administration details. It can be helpful to provide youth and families with handouts about treatments, such as those in MedlinePlus from the U.S. National Library of Medicine, available at http://www.nlm.nih.gov/medlineplus/.
4. Information about the importance of adherence and follow-up in depression treatment.
5. Information about risks specific to antidepressant medications. There are reports of increased suicidal ideation and behaviors in adolescents and young adults taking antidepressants, and the U.S. FDA has issued a black-box warning for all antidepressants recommending close monitoring of all individuals prescribed antidepressants. Youth and families should be aware of possible worsening of depression or increased suicidal thoughts, and should share any thoughts of suicide with the clinician. In addition, families and caregivers of adolescent patients are also encouraged to monitor for the emergence of other symptoms, such as agitation, irritability, unusual changes in behavior, and to report such symptoms immediately to health care providers. Clinicians will remain abreast of regulatory agencies as the field is changing, and integrate that in the treatment and explain the developments to patients.

The clinician can meet with parents to discuss how they can support the depressed youth. Parents can be encouraged to call a truce on "hot topics" or emotionally salient topics at home, as high expressed emotion has been shown to relate to poorer treatment response and increased risk of relapse. Also, the clinician can work with parents to address any preventable stressors as the child progresses in treatment. Finally, parents can support the child's treatment by taking him/her to treatment sessions and following treatment recommendations.

Treatment Planning

Factors to consider in treatment planning include the course and severity of depressive illness, presence of psychosocial difficulties, medical and/or psychiatric comorbidities, family and cultural factors, and caregiver and patient treatment preferences. Youths would likely benefit from referrals for psychotherapeutic intervention, which can be provided by psychologists, social workers, or licensed professional counselors. If the depression is deemed to be moderate to severe, a primary care clinician might begin pharmacological treatment or refer to child psychiatry for specialty care. To date, the combination of pharmacotherapy and psychotherapy, specifically treatment with selective serotonin reuptake inhibitors (SSRIs) and cognitive-behavioral therapy (CBT), appear to be the most efficacious treatment for moderate to severe depression in adolescents (TADS, 2004), though several effective treatment options are available for pediatric depression at this time (for reviews, see Maalouf & Brent, 2012; Sakolsky & Birmaher, 2012; Tompson, Boger, & Asarnow, 2012). The Association for Behavioral and Cognitive Therapies, and the Society of Clinical Child and Adolescent Psychology have developed a useful website for patients, caregivers, and professionals about evidence-based psychosocial mental health interventions (www.effectivechildtherapy.com).

SYSTEMATIC APPROACH TO TREATMENT OF DEPRESSION IN YOUTH

In promoting recovery and resilience, implementing effective treatment strategies to reduce depressive symptoms is a key priority. As noted in the previous section, providing teens and families with education about effective treatment options, potential side effects, and treatment expectations is important prior to beginning treatment. Youth presenting with mild or brief depression that does not significantly impact functioning and is not present with suicidal ideation or psychosis may be managed with complementary treatments, including education, case management, and supportive therapy. Treating moderate to severe pediatric depression, however, requires more specific types of psychotherapy and/or antidepressant medications. There are three phases of treatment to be considered: acute, continuation, and maintenance. Each phase has specific treatment targets, including symptom response/remission (acute), treatment consolidation and relapse prevention (continuation), and reducing the likelihood of recurrence (maintenance). Within this framework, both psychopharmacological and psychosocial treatment strategies should be considered.

Measurement-Based Care

Providers managing depression in youth often overlook use of a measurement-based approach to treatment. However, a measured approach to depression treatment that includes utilization of outcome assessments is one way to more systematically evaluate for symptom response and aid the clinician in treating the depressive episode. Adult literature suggests that these assessments are increasingly recommended as routine clinical care (Trivedi & Daly, 2007). In essence, a patient with hypertension would expect his physician to measure blood pressure at each visit to monitor changes and guide treatment decisions. Similarly, fully assessing all symptoms of depression at each visit is essential. Treatment response should ideally be determined using a combination of clinical assessment and validated tools.

Antidepressant Treatment

Acute Treatment

Current treatment guidelines recommend using SSRIs as first-line antidepressant treatment for youth with depression (Birmaher et al., 2007; Cheung et al., 2007; Hughes et al., 2007). These recommendations are based on antidepressant trials conducted in children and adolescents with MDD (Table 11.3). Of note, no double-blind, placebo-controlled studies have been conducted in youth with other depressive disorders (i.e. dysthymia, depression not otherwise specified (NOS), etc.). A 2007 meta-analysis of 27 randomized controlled trials (RCTs) for MDD in youth showed an average response rate of 61 percent (95% CI, 58–63%) for SSRI antidepressants and 50 percent (95% CI, 47–53%) for placebo. Pooled benefit versus risk differences favored antidepressants for the treatment of MDD with an NNT (number needed to treat) of 10 and NNH (number needed to harm) of 112. Efficacy was moderated by age, duration of depression, and number of sites in the trial. Fluoxetine showed a larger difference between medication and placebo than other antidepressants in children younger than age 12; the only drug to show benefit over placebo (Bridge et al., 2007). To date, fluoxetine is the only antidepressant with an FDA indication for treatment of both children and adolescents (ages 8 years and older) with MDD. Escitalopram has an FDA indication for adolescents (ages 12 years and older) with MDD. No other antidepressants have FDA indication for treatment of depression, although some have indications for other psychiatric conditions.

Once a decision is made to begin antidepressant treatment, additional consideration is needed to select which antidepressant to prescribe and dosing strategies. Most RCTs were conducted without prior dose finding studies in youth, and adult doses were generally used. Typically antidepressants are started at a fairly low dose, and then titrated to the target dose within a few weeks. Tao et al. examined timing of treatment response and found that youth who showed at least 50 percent improvement in their depressive symptoms by the fourth week of treatment were much more likely to achieve remission within 3 months than those who had limited response within the first month (2006). It should also be noted that it is important to have more frequent visits early in treatment and during antidepressant medication dose adjustments to engage the

TABLE 11.3   Antidepressant Randomized-Controlled Trials for Youth with MDD

Antidepressant	Total number of RCTs	Number of positive RCTs	References for RCTs
Citalopram	2	1	Von Knorring, Olsson, Thomsen, Lemming, and Hulten (2006), Wagner et al. (2004)
Escitalopram	2	1	Emslie, Ventura, Korotzer, and Tourkodimitris (2009), Wagner, Jonas, Findling, Ventura, and Saikali (2006)
Fluoxetine	4	3	Emslie et al. (2002); Emslie, Rush, Weinburg, Gullion, et al. (1997), March et al. (2004), Simeon, Dinicola, Ferguson, and Copping (1990)
Paroxetine	3	0	Berard, Fong, Carpenter, Thomason, and Wilkinson (2006), Emslie et al. (2006), Keller et al. (2001)
Sertraline	2	2 (pooled)	Wagner et al. (2003)
Bupropion	None	–	
Desvenlafaxine	1	0	Findling et al. (2014)
Duloxetine	2	0	Atkinson et al. (2014), Emslie et al. (2014)
Levomilnacipran	None	–	
Mirtazapine	2	0	Cheung, Emslie, and Mayes (2005)
Selegiline	1	0	DelBello et al. (2014)
Venlafaxine	2	0	Emslie, Findling, Yeung, Kunz, and Li (2007)
Vilazodone	Underway	–	
Vortioxetine	None	–	

youth in treatment and address any concerns or adverse effects including monitoring for suicidal ideation. Table 11.4 provides dosing information for antidepressants.

Treatment Refractory Depression

As noted, approximately 55 to 65 percent of youth will respond to treatment with an SSRI. However, remission rates are much lower (around 30 to 45 percent). In a review of three large studies examining psychopharmacological and psychosocial treatment, several clinical characteristics were linked to non-response to an antidepressant in all three studies, including

TABLE 11.4   Recommended Antidepressant Initial and Target Dose for Youth with MDD

Medication	Target dose, mg	Contraindications
Citalopram	Initial: 10 Children: 20 to 40 Adolescents: 20 to 40 Max: 40	MAOI use currently or within 2 wks of d/c; current linezolid use; prolonged QT interval
Escitalopram	Initial: 5 to 10 Children: 10 to 20 Adolescents: 10 to 20 Max: 20	MAOI use currently or within 2 wks of d/c; current linezolid use; prolonged QT interval
Fluoxetine	Initial: 10 Children: 20 Adolescents: 20 to 40 Max: 60	MAOI use currently or within 2 wks of d/c; current linezolid use
Paroxetine	Initial: 10 Children: 10 to 30 Adolescents: 20 to 40 Max: 50	MAOI use currently or within 2 wks of d/c; current thioridazine or pimozide use; allergy to peanuts
Sertraline	Initial: 12.5 to 25 Children: 50 to 200 Adolescents: 50 to 200 Max: 200	MAOI use currently or within 2 wks of d/c; current pimozide use
Bupropion	Initial: 100 Children: 150 to 300 Adolescents: 300 Max: 300	MAOI use currently or within 2 wks of d/c; current seizure disorder; CNS tumor; hx of bipolar disorder
Desvenlafaxine	Initial: 50 Children: 50 Adolescents: 50 to 100 Max: 100	MAOI use currently or within 2 wks of d/c
Duloxetine	Initial: 20 BID Children: 30 to 60 Adolescents: 40 to 60 Max: 60	MAOI use currently or within 2 wks of d/c; current fluvoxamine, ciprofloxacin or enoxacin use; severe renal/hepatic impairment
Levomilnacipran	Initial: 20 BID for 2 days then 40 Children: 40 to 120 Adolescents: 40 to 120 Max: 120	MAOI use currently or within 2 wks of d/c
Mirtazapine	Initial: 7.5 to 15 Children: 15 to 45 Adolescents: 15 to 45 Max: 45	MAOI use currently or within 2 wks of d/c

TABLE 11.4   Recommended Antidepressant Initial and Target Dose for Youth with MDD—cont'd

Medication	Target dose, mg	Contraindications
Venlafaxine	Initial: 37.5 Children: 150 to 225 Adolescents: 150 to 225 Max: 300	MAOI use currently or within 2 wks of d/c
Vilazodone	Initial: 10 Children: 15 to 30 Adolescents: 30 to 40 Max: 40	MAOI use currently or within 2 wks of d/c
Vortioxetine	Initial: 10 Children: 20 Adolescents: 20 Max: 20	MAOI use currently or within 2 wks of d/c

more severe depression, poorer functioning, higher rates of suicidal ideation and hopelessness, and comorbid psychiatric conditions, with several other characteristics identified in at least two of the studies (Emslie, Kennard, & Mayes, 2011).

For youth who do not respond to the first SSRI, guidelines recommend treatment with a second SSRI. No non-SSRI antidepressants have demonstrated efficacy for acute MDD, but some appear to be efficacious in anxiety disorders. Therefore, non-SSRIs are considered third line treatment options. Only one study has examined treatment-resistant depression in adolescents; this study found similar improvement rates for a second SSRI or a non-SSRI (venlafaxine), although there was a slightly better adverse event profile with the SSRIs (Brent et al., 2008). As a result of the limited evidence of efficacy and unfavorable side effect profile of tricyclic antidepressants (TCAs), they are also not considered a first-line treatment option. They too might be considered in cases where multiple agents have failed or when other family members have had a positive response.

Antidepressants and Suicidal Ideation

The controversy around increases in suicidal ideation in children and adolescents treated with antidepressants warrants special consideration. As initial reports suggesting increased activation, agitation, and suicidal behavior became available, inconsistency in the process of eliciting these events (spontaneous report) and defining the events (what constitutes a suicide attempt or increased suicidal ideation) became evident. This resulted in the FDA requesting an independent reanalysis of the adverse event data. Even with this reanalysis and the findings that suicidal ideation (not suicide) occurred in 4 percent of children on antidepressants compared with 2 percent on placebo on the basis of a spontaneous report, the prospectively collected rating scales from those studies did not demonstrate any difference in suicidal ideation between active treatment and placebo groups (Bridge et al., 2007; Hammad, Laughren, & Racoosin, 2006). These findings highlight the need to assess possible antidepressant-specific adverse events, side effects, and treatment response on an ongoing basis during acute treatment.

Continuation and Maintenance Treatment

While over 90 percent of children and adolescents recover from an initial episode of MDD within 1 to 2 years of onset (Emslie, Rush, Weinburg, Gullion, et al., 1997; Emslie, Rush, Weinburg, Kowatch, et al., 1997; Kovacs, Feinberg, Crouse-Novak, Paulauskas, & Finkelstein, 1984; Kovacs, Feinberg, Crouse-Novak, Paulauskas, Pollock, et al., 1984; McCauley et al., 1993; Strober, et al., 1993), recurrence rates are high. Factors contributing to recurrence of depression include comorbidity (Birmaher et al., 2000; Brent, Kolko, Birmaher, Baugher, & Bridge, 1999; Kovacs et al., 1984; Vostanis, Feehan, & Grattan, 1998); severity of depression (Birmaher, et al., 2000; Emslie, Rush, Weinburg, Gullion, et al., 1997; Emslie, Rush, Weinburg, Kowatch, et al., 1997); hopelessness (Birmaher, et al., 2000); low self-esteem at baseline and follow-up (Vostanis, et al., 1998); family dysfunction (Asarnow, Tompson, Hamilton, Goldstein, & Guthrie, 1994; Brent, et al., 1999; Goodyer, Herbert, Tamplin, Secher, & Pearson, 1997; Lewinsohn, Clarke, Hops, & Andrews, 1990); stress and life events (Garber & Hilsman, 1992; Goodyer, et al., 1997; Williamson et al., 1998); and suicidality at baseline (Emslie et al., 2001). In a recent longitudinal study investigating recurrence of MDD during adulthood (19 to 23 years of age) in formerly treated depressed adolescents, recurrence was predicted by multiple episodes of depression, family history of recurrence of major depression, borderline personality disorder symptoms, and increased conflict with parents (for females only) (Lewinsohn, Joiner, & Rohde, 2001). Youth who do not achieve remission or who have continuing residual symptoms following acute treatment are also at increased risk for relapse or recurrence (Curry et al., 2010; Emslie et al., 2008, 2010; Vitiello et al., 2011).

Few studies have focused on continuation treatment, either psychotherapy or pharmacotherapy. As noted in the previous section, studies suggest that youth who do not continue treatment, particularly those with residual symptoms, experience higher rates of relapse. It is therefore recommended that all youth continue treatment, with psychotherapy and/or antidepressants for at least 6 to 12 months following acute response. If prescribed antidepressants youth should be followed at regular intervals with emphasis on optimizing medication dose and adherence and evaluating side effects (Birmaher et al., 2007).

The burden of determining the need for maintenance pharmacotherapy falls to the clinician who must consider if the therapy is indicated, and which type of therapy and for how long. It is generally held that youth with chronic/severe depression or more than two depressive episodes continue in maintenance treatment for at least 1 year. Many additional factors may support the need for maintenance treatment include suicidal ideation, family mental illness, and lack of community resources.

Discontinuing Antidepressant Treatment

When discontinuing treatment, providers should consider psychosocial stressors and protective factors, such as family support and school requirements. In addition, following discontinuation of medication, youth should be reassessed within 1–2 weeks to assess for side effects and return of depressive symptoms.

Other Considerations to Enhance Recovery

Comorbid Psychiatric Conditions

Comorbid conditions are common in depression; 40 to 90 percent of youth with a depressive disorder will also experience anxiety disorders, attention-deficit hyperactivity disorder (ADHD), or other disruptive behavior disorders. Substance abuse disorders are common in depressed adolescents. Comorbidities impact the genesis and perpetuation of depressive symptoms as well as contribute to increased disease burden including suicide risk, academic dysfunction, and interpersonal ineffectiveness. Generally, the primary condition, that is the condition that is causing the most impairment and distress, is treated first. If the comorbid condition inhibits recovery from depression, then it is addressed preferentially. Pharmacological and psychosocial treatments that are efficacious in depression may also be useful in the treatment of comorbid conditions, specifically anxiety disorders (Birmaher et al., 2003).

Associated Symptoms of Depression

Suicidal ideation and behavior, symptoms that commonly accompany major depression, warrant special consideration. The presence of disruptive behavior disorders, substance use disorders, and impulsivity, as well as history of physical or sexual abuse, suicide attempts, and family suicidal behavior increases risk (Gould et al., 1998; Gould, Fisher, Parides, Flory, & Shaffer, 1996). The suicidal depressed patient requires frequent safety assessment, enhanced supervision including minimizing access to means (firearms, medications, etc.), and a safety plan that ideally addresses triggers, warning signs, coping, and where and how to seek help. Other depression-associated symptoms may require additional treatment, for example insomnia. Treatments both pharmacological and non-pharmacological that target improved sleep and reduced levels of aggression, agitation, and/or anxiety are expected to be used temporarily, and are added to assist the patient until antidepressant treatment takes effect.

Drug–Drug Interactions and Side Effects

Consideration of potential drug interactions is important when treating depression. Side effects associated with the antidepressants are also important, as these medications may be selected to prevent or counteract side effects associated with other treatments. For example, in patients experiencing weight loss as a result of a medical condition or another medication, an antidepressant known to reduce weight loss may be selected. Generally, the most common side effects associated with antidepressants are nausea, headaches, changes in appetite, sleep disturbance, dry mouth, nervousness, and dizziness. Sexual side effects, increased bruising and/or bleeding, and mania are also important, albeit less common, side effects.

Role of Therapy in Managing Depression

Psychotherapy as a treatment for depression can be used in combination with antidepressant medications, or as a stand-alone, monotherapy. In general, the combination of psychotherapy and medication has been found to be more effective than psychotherapy for those with more severe depression (TADS, 2004). Acute treatment studies of psychotherapy alone for the treatment of pediatric depression show mixed results. While some studies in a meta-analysis of 35 RCTs showed robust effects, the overall effect of psychotherapy for the acute management of depression in youth was modest. There was no difference in efficacy between age groups, delivery modality, or type of therapy. Also no correlation between treatment duration and response was found (Weisz, McCarty, & Valeri, 2006). Of the various therapeutic modalities, only CBT and interpersonal psychotherapy (IPT) have demonstrated efficacy in RTCs. Although widely utilized in clinical settings, psychodynamic psychotherapy lacks evidence. CBT is the most widely studied psychotherapy for the treatment of pediatric depression. Several studies have shown CBT to be effective even when dealing with comorbid conditions and suicidal ideation. Conversely, there are findings from RCTs (March et al., 2004; March, Silva, Vitiello, & Team, 2006) in which CBT does not differentiate from placebo. Combined treatment of CBT and medication (fluoxetine) resulted in more rapid symptom reduction but results were no different at endpoint between combination treatment and medication alone (Curry et al., 2006). A remission rate of 37 percent, the greatest of any treatment, was reported in the combination treatment group (Kennard et al., 2006). While the superiority of combined treatment approaches seems obvious, in the Treatment for Adolescents with Depression Study (TADS), the differences between combination and medication alone were modest. Remission rates were the highest in the combination group, but still discouragingly low (37 percent in combination group versus 23 percent in medication alone March et al., 2006). In treatment resistant depression, however, the gains of the combination approach of CBT and medication were considerably stronger, with a higher response rate in those who got the combination treatment compared to those on medication alone (55 percent versus 41 percent) (Brent et al., 2008). Other therapeutic modalities have even less robust efficacy data available. A study by Rossello and Bernal (1999) showed that IPT was at least as efficacious as CBT in the management of adolescent depression. There have been no studies in adolescent depression comparing IPT to pharmacological treatments or evaluating the efficacy of a combination approach versus a mono-therapy.

PROMOTING WELLNESS AND POSITIVE MENTAL HEALTH

The bulk of the literature in child and adolescent psychiatry has focused on the treatment of illness. This is especially true for major depressive illness, where much progress has been made in establishing the efficacy of acute-phase treatments. Considerably less work has been done on the promotion of wellness and resilience. The positive psychology movement has spearheaded some of the early important work in this area (Seligman & Csikszentmihalyi, 2000). This research emphasizes the need for practitioners to focus more attention on amplifying strengths and building positive traits (eg, optimism) as a means of preventing illness (Duckworth, Steen, & Seligman, 2005; Kobau et al., 2011).

There have been effective preventative programs in youth at risk for depression (Clarke et al., 2001; Stice, Shaw, Bohon, Marti, & Rohde, 2009). Working with at-risk populations of children and young adults preventative interventions have focused on changing explanatory style and developing social problem-solving skills as a means of preventing the future moderate depressive episodes (Gillham et al., 2012; Jaycox, Reivich, Gillham, & Seligman, 1994; Seligman, Schulman, DeRubeis, & Hollon, 1999). In a recent multi-site study, children of parents who have been diagnosed with depression, thus who at risk for depression onset, received an 8-week (weekly sessions) prevention CBT program. At 9-month follow-up, those who received the CBT preventative program had reduced rates of depression onset compared to usual care

(Garber et al., 2009). Furthermore, these rates were sustained at up to 3-year follow-up, with lower rates of depression diagnosis in those who were treated with the prevention program (Beardslee, Solantaus, Morgan, Gladstone, & Kowalenko, 2013).

Recently psychosocial treatments have included more focus on building strengths as opposed to addressing deficits (ie, decreasing negative mood and cognitions). A positive approach includes the enhancement of strengths, positive experiences, mood, and cognitions. The focus of treatment is to not only achieve the absence of illness but to promote the presence of wellness. Strategies that promote health and well-being include mastery, positive self-regard, goal setting, quality relations/ social problem-solving, and optimism (Jaycox et al., 1994; Ryff & Singer, 1996; Segal, Williams, & Teasdale, 2002; Seligman & Csikszentmihalyi, 2000; Snyder & Lopez, 2005). Attributions for positive events can help build positive self-worth and optimistic explanatory style (Curry & Craighead, 1990).

Ryff and Singer (1996) provide a model for defining dimensions of wellness in adults, which was later adapted into intervention strategies for relapse prevention in adults remitted for depression, also known as well-being therapy (Fava, Rafanelli, Grandi, Canestrari, & Morphy, 1998). Cognitive-behavioral strategies used in the continuation treatment phase of depression in adults have been found to prevent relapse of depression (Jarrett, Minhajuddin, Gershenfeld, Friedman, & Thase, 2013; Nierenberg, 2001). In addition, adult studies indicate that relapse rates can be significantly reduced by augmenting psycho-pharmacotherapies with CBT in the continuation phase of treatment for major depression (Fava, Grandi, Zielezny, Canestrari, & Morphy, 1994; Fava, Grandi, Zielezny, Rafanelli, & Canestrari, 1996; Fava et al., 1998; Fava et al., 2004; Guidi, Fava, Fava, & Papakostas, 2011; Nierenberg, 2001; Paykel, 2007; Paykel et al., 1999; Teasdale et al., 2000).

A meta-analysis of treatment studies using positive psychology interventions in both pediatric and adult populations, show promising results for the treatment of depression (Sin & Lyubomirsky, 2009). In youth, more recent work has been done to promote wellness along with adaptive coping strategies to enhance well-being in youth who were successfully treated for depression (Kennard et al., 2014; Kennard et al., 2008). Using a continuation CBT approach which included a wellness, strengths-based approach (Relapse Prevention-CBT; RP-CBT), those who were treated with the RP-CBT, plus continued antidepressant medication, had lower relapse rates over a 30-week treatment period compared to those treated with medication only (9 percent versus 26.5 percent). The study also concluded that those who were treated with CBT had higher percentage of time well, and required a dose of lower antidepressant (Kennard et al., 2014).

Positive Health: Sleep, Exercise

Treatment studies in adults have demonstrated that high dose exercise programs can be effective in the treatment of depression (Dunn, Trivedi, Kampert, Clark, & Chambliss, 2005; Dunn, Trivedi, Kampert, Clark, & Chambliss, 2002). Recent evidence suggests that exercise is associated with lower rates of depressive symptoms in youth. In a prospective, longitudinal study of a community sample, those youth with greater levels of exercise demonstrated lower levels of depressive symptoms (Rothon et al., 2010). In clinical samples, exercise has been shown to be a promising alternative treatment strategy for depression (Dopp, Mooney, Armitage, & King, 2012; Hughes et al., 2013, 2009). In an RCT of adolescent depression, those treated with exercise versus a stretch only control group, had a 100 percent remission rate at week 26 and 52, compared to a 70 percent remission rate in the stretch control group (Hughes et al., 2013, 2009).

Insomnia is frequently comorbid with depression, with approximately 75 percent of those with depression reporting symptoms of sleep disturbance (Ivanenko, Crabtree, & Gozal, 2004). Insomnia can persist even after treatment, as it is one of the most common residual symptoms in those treated for depression (Kennard et al., 2006). Insomnia has been found to be associated with poorer treatment outcomes in depressed youth. Emslie et al. (2012) found that adolescents who reported having both insomnia and depression were less likely to respond to antidepressant treatment than those without insomnia. Insomnia has also been linked to death by suicide in adolescents (Goldstein, Bridge, & Brent, 2008). Recent treatments for depression which target insomnia have been found to be effective in adults, and have recently been adapted for depressed adolescents (Manber et al., 2008; Clarke & Harvey, 2012). These treatments address dysfunctional thoughts related to sleep, as well as provide stimulus control (ie, associate the bed with sleep) and sleep restriction (ie, regulate sleep-wake cycle) strategies to reduce stimulation and promote sleep. Motivational enhancement strategies are also employed. CBT-I for the treatment of depression and insomnia is currently being tested for efficacy in a randomized-controlled trial (Clarke & Harvey, 2012).

Wellness and Promotion of Strength

More recently, psychosocial treatments for depression have focused on assessing and building on strengths in the child and family. It is important for clinicians to assess strengths, both current and prior to the onset of illness, in youth with depression. This will allow the clinician to collaborate with the child and family to build on current strengths, as well as to revisit former behaviors and activities that may promote wellness. This approach was included in the wellness component of RP-CBT, where the focus was to assess and build on the current wellness-related skills/ strengths that the youth and family bring to the treatment (Kennard et al., 2008). In particular, the RP-CBT program emphasized strategies that promoted health and wellness (Ryff & Singer, 1996). These strategies included "the Six S's:" (1) self-acceptance; (2) social wellness; (3) success; (4) self-goals; (5) soothing; and (6) spiritual. Self-acceptance includes strategies to develop positive self-schema and a positive explanatory style. Social wellness includes a focus on planning and engaging in social activities, as well as enhanced social skills and social problem-solving. The success component emphasizes autonomy and mastery, while the self-goals component focuses on purpose. The soothing component of wellness emphasizes planned relaxation and rest. Lastly, the spirituality component within the wellness program is broadly defined and individualized for each patient, and may include meditation, altruism, gratitude, and values, as well as more traditional forms of spirituality such as religious beliefs (Pargament & Mahoney, 2002). RP-CBT is designed to identify the unique strengths, or in this case, sources of spirituality that the patient already has, and to reinforce those aspects of spirituality already present in the patient. Although there are few empirical studies using spirituality in treatment, preliminary data from the field of positive psychology suggests that including this component can be an effective intervention (Frisch, 2006; McCullough & Worthington, 1999; Propst, Ostrom, Watkins, Dean, & Mashburn, 1992).

CONCLUSIONS

Depression in children and adolescents continues to go unrecognized and definitely undertreated. As noted, both stigma and access to care are barriers to recognition and treatment. Screening for depression in at-risk youth is an important first step to identification, and this can be implemented in primary care settings. Resistance to screening in part comes from concerns about how to manage patients who are identified. A continuum of effective treatments is available, from general health advice (eg, improved health habits, sleep-wake schedule improvements, and exercise) to intensive treatment with medication and specific psychotherapies. The need to individualize the treatment based on severity, psychosocial stressors, and family circumstances will inform treatment decisions. Continued work is necessary on identifying barriers from identification to adequate treatment, including accessible, culturally sensitive care, and dealing with limited numbers of adequately trained professionals.

Effective treatments (psychotherapies and antidepressants) are available, and the primary goal of acute treatment is remission of symptoms. Utilizing ongoing measurement of response in addition to clinical assessment helps achieve that goal. Remission is essentially few or no remaining symptoms of depression. However, this does not guarantee that patients are back to optimal functioning (ie, well). Recognition of strengths and skills that can be developed is an important part of treatment at this stage to lead to optimal functioning and increase resistance to future episodes of depression.

References

Arkowitz, H., & Burke, B. L. (2008). MI as a framework for the treatment of depression. In H. Arkowitz, H. A. Westra, W. R. Miller, & S. Rollnick (Eds.), *Motivational interviewing in the treatment of psychological problems* (pp. 145–172). New York: Guilford Press.

Asarnow, J. R., & Bates, S. (1988). Depression in child psychiatric inpatients: cognitive and attributional patterns. [Research Support, Non-U.S. Gov't]. *Journal of Abnormal Child Psychology, 16*(6), 601–615.

Asarnow, J. R., Tompson, M., Hamilton, E. B., Goldstein, M. J., & Guthrie, D. (1994). Family-expressed emotion, childhood-onset depression, and childhood-onset schizophrenia spectrum disorders: is expressed emotion a nonspecific correlate of child psychopathology or a specific risk factor for depression? *Journal of Abnormal Child Psychology, 22*(2), 129–146.

Atkinson, S. D., Prakash, A., Zhang, Q., Pangallo, B. A., Bangs, M. E., Emslie, G. J., ... March, J. S. (2014). A double-blind efficacy and safety study of duloxetine flexible dosing in children and adolescents with major depressive disorder. [Clinical Trial, Phase III Comparative Study Randomized Controlled Trial Research Support, Non-U.S. Gov't]. *Journal of Child and Adolescent Psychopharmacology, 24*(4), 180–189. http://dx.doi.org/10.1089/cap.2013.0146.

Avenevoli, S., Swendsen, J., He, J. P., Burstein, M., & Merikangas, K. R. (2015). Major depression in the national comorbidity survey-adolescent supplement: prevalence, correlates, and treatment. [Research Support, N.I.H., Extramural]. *Journal of the American Academy of Child and Adolescent Psychiatry, 54*(1), 37–44. http://dx.doi.org/10.1016/j.jaac.2014.10.010, e32.

Barraclough, B. H. (1981). Suicide and epilepsy. In E. H. Reynolds, & M. R. Trimble (Eds.), *Epilepsy and psychiatry* (pp. 72–76) Edinburgh.

Beardslee, W. R., Solantaus, T. S., Morgan, B. S., Gladstone, T. R., & Kowalenko, N. M. (2013). Preventive interventions for children of parents with depression: international perspectives. *The Medical Journal of Australia, 199*(3 Suppl.), S23–S25.

Beck, A. T., Epstein, N., Brown, G., & Steer, R. A. (1988). An inventory for measuring clinical anxiety: psychometric properties. [Research Support, Non-U.S. Gov't Research Support, U.S. Gov't, P.H.S.]. *Journal of Consulting and Clinical Psychology, 56*(6), 893–897.

Beevers, C. G., Keitner, G. I., Ryan, C. E., & Miller, I. W. (2003). Cognitive predictors of symptom return following depression treatment. *Journal of Abnormal Psychology, 112*(3), 488–496.

Berard, R., Fong, R., Carpenter, D. J., Thomason, C., & Wilkinson, C. (2006). An international, multicenter, placebo-controlled trial of paroxetine in adolescents with major depressive disorder. *Journal of Child and Adolescent Psychopharmacology, 16*(1/2), 59–75.

Birmaher, B., Axelson, D. A., Monk, K., Kalas, C., Clark, D. B., Ehmann, M., ... Brent, D. A. (2003). Fluoxetine for the treatment of childhood anxiety disorders. *Journal of the American Academy of Child and Adolescent Psychiatry, 42*(4), 415–423. http://dx.doi.org/10.1097/01.chi.0000037049.04952.9f.

Birmaher, B., Brent, D., Bernet, W., Bukstein, O., Walter, H., Benson, R., ... Medicus, J. (2007). Practice parameter for the assessment and treatment of children and adolescents with depressive disorders. *Journal of the American Academy of Child and Adolescent Psychiatry, 46*(11), 1503–1526. http://dx.doi.org/10.1097/chi.0b013e318145ae1c0, 0004583-200711000-00018 [pii].

Birmaher, B., Brent, D. A., Kolko, D. J., Baugher, M., Bridge, J., Holder, D., ... Ulloa, R. E. (2000). Clinical outcome after short-term psychotherapy for adolescents with major depressive disorder. *Archives of General Psychiatry, 57*, 8.

Brent, D., Emslie, G., Clarke, G., Wagner, K. D., Asarnow, J. R., Keller, M., ... Zelazny, J. (2008). Switching to another SSRI or to venlafaxine with or without cognitive behavioral therapy for adolescents with SSRI-resistant depression: the TORDIA randomized controlled trial. *JAMA, 299*(8), 901–913. http://dx.doi.org/10.1001/jama.299.8.901, 299/8/901 [pii].

Brent, D. A., Kolko, D. J., Birmaher, B., Baugher, M., & Bridge, J. (1999). A clinical trial for adolescent depression: predictors of additional treatment in the acute and follow-up phases of the trial. *Journal of the American Academy of Child & Adolescent Psychiatry, 38*(3), 263–270.

Bridge, J. A., Iyengar, S., Salary, C. B., Barbe, R. P., Birmaher, B., Pincus, H. A., ... Brent, D. A. (2007). Clinical response and risk for reported suicidal ideation and suicide attempts in pediatric antidepressant treatment: a meta-analysis of randomized controlled trials. [Meta-Analysis Research Support, N.I.H., Extramural Research Support, Non-U.S. Gov't]. *JAMA, 297*(15), 1683–1696. http://dx.doi.org/10.1001/jama.297.15.1683.

Brody, A. E. (2009). Motivational interviewing with a depressed adolescent. *Journal of Clinical Psychology, 65*(11), 1168–1179. http://dx.doi.org/10.1002/jclp.20636.

Brumback, R. A., & Weinberg, W. A. (1990). Pediatric behavioral neurology: an update on the neurologic aspects of depression, hyperactivity, and learning disabilities. *Neurologic Clinics, 8*(3), 677–703.

Cantwell, D. P., Baker, L., & Mattison, R. E. (1980). Psychiatric disorders in children with speech and language retardation. Factors associated with development. *Archives of General Psychiatry, 37*(4), 423–426.

Charmaz, K. (1993). *Good days, bad days: The self in chronic illness and time.* New Brunswick, NJ: Rutgers University Press.

Cheung, A., Emslie, G. J., & Mayes, T. L. (2005). Review of the efficacy and safety of antidepressants in youth depression. *Journal of Child Psychology & Psychiatry, 46*(7), 735–754.

Cheung, A., Zuckerbrot, R. A., Jensen, P. S., Ghalib, K., Laraque, D., Stein, R. E. K., ... GLAD-PC Steering Group (2007). Guidelines for adolescent depression in primary care (GLAD-PC): II. Treatment and ongoing management [guideline]. *Pediatrics, 120*(5), 14.

Clarke, G., & Harvey, A. G. (2012). The complex role of sleep in adolescent depression. *Child and Adolescent Psychiatric Clinics of North America, 21*(2), 385–400. http://dx.doi.org/10.1016/j.chc.2012.01.006.

Clarke, G. N., Hornbrook, M., Lynch, F., Polen, M., Beardslee, W. R., O'Connor, E., ... Seeley, J. R. (2001). A randomized trial of a group cognitive intervention for preventing depression in adolescent offspring of depressed parents. *Archives of General Psychiatry, 58*(12), 1127–1134.

Connolly, J., Geller, S., Marton, P., & Kutcher, S. (1992). Peer responses to social interaction with depressed adolescents. *Journal of Clinical Child Psychology, 21*(5), 365–370.

Curry, J. F., & Craighead, W. E. (1990). Attributional style in clinically depressed and conduct disordered adolescents. *Journal of Consulting and Clinical Psychology, 58*(1), 109–115.

Curry, J. F., Rohde, P., Simons, A. D., Silva, S., Vitiello, B., Kratochvil, C., ... Team, T. T. (2006). Predictors and moderators of acute outcome in the treatment for adolescents with depression study (TADS). *Journal of the American Academy of Child & Adolescent Psychiatry, 45*(12), 1427–1439.

Curry, J., Silva, S., Rohde, P., Ginsburg, G., Kratochvil, C., Simons, A., ... March, J. (2010). Recovery and recurrence following treatment for adolescent major depression. *Archives of General Psychiatry, 68*(3), 263–269. http://dx.doi.org/10.1001/archgenpsychiatry.2010.150, archgenpsychiatry2010.150 [pii].

Daviss, W. B., Birmaher, B., Melhem, N. A., Axelson, D. A., Michaels, S. M., & Brent, D. A. (2006). Criterion validity of the mood and feelings questionnaire for depressive episodes in clinic and non-clinic subjects. *Journal of Child Psychology & Psychiatry, 47*(9), 927–934.

III. INTERVENTIONS AND TREATMENTS

DelBello, M. P., Hochadel, T. J., Portland, K. B., Azzaro, A. J., Katic, A., Khan, A., & Emslie, G. (2014). A double-blind, placebo-controlled study of selegiline transdermal system in depressed adolescents. *Journal of Child and Adolescent Psychopharmacology, 24*(6), 311–317. http://dx.doi.org/10.1089/cap.2013.0138.

Dopp, R. R., Mooney, A. J., Armitage, R., & King, C. (2012). Exercise for adolescents with depressive disorders: a feasibility study. *Depression Research and Treatment, 2012*, 257472. http://dx.doi.org/10.1155/2012/257472.

Duckworth, A. L., Steen, T. A., & Seligman, M. E. (2005). Positive psychology in clinical practice. *Annual Review of Clinical Psychology, 1*, 629–651. http://dx.doi.org/10.1146/annurev.clinpsy.1.102803.144154.

Dunn, A. L., Trivedi, M. H., Kampert, J. B., Clark, C. G., & Chambliss, H. O. (2005). Exercise treatment for depression. *American Journal of Preventive Medicine, 28*(1), 1–8.

Dunn, A. L., Trivedi, M. H., Kampert, J. B., Clark, C. G., & Chambliss, H. O. (2002). The DOSE study: a clinical trial to examine efficacy and dose-response of exercise as treatment for depression. *Controlled Clinical Trials, 23*, 584–603.

Eaton, W., Muntaner, C., Smith, C., Tien, A., & Ybarra, M. (2004). Center for Epidemiologic studies depression scale: review and revision (CESD and CESD-R). In M. Maruish (Ed.), *The use of psychological testing for treatment planning and outcome assessment* (3rd ed.) (pp. 363–377). Mahway, NJ: Lawrence Erlbaum.

Emslie, G. J. (2008). Improving outcome in pediatric depression. *The American Journal of Psychiatry, 165*(1), 1–3. http://dx.doi.org/10.1176/appi.ajp.2007.07101647, 165/1/1 [pii].

Emslie, G. J., Armitage, R., Weinberg, W. A., Rush, A. J., Mayes, T. L., & Hoffmann, R. F. (2001). Sleep polysomnography as a predictor of recurrence in children and adolescents with major depressive disorder. *The International Journal of Neuropsychopharmacology, 4*(2), 159–168. http://dx.doi.org/10.1017/S1461145701002383, S1461145701002383 [pii].

Emslie, G. J., Findling, R. L., Yeung, P. P., Kunz, N. R., & Li, Y. (2007). Venlafaxine ER for the treatment of pediatric subjects with depression: results of two placebo-controlled trials. *Journal of the American Academy of Child & Adolescent Psychiatry, 46*(4), 479–488.

Emslie, G. J., Heiligenstein, J. H., Wagner, K. D., Hoog, S. L., Ernest, D. E., Brown, E., ... Jacobson, J. G. (2002). Fluoxetine for acute treatment of depression in children and adolescents: a placebo-controlled, randomized clinical trial. *Journal of the American Academy of Child and Adolescent Psychiatry, 41*(10), 1205–1215. http://dx.doi.org/10.1097/00004583-200210000-00010 S0890-8567(09)60765-6 [pii].

Emslie, G. J., Kennard, B. D., & Kowatch, R. A. (1995). Affective disorders in children: diagnosis and management. *Journal of Child Neurology, 10*(Suppl. 1), S42–S49.

Emslie, G. J., Kennard, B. D., & Mayes, T. L. (2011). Predictors of treatment response in adolescent depression. *Pediatric Annals, 40*(6), 300–306. http://dx.doi.org/10.3928/00904481-20110512-05.

Emslie, G. J., Kennard, B. D., Mayes, T. L., Nakonezny, P. A., Zhu, L., Tao, R., ... Croarkin, P. (2012). Insomnia moderates outcome of serotonin-selective reuptake inhibitor treatment in depressed youth. *Journal of Child and Adolescent Psychopharmacology, 22*(1), 21–28. http://dx.doi.org/10.1089/cap.2011.0096.

Emslie, G. J., Kennard, B. D., Mayes, T. L., Nightingale-Teresi, J., Carmody, T., Hughes, C. W., ... Rintelmann, J. W. (2008). Fluoxetine versus placebo in preventing relapse of major depression in children and adolescents. *The American Journal of Psychiatry, 165*(4), 459–467. http://dx.doi.org/10.1176/appi.ajp.2007.07091453, appi.ajp.2007.07091453 [pii].

Emslie, G. J., Mayes, T., Porta, G., Vitiello, B., Clarke, G., Wagner, K. D., ... Brent, D. (2010). Treatment of resistant depression in adolescents (TORDIA): week 24 outcomes. *The American Journal of Psychiatry, 167*(7), 782–791. http://dx.doi.org/10.1176/appi.ajp.2010.09040552, appi.ajp.2010.09040552 [pii].

III. INTERVENTIONS AND TREATMENTS

Emslie, G. J., Prakash, A., Zhang, Q., Pangallo, B. A., Bangs, M. E., & March, J. S. (2014). A double-blind efficacy and safety study of duloxetine fixed doses in children and adolescents with major depressive disorder. [Clinical Trial, Phase III Comparative Study Randomized Controlled Trial Research Support, Non-U.S. Gov't]. *Journal of Child and Adolescent Psychopharmacology, 24*(4), 170–179. http://dx.doi.org/10.1089/cap.2013.0096.

Emslie, G. J., Rush, A. J., Weinberg, W. A., Gullion, C. M., Rintelmann, J., & Hughes, C. W. (1997). Recurrence of major depressive disorder in hospitalized children and adolescents. *Journal of the American Academy of Child & Adolescent Psychiatry, 36*(6), 785–792.

Emslie, G. J., Rush, A. J., Weinberg, W. A., Kowatch, R. A., Hughes, C. W., Carmody, T., ... Rintelmann, J. (1997). A double-blind, randomized, placebo-controlled trial of fluoxetine in children and adolescents with depression. *Archives of General Psychiatry, 54*(11), 1031–1037.

Emslie, G. J., Ventura, D., Korotzer, A., & Tourkodimitris, S. (2009). Escitalopram in the treatment of adolescent depression: a randomized placebo-controlled multisite trial. *Journal of the American Academy of Child and Adolescent Psychiatry, 48*(7), 721–729. http://dx.doi.org/10.1097/CHI.0b013e3181a2b304, S0890-8567(09)60109-X [pii].

Emslie, G. J., Wagner, K. D., Kutcher, S., Kruelewicz, S. P., Fong, R., Carpenter, D. J., & Wilkinson, C. (2006). Paroxetine treatment in children and adolescents with major depressive disorder: a randomized, multicenter, double-blind, placebo-controlled trial. *Journal of the American Academy of Child & Adolescent Psychiatry, 45*(6), 709–719.

Fava, G., Grandi, S., Zielezny, M., Canestrari, R., & Morphy, M. A. (1994). Cognitive behavioral treatment of residual symptoms in primary major depressive disorder. *American Journal of Psychiatry, 151*(9), 1295–1299.

Fava, G., Grandi, S., Zielezny, M., Rafanelli, C., & Canestrari, R. (1996). Four-year outcome for cognitive behavioral treatment of residual symptoms in major depression. *American Journal of Psychiatry, 153*(7), 945–947.

Fava, G., Rafanelli, C., Grandi, S., Canestrari, R., & Morphy, M. A. (1998). Six-year outcome for cognitive behavioral treatment of residual symptoms in major depression. *American Journal of Psychiatry, 155*(10), 1443–1445.

Fava, G. A., Ruini, C., Rafanelli, C., Finos, L., Conti, S., & Grandi, S. (2004). Six-year outcome of cognitive behavior therapy for prevention of recurrent depression. *The American Journal of Psychiatry, 161*(10), 1872–1876. http://dx.doi.org/10.1176/appi.ajp.161.10.1872.

Findling, R. L., Groark, J., Chiles, D., Ramaker, S., Yang, L., & Tourian, K. A. (2014). Safety and tolerability of desvenlafaxine in children and adolescents with major depressive disorder. [Multicenter study randomized controlled trial research support, Non-U.S. Gov't]. *Journal of Child and Adolescent Psychopharmacology, 24*(4), 201–209. http://dx.doi.org/10.1089/cap.2012.0126.

Frisch, M. B. (2006). *Quality of life therapy: Applying a life satisfaction approach to positive psychology and cognitive therapy.* Hoboken, NJ: John Wiley and Sons.

Garber, J., Clarke, G. N., Weersing, V. R., Beardslee, W. R., Brent, D. A., Gladstone, T. R., ... Iyengar, S. (2009). Prevention of depression in at-risk adolescents: a randomized controlled trial. *JAMA, 301*(21), 2215–2224. http://dx.doi.org/10.1001/jama.2009.788 301/21/2215 [pii].

Garber, J., & Hilsman, R. (1992). Cognitions, stress, and depression in children and adolescents. *Child and Adolescent Psychiatric Clinics of North America, 1*(8), 129–167.

Garber, J., Weiss, B., & Shanley, N. (1993). Cognitions, depressive symptoms, and development in adolescents. *Journal of Abnormal Psychology, 102*(1), 47–57.

Gillham, J. E., Reivich, K. J., Brunwasser, S. M., Freres, D. R., Chajon, N. D., Kash-Macdonald, V. M., ... Seligman, M. E. (2012). Evaluation of a group cognitive-behavioral depression prevention program for young adolescents: a randomized effectiveness trial. *Journal of Clinical Child and Adolescent Psychology: The Official Journal for the Society of Clinical Child and Adolescent Psychology, American Psychological Association, Division 53, 41*(5), 621–639. http://dx.doi.org/10.1080/15374416.2012.706517.

Goldstein, T. R., Bridge, J. A., & Brent, D. A. (2008). Sleep disturbance preceding completed suicide in adolescents. *Journal of Consulting and Clinical Psychology, 76*(1), 84–91. http://dx.doi.org/10.1037/0022-006X.76.1.84, 2008-00950-011 [pii].

Goodyer, I. M., Herbert, J., Tamplin, A., Secher, S. M., & Pearson, J. (1997). Short-term outcome of major depression II. Life events, family dysfunction, and friendship difficulties as predictors of persistent disorder. *Journal of the American Academy of Child & Adolescent Psychiatry, 36*, 474–480.

Gould, M. S., Fisher, P., Parides, M., Flory, M., & Shaffer, D. (1996). Psychosocial risk factors of child and adolescent completed suicide. *Archives of General Psychiatry, 53*(12), 1155–1162.

Gould, M., King, R., Greenwald, S., Fisher, P., Schwab-Stone, M., Kramer, R., ... Shaffer, D. (1998). Psychopathology associated with suicidal ideation and attempts among children and adolescents. *Journal of the American Academy of Child & Adolescent Psychiatry, 37*(9), 915–923.

Guidi, J., Fava, G. A., Fava, M., & Papakostas, G. I. (2011). Efficacy of the sequential integration of psychotherapy and pharmacotherapy in major depressive disorder: a preliminary meta-analysis. *Psychological Medicine, 41*(2), 321–331. http://dx.doi.org/10.1017/S0033291710000826.

Hamilton, E. B., Asarnow, J. R., & Tompson, M. C. (1997). Social, academic, and behavioral competence of depressed children: relationship to diagnostic status and family interaction style. *Journal of Youth and Adolescence, 26*(1), 77–87.

Hammad, T. A., Laughren, T., & Racoosin, J. (2006). Suicidality in pediatric patients treated with antidepressant drugs. *Archives of General Psychiatry, 63*, 332–339.

Herjanic, B., & Reich, W. (1997). Development of a structured psychiatric interview for children: agreement between child and parent on individual symptoms. *Journal of Abnormal Child Psychology, 25*(1), 21–31.

Hoek, W., Marko, M., Fogel, J., Schuurmans, J., Gladstone, T., Bradford, N., ... Van Voorhees, B. W. (2011). Randomized controlled trial of primary care physician motivational interviewing versus brief advice to engage adolescents with an internet-based depression prevention intervention: 6-month outcomes and predictors of improvement. [Randomized Controlled Trial Research Support, N.I.H., Extramural Research Support, Non-U.S. Gov't]. *Translational Research: The Journal of Laboratory and Clinical Medicine, 158*(6), 315–325. http://dx.doi.org/10.1016/j.trsl.2011.07.006.

Hope, T. L., Adams, C., Reynolds, L., Powers, D., Perez, R. A., & Kelley, M. L. (1999). Parent vs. self-report: contributions toward diagnosis of adolescent psychopathology. *Journal of Psychopathology and Behavioral Assessment, 21*(4), 349–363.

Hops, H., Lewinsohn, P. M., Andrews, J. A., & Roberts, R. E. (1990). Psychosocial correlates of depressive symptomatology among high school students. *Journal of Clinical Child Psychology, 19*(3), 211–220.

Hughes, C. W., Barnes, S., Barnes, C., Defina, L. F., Nakonezny, P., & Emslie, G. J. (2013). Depressed adolescents treated with exercise (DATE): a pilot randomized controlled trial to test feasibility and establish preliminary effect sizes. *Mental Health and Physical Activity, 6*(2). http://dx.doi.org/10.1016/j.mhpa.2013.06.006.

Hughes, C. W., Emslie, G. J., Crismon, M. L., Posner, K., Birmaher, B., Ryan, N., ... Trivedi, M. H. (2007). Texas Children's Medication Algorithm Project: update from Texas Consensus Conference Panel on medication treatment of childhood major depressive disorder. [Consensus development Conference research support, Non-U.S. Gov't]. *Journal of the American Academy of Child and Adolescent Psychiatry, 46*(6), 667–686. http://dx.doi.org/10.1097/chi.0b013e31804a859b.

Hughes, C. W., Trivedi, M. H., Cleaver, J., Greer, T. L., Emslie, G. J., Kennard, B., ... Barnes, C. (2009). DATE: depressed adolescents treated with exercise: study rationale and design for a pilot study. *Mental Health Physical Activity, 2*(2), 76–85. http://dx.doi.org/10.1016/j.mhpa.2009.09.005.

Ivanenko, A., Crabtree, V. M., & Gozal, D. (2004). Sleep in children with psychiatric disorders. *Pediatric Clinics of North America, 51*(1), 51–68.

III. INTERVENTIONS AND TREATMENTS

Jacobs, R. H., Klein, J. B., Reinecke, M. A., Silva, S. G., Tonev, S., Breland-Noble, A., ... March, J. S. (2008). Ethnic differences in attributions and treatment expectancies for adolescent depression. *International Journal of Cognitive Therapy, 1*(2), 163–178. http://dx.doi.org/10.1680/ijct.2008.1.2.163.

Jarrett, R. B., Minhajuddin, A., Gershenfeld, H., Friedman, E. S., & Thase, M. E. (2013). Preventing depressive relapse and recurrence in higher-risk cognitive therapy responders: a randomized trial of continuation phase cognitive therapy, fluoxetine, or matched pill placebo. *JAMA Psychiatry.* http://dx.doi.org/10.1001/jamapsychiatry.2013.1969, 1733252 [pii].

Jaycox, L. H., Reivich, K. J., Gillham, J. E., & Seligman, M. E. (1994). Prevention of depressive symptoms in school children. *Behavior Research & Therapy, 32*, 801–816.

Jensen, P. S., Rubio-Stipec, M., Canino, G., Bird, H., Dulcan, M., Schwab-Stone, M. E., & Lahey, B. B. (1999). Parent and child contributions to diagnosis of mental disorder: are both informants always necessary? *Journal of the American Academy of Child & Adolescent Psychiatry, 38*(12), 1569–1579.

Johnson, J. G., Harris, E. S., Spitzer, R. L., & Williams, J. B. W. (2002). The patient health questionnaire for adolescents: validation of an instrument for the assessment of mental disorders among adolescent primary care patients. *Journal of Adolescent Health, 30*(3), 196–204.

Kanter, J. W., Rusch, L. C., & Brondino, M. J. (2008). Depression self-stigma: a new measure and preliminary findings. [Research Support, Non-U.S. Gov't]. *The Journal of Nervous and Mental Disease, 196*(9), 663–670. http://dx.doi.org/10.1097/NMD.0b013e318183f8af.

Kashani, J. H., Burbach, D. J., & Rosenberg, D. R. (1988). Perception of family conflict resolution and depressive symptomatology in adolescents. *Journal of the American Academy of Child & Adolescent Psychiatry, 27*(1), 42–48.

Keller, M. B., Ryan, N. D., Strober, M., Klein, R. G., Kutcher, S. P., Birmaher, B., ... McCafferty, J. P. (2001). Efficacy of paroxetine in the treatment of adolescent major depression: a randomized, controlled trial. *Journal of the American Academy of Child and Adolescent Psychiatry, 40*(7), 762–772. http://dx.doi.org/10.1097/00004583-200107000-00010, S0890-8567(09)60309-9 [pii].

Kennard, B. D., Emslie, G. J., Mayes, T. L., Nakonezny, P. A., Jones, J. M., Foxwell, A. A., & King, J. (2014). Sequential treatment with fluoxetine and relapse–prevention CBT to improve outcomes in pediatric depression. *The American Journal of Psychiatry, 171*(10), 1083–1090. http://dx.doi.org/10.1176/appi.ajp.2014.13111460.

Kennard, B. D., Emslie, G. J., Mayes, T. L., Nightingale-Teresi, J., Nakonezny, P. A., Hughes, J. L., ... Jarrett, R. B. (2008). Cognitive-behavioral therapy to prevent relapse in pediatric responders to pharmacotherapy for major depressive disorder. *Journal of the American Academy of Child and Adolescent Psychiatry, 47*(12), 1395–1404. http://dx.doi.org/10.1097/CHI.0b013e31818914a1, S0890-8567(08)60140-9 [pii].

Kennard, B. D., Silva, S. G., Tonev, S., Rohde, P., Hughes, J. L., Vitiello, B., ... March, J. (2009). Remission and recovery in the treatment for adolescents with depression study (TADS): acute and long-term outcomes. *Journal of the American Academy of Child and Adolescent Psychiatry, 48*(2), 186–195. http://dx.doi.org/10.1097/CHI.0b013e31819176f9, S0890-8567(09)60012-5 [pii].

Kennard, B., Silva, S., Vitiello, B., Curry, J., Kratochvil, C., Simons, A., ... March, J. (2006). Remission and residual symptoms after short-term treatment in the treatment of adolescents with depression study (TADS). *Journal of the American Academy of Child and Adolescent Psychiatry, 45*(12), 1404–1411. http://dx.doi.org/10.1097/01.chi.0000242228.75516.21, 00004583-200612000-00002 [pii].

Kobau, R., Seligman, M. E., Peterson, C., Diener, E., Zack, M. M., Chapman, D., ... Thompson, W. (2011). Mental health promotion in public health: perspectives and strategies from positive psychology. *American Journal of Public Health, 101*(8), e1–9. http://dx.doi.org/10.2105/ajph.2010.300083.

Kovacs, M. (1985). The Children's depression, inventory (CDI). *Psychopharmacology, 21*(4), 995–998.

Kovacs, M., Feinberg, T. L., Crouse-Novak, M. A., Paulauskas, S. L., & Finkelstein, R. (1984). Depressive disorders in childhood I. A longitudinal prospective study of characteristics and recovery. *Archives of General Psychiatry, 41,* 229–237.

Kovacs, M., Feinberg, T. L., Crouse-Novak, M. A., Paulauskas, S. L., Pollock, M., & Finkelstein, R. (1984). Depressive disorders in childhood II. A longitudinal study of the risk for a subsequent major depression. *Archives of General Psychiatry, 41,* 643–649.

Lewinsohn, P. M., & Clarke, G. N. (1999). Psychosocial treatments for adolescent depression. *Clinical Psychology Review, 19*(3), 329–342.

Lewinsohn, P. M., Clarke, G. N., Hops, H., & Andrews, J. A. (1990). Cognitive-behavioral treatment for depressed adolescents. *Behavior Therapy, 21,* 385–401.

Lewinsohn, P. M., Joiner, T. E., Jr., & Rohde, P. (2001). Evaluation of cognitive diathesis-stress models in predicting major depressive disorder in adolescents. *Journal of Abnormal Psychology, 110*(2), 203–215.

Ling, W., Oftedal, G., & Weinberg, W. A. (1970). Depressive illness in childhood presenting as severe headache. *American Journal of Diseases of Children, 120,* 122–124.

Link, B. G., & Phelan, J. C. (2001). Conceptualizing stigma. *Annual Review of Sociology, 27,* 363–385.

Link, B. G., Phelan, J. C., Bresnahan, M., Stueve, A., & Pescosolido, B. A. (1999). Public conceptions of mental illness: labels, causes, dangerousness, and social distance. *American Journal of Public Health, 89*(9), 1328–1333.

Livingston, R. (1985). Depressive illness and learning difficulties: research needs and practical implications. *Journal of Learning Disabilities, 18*(9), 518–520.

Maalouf, F. T., & Brent, D. A. (2012). Child and adolescent depression intervention overview: what works, for whom and how well? *Child and Adolescent Psychiatric Clinics of North America, 21*(2), 299–312. http://dx.doi.org/10.1016/j.chc.2012.01.001, viii.

Manber, R., Edinger, J. D., Gress, J. L., San Pedro-Salcedo, M. G., Kuo, T. F., & Kalista, T. (2008). Cognitive behavioral therapy for insomnia enhances depression outcome in patients with comorbid major depressive disorder and insomnia. *Sleep, 31*(4), 489–495.

March, J., Silva, S., Petrycki, S., Curry, J., Wells, K., Fairbank, J., ... Severe, J. (2004). Fluoxetine, cognitive-behavioral therapy, and their combination for adolescents with depression: treatment for adolescents with depression study (TADS) randomized controlled trial. *JAMA, 292*(7), 807–820. http://dx.doi.org/10.1001/jama.292.7.807, 292/7/807 [pii].

March, J. S., Silva, S., Vitiello, B., & Team, T. T. (2006). The treatment for adolescents with depression study (TADS): methods and message at 12 weeks. [TADS]. *Journal of the American Academy of Child & Adolescent Psychiatry, 45*(12), 1393–1403.

Markowitz, F. E. (1998). The effects of stigma on the psychological well-being and life satisfaction of persons with mental illness. [Research Support, Non-U.S. Gov't Research Support, U.S. Gov't, P.H.S.]. *Journal of Health and Social Behavior, 39*(4), 335–347.

Marton, P., & Kutcher, S. (1995). The prevalence of cognitive distortion in depressed adolescents. [Research Support, Non-U.S. Gov't]. *Journal of Psychiatry & Neuroscience, 20*(1), 33–38.

McCauley, E., Myers, K., Mitchell, J., Calderon, R., Schloredt, K., & Treder, R. (1993). Depression in young people: initial presentation and clinical course. *Journal of the American Academy of Child & Adolescent Psychiatry, 32*(4), 714–722.

McCullough, M. E., & Worthington, E. L., Jr. (1999). Religion and the forgiving personality. *Journal of Personality, 67*(6), 1141–1164.

Meredith, L. S., Stein, B. D., Paddock, S. M., Jaycox, L. H., Quinn, V. P., Chandra, A., ... Burnam, A. (2009). Perceived barriers to treatment for adolescent depression. *Medical Care, 47*(6), 677–685.

Mesman, J., & Koot, H. M. (2000). Child-reported depression and anxiety in preadolescence: I. Associations with parent- and teacher-reported problems. *Journal of the American Academy of Child & Adolescent Psychiatry, 39*(11), 1371–1378.

Miller, W. R., & Rollnick, S. (2002). *Motivational interviewing: Preparing people for change* (2nd ed.). New York: Guilford Press.

Miller, W. R., & Rollnick, S. (2012). Meeting in the middle: motivational interviewing and self-determination theory. *The International Journal of Behavioral Nutrition and Physical Activity, 9*, 25. http://dx.doi.org/10.1186/1479-5868-9-25.

Moore, H. K., Hughes, C. W., Mundt, J. C., Rush, A. J., Macleod, L., Emslie, G. J., ... Greist, J. H. (2007). A pilot study of an electronic, adolescent version of the quick inventory of depressive symptomatology. *The Journal of Clinical Psychiatry, 68*(9), 1436–1440.

Nierenberg, A. A. (2001). Long-term management of chronic depression. *The Journal of Clinical Psychiatry, 62*(Suppl. 6), 17–21.

Osman, A., Gutierrez, P. M., Bagge, C. L., Fang, Q., & Emmerich, A. (2010). Reynolds adolescent depression scale-second edition: a reliable and useful instrument. [validation studies]. *Journal of Clinical Psychology, 66*(12), 1324–1345. http://dx.doi.org/10.1002/jclp.20727.

Pargament, K., & Mahoney, A. (2002). Spirituality: discovering and conserving the sacred. In C. R. Snyder, & S. J. Lopez (Eds.), *Handbook of positive psychology*. New York: Oxford University Press.

Paykel, E. S. (2007). Cognitive therapy in relapse prevention in depression. *The International Journal of Neuropsychopharmacology, 10*(1), 131–136. http://dx.doi.org/10.1017/s1461145706006912.

Paykel, E. S., Scott, J., Teasdale, J. D., Johnson, A. L., Garland, A., Moore, R., ... Pope, M. (1999). Prevention of relapse in residual depression by cognitive therapy a controlled trial. *Archives of General Psychiatry, 56*, 829–835.

Poznanski, E., & Mokros, H. (1996). *Children's depression rating scale revised (CDRS-R) manual.* Los Angeles, CA: Western Psychological Services.

Propst, L. R., Ostrom, R., Watkins, P., Dean, T., & Mashburn, D. (1992). Comparative efficacy of religious and nonreligious cognitive-behavioral therapy for the treatment of clinical depression in religious individuals. *Journal of Consulting and Clinical Psychology, 60*(1), 94–103.

Puig-Antich, J., Kaufman, J., Ryan, N. D., Williamson, D. E., Dahl, R. E., Lukens, E., ... Nelson, B. (1993). The psychosocial functioning and family environment of depressed adolescents. [Research Support, U.S. Gov't, P.H.S.]. *Journal of the American Academy of Child and Adolescent Psychiatry, 32*(2), 244–253. http://dx.doi.org/10.1097/00004583-199303000-00003.

Puig-Antich, J., Lukens, E., Davies, M., Goetz, D., Brennan-Quattrock, M., & Todak, G. (1985a). Psychosocial functioning in prepubertal major depressive disorders I. Interpersonal relationships during the depressive episode. *Archives of General Psychiatry, 42*, 500–507.

Puig-Antich, J., Lukens, E., Davies, M., Goetz, D., Brennan-Quattrock, M., & Todak, G. (1985b). Psychosocial functioning in prepubertal major depressive disorders II. Interpersonal relationships after sustained recovery from affective episode. *Journal of Affective Disorders, 42*, 511–517.

Radloff, L. (1977). The CES-D scale: a self-report depression scale for research in the general population. *Applied Psychological Measurement, 1*, 385–401.

Richardson, L. P., McCauley, E., Grossman, D. C., McCarty, C. A., Richards, J., Russo, J. E., ... Katon, W. (2010). Evaluation of the patient health questionnaire-9 item for detecting major depression among adolescents. *Pediatrics, 126*(6), 1117–1123. http://dx.doi.org/10.1542/peds.2010-0852, peds.2010-0852 [pii].

Ring, H. A., & Trimble, M. R. (1993). Depression in epilepsy. In S. E. Starkstein, & R. G. Robinson (Eds.), *Depression in neurological disease* (pp. 63–83). Baltimore, MD: Johns Hopkins University Press.

Robertson, M. M. (1989). The organic contribution to depressive illness in patients with epilepsy. *Journal of Epilepsy, 2*, 189–230.

Robinson, R. G., Boston, J. D., Starkstein, S. E., & Price, T. R. (1988). Comparison of mania and depression after brain injury: causal factors. [Research Support, Non-U.S. Gov't Research Support, U.S. Gov't, P.H.S.]. *The American Journal of Psychiatry, 145*(2), 172–178.

Robinson, R. G., & Starkstein, S. E. (1990). Current research in affective disorders following stroke. [Research Support, Non-U.S. Gov't Research Support, U.S. Gov't, P.H.S. Review]. *The Journal of Neuropsychiatry and Clinical Neurosciences, 2*(1), 1–14.

Rossello, J., & Bernal, G. (1999). The efficacy of cognitive-behavioral and interpersonal treatments for depression in Puerto Rican adolescents. *Journal of Consulting and Clinical Psychology, 67*(5), 734–745.

Rothon, C., Edwards, P., Bhui, K., Viner, R. M., Taylor, S., & Stansfeld, S. A. (2010). Physical activity and depressive symptoms in adolescents: a prospective study. *BMC Medicine, 8*, 32. http://dx.doi.org/10.1186/1741-7015-8-32.

Rutter, M. L. (1970). Psycho-social disorders in childhood, and their outcome in adult life. *Journal of the Royal College of Physicians of London, 4*(3), 211–218.

Rutter, M., Tizard, J., Yule, W., Graham, P., & Whitmore, K. (1976). Research report: Isle of Wight studies, 1964–1974. *Psychological Medicine, 6*(2), 313–332.

Ryff, C. D., & Singer, B. (1996). Psychological well-being: meaning, measurement, and implications for psychotherapy research. *Psychotherapy and Psychosomatics, 65*(1), 14–23.

Sakolsky, D., & Birmaher, B. (2012). Developmentally informed pharmacotherapy for child and adolescent depressive disorders. *Child and Adolescent Psychiatric Clinics of North America, 21*(2), 313–325. http://dx.doi.org/10.1016/j.chc.2012.01.005, viii.

Segal, Z. V., Williams, J. M. G., & Teasdale, J. D. (2002). In G. Press (Ed.), *Mindfulness-based cognitive therapy for depression* (New York).

Seligman, M., & Csikszentmihalyi, M. (2000). Positive psychology: an introduction. *American Psychologist, 55*, 5–14.

Seligman, M. E., Schulman, P., DeRubeis, R. J., & Hollon, S. D. (1999). The prevention of depression and anxiety. *Prevention and Treatment, 2*. Article 8. Retrieved from: http://journals.apa.org/prevention/volume2/pre0020008a.html.

Simeon, J. G., Dinicola, V. F., Ferguson, H. B., & Copping, W. (1990). Adolescent depression: a placebo-controlled fluoxetine treatment study and follow-up. *Progressive Neuro-Psychopharmacology & Biological Psychiatry, 14*(5), 791–795.

Sin, N. L., & Lyubomirsky, S. (2009). Enhancing well-being and alleviating depressive symptoms with positive psychology interventions: a practice-friendly meta-analysis. *Journal of Clinical Psychology, 65*(5), 467–487. http://dx.doi.org/10.1002/jclp.20593.

Snyder, C. R., & Lopez, S. J. (2005). *Handbook of positive psychology.* New York: Oxford University Press.

Starkstein, S. E., Mayberg, H. S., Berthier, M. L., Fedoroff, P., Price, T. R., Dannals, R. F., … Robinson, R. G. (1990). Mania after brain injury: neuroradiological and metabolic findings. [Case reports research support, Non-U.S. Gov't research support, U.S. Gov't, P.H.S.]. *Annals of Neurology, 27*(6), 652–659. http://dx.doi.org/10.1002/ana.410270612.

Stewart, S. M., Lee, P. W. H., Ho, L. M., Kennard, B. D., Hughes, C., & Emslie, G. (2002). Symptom patterns in depression and "subthreshold" depression among adolescents in Hong Kong and the United States. *Journal of Cross-Cultural Psychology, 33*, 559–576.

Stewart, S. M., Simmons, A., & Habibpour, E. (2012). Treatment of culturally diverse children and adolescents with depression. [Review]. *Journal of Child and Adolescent Psychopharmacology, 22*(1), 72–79. http://dx.doi.org/10.1089/cap.2011.0051.

Stice, E., Shaw, H., Bohon, C., Marti, C. N., & Rohde, P. (2009). A meta-analytic review of depression prevention programs for children and adolescents: factors that predict magnitude of intervention effects. *Journal of Consulting and Clinical Psychology, 77*(3), 486–503. http://dx.doi.org/10.1037/a0015168.

Strober, M., Lampert, C., Schmidt-Lackner, S., & Morrell, W. (1993). The course of major depressive disorder in adolescents: I. Recovery and risk of manic switching in a follow-up of psychotic and nonpsychotic subtypes. *Journal of the American Academy of Child & Adolescent Psychiatry, 32*(1), 34–42.

Teasdale, J. D., Williams, J. M. G., Soulsby, J. M., Segal, Z. V., Ridgeway, V. A., & Lau, M. A. (2000). Prevention of relapse/recurrence in major depression by mindfulness-based cognitive therapy. *Journal of Consulting and Clinical Psychology, 68*(4), 615–625.

Tompson, M. C., Boger, K. D., & Asarnow, J. R. (2012). Enhancing the developmental appropriateness of treatment for depression in youth: integrating the family in treatment. *Child and Adolescent Psychiatric Clinics of North America, 21*(2), 345–384. http://dx.doi.org/10.1016/j.chc.2012.01.003.

Treatment for Adolescents with Depression Study (TADS). (2004). Fluoxetine, cognitive-behavioral therapy, and their combination for adolescents with depression treatment for adolescents with depression study (TADS) randomized controlled trial. *Journal of the American Medical Association, 292*(7), 807–820.

Trivedi, M. H., & Daly, E. J. (2007). Measurement-based care for refractory depression: a clinical decision support model for clinical research and practice. *Drug and Alcohol Dependence, 88*(Suppl.), 11.

Van Voorhees, B. W., Fogel, J., Pomper, B. E., Marko, M., Reid, N., Watson, N., ... Domanico, R. (2009). Adolescent dose and ratings of an internet-based depression prevention program: a randomized trial of primary care physician brief advice versus a motivational interview. *Journal of Cognitive and Behavioral Psychotherapies: The Official Journal of the International Institute for the Advanced Studies of Psychotherapy and Applied Mental Health, 9*(1), 1–19.

Vitiello, B., Emslie, G., Clarke, G., Wagner, K. D., Asarnow, J. R., Keller, M. B., ... Brent, D. A. (2011). Long-term outcome of adolescent depression initially resistant to selective serotonin reuptake inhibitor treatment: a follow-up study of the TORDIA sample. *The Journal of Clinical Psychiatry, 72*(3), 388–396. http://dx.doi.org/10.4088/JCP.09m05885blu.

Von Knorring, A.-L., Olsson, G. I., Thomsen, P. H., Lemming, O. M., & Hulten, A. (2006). A randomized, double-blind, placebo-controlled study of citalopram in adolescents with major depressive disorder. *Journal of Clinical Psychopharmacology, 26*(3), 311–315.

Vostanis, P., Feehan, C., & Grattan, E. F. (1998). Two-year outcome of children treated for depression. *European Child & Adolescent Psychiatry, 7*(1), 7.

Wagner, K. D., Ambrosini, P. J., Rynn, M., Wohlberg, C., Ruoyong, Y., Greenbaum, M. S., ... Deas-Nesmith, D. (2003). Efficacy of sertraline in the treatment of children and adolescents with major depressive disorder two randomized controlled trials. *Journal of the American Medical Association, 290*(8), 1033–1041.

Wagner, K. D., Jonas, J., Findling, R. L., Ventura, D., & Saikali, K. (2006). A double-blind, randomized, placebo-controlled trial of escitalopram in the treatment of pediatric depression. [Randomized Controlled Trial Research Support, N.I.H., Extramural Research Support, Non-U.S. Gov't]. *Journal of the American Academy of Child and Adolescent Psychiatry, 45*(3), 280–288. http://dx.doi.org/10.1097/01.chi.0000192250.38400.9e.

Wagner, K. D., Robb, A. S., Findling, R. L., Jin, J., Gutierrez, M. M., & Heydorn, W. E. (2004). A randomized, placebo-controlled trial of citalopram for the treatment of major depression in children and adolescents. *American Journal of Psychiatry, 161*(6), 1079–1083.

Walker, J. S., Coleman, D., Lee, J., Squire, P. N., & Friesen, B. J. (2008). Children's stigmatization of childhood depression and ADHD: magnitude and demographic variation in a national sample. [Research Support, U.S. Gov't, Non-P.H.S. Research Support, U.S. Gov't, P.H.S.]. *Journal of the American Academy of Child and Adolescent Psychiatry, 47*(8), 912–920. http://dx.doi.org/10.1097/CHI.0b013e318179961a.

Wang, P. S., Berglund, P. A., Olfson, M., & Kessler, R. C. (2004). Delays in initial treatment contact after first onset of a mental disorder. [Comparative Study]. *Health Services Research, 39*(2), 393–415. http://dx.doi.org/10.1111/j.1475-6773.2004.00234.x.

Weinberg, W. A., & Rehmet, A. (1983). Childhood affective disorder and school problems. In D. P. Cantwell, & G. Carlson (Eds.), *Affective disorders in childhood and adolescence: An update* (pp. 109–128). Jamaica, NY: Spectrum Publications.

Weinberg, W. A., Rutman, J., Sullivan, L., Penick, E. C., & Dietz, S. G. (1973). Depression in children referred to an educational diagnostic center: diagnosis and treatment. Preliminary report. [Clinical Trial]. *The Journal of Pediatrics, 83*(6), 1065–1072.

Weisz, J. R., McCarty, C. A., & Valeri, S. M. (2006). Effects of psychotherapy for depression in children and adolescents: a meta-analysis. *Psychological Bulletin, 132*(1), 132–149.

Williamson, D. E., Birmaher, B., Frank, E., Anderson, B. P., Matty, M. K., & Kupfer, D. J. (1998). Nature of life events and difficulties in depressed adolescents. *Journal of the American Academy of Child & Adolescent Psychiatry, 37*(10), 1049–1057.

Wisdom, J. P., Clarke, G. N., & Green, C. A. (2006). What teens want: barriers to seeking care for depression. [Research Support, Non-U.S. Gov't Research Support, U.S. Gov't, P.H.S.]. *Administration and Policy in Mental Health, 33*(2), 133–145. http://dx.doi.org/10.1007/s10488-006-0036-4.

III. INTERVENTIONS AND TREATMENTS

12

Treatment of Eating Disorders in Children and Adolescents

J. Derenne, J. Lock

Stanford University School of Medicine, Stanford, CA, United States

INTRODUCTION

Once thought to affect mostly affluent Western caucasian teenage females, eating disorders are chronic, biologically based illnesses now known to affect individuals across the lifespan. Due to severe medical sequelae in every organ system of the body (Golden, 2015), they cause significant morbidity and possess the dubious honor of having the highest mortality rates of any mental illness other than the substance use disorders (Birmingham, 2005). They are found in all cultures, socioeconomic groups, and are increasingly being seen in males [ratio thought to be 1:10, (Hudson, 2007) but may be changing as screening improves and stigma decreases (Lock, 2008)], as well as in their female counterparts. Eating disorder symptoms can arise at any time in the life cycle, with the most common presentation occurring in the adolescent years.

Anorexia nervosa (AN), a disorder of inadequate and restricted energy intake, results in low weight, distorted perception of one's weight and shape, and fear of weight gain or becoming fat (or behavior that interferes with weight gain) (American Psychiatric Association, 2013). While often considered "rare," it is thought to affect approximately 0.5–1.5% (Smink, van Hoeken, Oldehinkel, & Hoek, 2014) of adolescent females, which is similar to the incidence of schizophrenia and bipolar affective disorder. In DSM-5, diagnostic criteria were modified to be more inclusive of males (removing the requirement for amenorrhea), and to use less stigmatizing language to describe behavioral manifestations of the illness, which previously could be construed as being rather judgmental and suggesting that AN is a voluntary illness.

Positive Mental Health, Fighting Stigma and Promoting Resiliency for Children and Adolescents
http://dx.doi.org/10.1016/B978-0-12-804394-3.00012-7

Bulimia nervosa (BN) is characterized by binge eating episodes followed by compensatory purging mechanisms such as vomiting, or laxative or diuretic use. Individuals may also use fasting, compulsive exercise, or omission of insulin to counteract the effects of objective or subjective binge episodes, which occur weekly (new DSM-5 criteria) for at least three months. DSM-IV had required twice weekly episodes to meet diagnostic criteria. Self-evaluation is excessively influenced by weight and shape, and patients often experience a maladaptive cycle of high dietary restriction, followed by binge eating and purging (American Psychiatric Association, 2013). BN is thought to affect 1–2% of adolescent females (Smink et al., 2014), although it is difficult to accurately pinpoint the true number of individuals afflicted due to concerns about stigma and shame that may limit reporting.

Binge eating disorder (BED) was included in DSM-5 for the first time. It was previously only diagnosable under the now-defunct eating disorder not otherwise specified (EDNOS) umbrella. BED is estimated to affect 2.3% of female adolescents and 0.8% of male adolescents (Swanson, 2011). BED is characterized by the presence of objective binge eating episodes (eating large amounts of food rapidly, secretly, to the point of feeling overly full or ill, and experiencing a feeling of loss of control of food intake) without compensatory purgative behaviors. Similar to BN, episodes occur weekly for three months (American Psychiatric Association, 2013).

Avoidant restrictive food intake disorder (ARFID) is another new inclusion in DSM-5, although the behaviors have been observed for quite some time. ARFID is typically seen in younger children and teens, and may present as vomiting or choking phobia, overly restrictive intake related to texture or flavor preferences, or avoidance of eating due to discomfort or pain (such as that seen in functional abdominal pain). Patients do not report weight and shape concerns. There is a strong overlap with other anxiety disorders and it is often seen in children with autism spectrum illnesses (American Psychiatric Association, 2013).

Other specified feeding and eating disorders (OSFED) is the DSM-5 diagnosis previously described disordered eating that does not fit cleanly into the previously described diagnostic categories (eg, night eating syndrome, purging disorder, and subclinical restrictive and binge-purge behaviors) (American Psychiatric Association, 2013). These syndromes were previously captured under the EDNOS diagnosis.

ETIOLOGY

While it can be tempting for patients, families, and clinicians to try to isolate a causative trigger for the development of disordered eating, this approach is rarely fruitful. Rather, it is generally more effective to conceptualize it as a "perfect storm" of factors that make conditions ideal for the development of disordered eating. Factors may include biological vulnerabilities to anxiety disorders, particularly obsessive-compulsive disorder (OCD), temperament (avoidant, perfectionistic, self-doubting, and risk-averse individuals appear to be more at risk) (Anderluh, Tchanturia, Rabe-Hesketh, & Treasure, 2003), and difficult stresses in one's life. It is common to see eating disorders arise in the context of life transition (puberty, matriculation at college, marriage and child-bearing, menopause). Family dynamics may make it challenging for an individual to recover from disordered eating, and stresses clearly have an impact on symptom severity, but it is not helpful to blame the development of the disorder on difficult families. Eating disorders can and do arise in individuals with very loving and supportive family and social networks. Finally, societal pressure to achieve the thin ideal perpetuated by many media outlets may be a factor in the development of the drive for thinness that commonly triggers disordered eating (Jones, 2004). Individuals and their families often report that the disorder started as an innocent attempt at modifying one's diet to eat healthful foods, minimize intake of sugar and fat-laden snacks, and increase physical activity. Weight loss is a well-known trigger and may result from dieting as well as unintentional weight loss stemming from gastrointestinal illness, orthodontia, medication side effects, or loss of appetite related to psychiatric illness such as depression, anxiety, or psychosis.

COMORBIDITY

A significant number of individuals with eating disorders have co-occurring mood (Holtkamp, Muller, et al., 2005), anxiety (Strober, 2007), substance use (Becker, 2015), attention deficit (Seitz et al., 2013), and personality disorders (Friborg & Kaiser, 2014). In order to develop an effective, evidence-based treatment plan, and to consider the potential utility of psychotropic medications versus re-nourishment alone, it is important to take a very careful history to establish the timeline of development of all symptoms.

Disordered eating often results in an inadequate caloric intake, and may cause malnutrition, which produces a constellation of symptoms that are quite similar to the neuro-vegetative symptoms of depression. Insufficient fuel to the brain can cause dysphoria, irritability, difficulties with sleep, anhedonia, guilty ruminations, anergia, poor concentration, poor focus, and feelings of hopelessness and helplessness. However, premorbid depression may complicate the picture by causing low appetite and anhedonia, which can, in turn, trigger the development of disordered eating, and may perpetuate a vicious cycle of low mood and inadequate nutritional intake. Clinicians must be willing to differentiate the timeline of symptom appearance in order to specify the most accurate diagnosis. Similarly, providers must be alert and monitor for the development of suicidal ideation, as an alarming number of individuals struggling with these disorders die by suicide. In fact, 50% of eating disorder-related deaths are thought to be due to suicide (Birmingham, 2005).

A starving brain may also present symptoms of anxiety or inattention that can be misdiagnosed, but are actually directly related to the eating disorder itself. One must always assess for the presence of premorbid symptoms, as the treatment of choice for eating disorders is to re-nourish the individual by regulating eating patterns and increasing caloric intake. Treatment of comorbid depression, anxiety, OCD, or attention-deficit hyperactivity disorder (ADHD) may be necessary, but is likely to be more effective once the malnutrition has been reversed. In addition, medications used to treat these conditions may interfere with the re-nourishment process (eg, stimulant medications for ADHD may worsen appetite). Other common comorbid conditions include substance use disorders (alcohol and narcotics in patients with BN; cocaine, stimulants, methamphetamine in individuals with AN) and personality disorders (avoidant, borderline, histrionic, obsessive compulsive) in those over the age of 18 years.

MEDICAL COMPLICATIONS

In addition to their very real impact on mood, anxiety, and other psychological symptoms, eating disorders have significant effects on every organ system in the body (Golden, 2015). Malnutrition triggers energy conservation through diminished metabolic rate, which results in the widespread slowing of bodily functions.

The most concerning of these relates to the cardiovascular effects of inadequate nutritional intake, as these can be fatal and account for a large percentage of eating disorder-related deaths. Slowed heart rate and prolonged and delayed conduction of electrical impulses through the heart muscle can cause fatal arrhythmia. These can be worsened by electrolyte abnormalities (dysregulated levels of potassium, phosphorus, and magnesium) that may be related to starvation, purging, or inappropriate rate of re-nourishment after starvation (Jauregui-Garrido & Jauregui-Lobera, 2012). Medical hospitalization typically focuses on cardiac stability, with close monitoring of heart rates, blood pressures, and electrolyte levels (Freeman, 2011).

The medical team must also be very aware of the dangers of "refeeding" syndrome in the initial days and weeks of treatment of malnourished individuals who present for re-nourishment. Refeeding syndrome was initially observed in the famous Keys experiments, which used conscientious objectors during WWII to study the effects of starvation and refeeding in otherwise healthy young men (Keys, 1950). Unlimited access to food after a period of extreme deprivation increases blood sugar, which stimulates insulin production and gluconeogenesis. This process requires phosphorus, potassium, and magnesium, which have been depleted by malnutrition; intracellular shifts result in plummeting serum levels of these substances, which put the heart at risk of fatal arrhythmia. Phosphorus is particularly important in human physiology; all muscle, including cardiac muscle, requires adenosine triphosphate in order to contract appropriately (Skipper, 2012); and 2,3 diphosphoglycerate, which is present in red blood cells, allows oxygen to be appropriately released near necessary organs. Furthermore, cardiac muscle atrophies in response to malnutrition. When increased food and hydration is introduced during refeeding, the weakened heart may have diminished capacity to handle the increased load, resulting in increased risk of congestive heart failure. Therefore, the common consensus is that refeeding should proceed in a relatively cautious manner; calories should be increased steadily and not too slowly, and electrolytes should be monitored regularly (Golden, Keane-Miller, Sainani, & Kapphahn, 2013).

The gastrointestinal system is almost universally affected by malnutrition. Decreased metabolic rate leads to slowed gut motility and increased transit time. Gastroparesis can lead to early satiety, abdominal discomfort, and very uncomfortable bloating (Kamal et al., 1991); all of these can limit an individual's willingness to increase intake, which interferes with treatment. Chronic constipation is an issue in the majority of patients, and can be exacerbated by poor hydration, which is also common in patients restricting intake. Chronic laxative abuse may also adversely effect transit time, and stopping laxative use can be dangerous; patients often require laxative taper and may need additional treatment as stimulant laxatives may damage enteric nerves over time (Wald, 2003). Retching with vomiting can cause hematemesis secondary to Mallory-Weiss tears, and severe bingeing can result in gastric rupture and death (Takehiro, 2012). An abrupt cessation of purging can actually lead to significant fluid shifts due to changes in baseline levels of antidiuretic hormone, which, in turn, can be quite emotionally distressing (Bahia, 2012). Patients often interpret increased body weight (even when related to fluid shifts) as a rapid gain of adipose tissue. Abdominal discomfort makes it challenging for patients to push forward with increasing intake, but it is essential that they do so, as oral re-nourishment allows the gastrointestinal tract to practice processing food, and allows the individual to re-establish normal eating patterns and hunger and satiety cues.

In female patients, amenorrhea is a significant health concern indicating inadequate production of estrogen and progesterone, generally resulting from hypothalamic suppression (Golden, 1993). In addition to implications for future fertility, low estrogen levels can have a concerning impact on bone composition, which is critical during adolescence as there is limited time during which bone can be built. Even those who have fully recovered from their eating disorder may not be able to correct damage done to bone density, which can increase the likelihood of osteoporosis and related complications later in life (Bailey, 2000). In males, hypothalamic suppression of testosterone can lead to difficulty with pubertal development, low libido, and erectile dysfunction (Hatchman, 2005).

Malnutrition also causes dry skin and hair, hair loss, skin breakdown, and cold intolerance. Downy, furry hair (lanugo) may appear in areas not typically associated with hair growth, and serves to keep the body warm when fat stores are inadequate (Strumia, 2013). Malnutrition may also interfere with the body's ability to manufacture blood cells across all lines, resulting in anemia and putting yet another stress on the circulatory system. It can suppress the immune system, leading to increased susceptibility to illness and impaired healing as well as prolonged recovery from malnutrition itself (Mehler, 2015).

NATURAL HISTORY

For many patients, eating disorders are chronic, with relapsing and remitting courses. The ego-syntonic nature of symptoms can make them difficult to treat, particularly as the behaviors and distorted thinking are more firmly entrenched over time. However, when eating disorders are identified early and treated aggressively by specialty providers who focus on re-nourishment, the prognosis can be quite good, with one family-based treatment (FBT) study demonstrating that a large number of patients showed continued evidence of recovery at a mean of 3.96 years post-treatment (89% of patients remained at greater than 90% ideal body weight, 74% had eating disorder evaluation (EDE) scores within the normal range, and 91% of post-menarchal females not taking birth control pills had return of menses) (Lock, Couturier, & Agras, 2006). Medical stabilization, re-nourishment, and weight restoration are typically the initial goals of treatment. Structure and support of family and the treatment team providers can promote this and allow the individual to demonstrate regular, normal eating patterns, and the cessation of maladaptive behaviors such as restrictive eating, binge eating, purging, and compulsive exercise. As these behaviors cease, and the individual is able to resist urges to return to them, there is then more time and mental space to focus on psychological recovery. This may include attention to mood, anxiety, or impulse control disorders, and may also focus on resuming a normal developmental trajectory (separation and individuation, school, work, social and romantic relationships, and leisure activities not involving dieting and exercise).

TREATMENT APPROACHES AND EVIDENCE BASE

Role of the Multidisciplinary Treatment Team: Medical Provider, Registered Dietician, Individual/Group/Family Therapy

A multidisciplinary team approach is the standard of care for eating disorders. Given the significant overlap between medical and psychological aspects of the illness, patients benefit from the involvement of subspecialist clinicians with clearly defined roles, who communicate closely to minimize confusion and to insure that the patient and family are receiving consistent messages from all team members. In the United States, the team is generally composed of a medical provider (typically a pediatrician or adolescent medicine specialist), a dietitian (who may consult only to parents, depending on the treatment modality employed), and a psychotherapist trained in evidence-based psychotherapies. Depending on the treatment approach and setting, the therapist may utilize family, individual, and group therapy sessions. A psychiatrist may be involved in cases warranting a medication intervention, often targeting psychiatric comorbidities that may be affecting eating disorder recovery (Lock, 2015b).

Family-Based Treatment

Family-based treatment (FBT), sometimes known as "The Maudsley Model" (named after the Maudsley Hospital, London, where earlier innovative work was carried out), is the gold standard treatment intervention for adolescent AN (Lock, 2015a). It is being studied in BN (Forsberg & Lock, 2015) as well, and may be modified for use in young adults who are willing to have parents more actively involved in their care. This approach assumes that parents and siblings are assets in treatment, rather than "problems" who need to be separated from the identified patient. As such, all members of the family are valued members of the treatment team and are expected to attend each session. The goal of this agnostic therapy is to re-nourish the patient, and to help him or her abstain from unhealthy eating and exercise patterns rather than to try to uncover the reason for disordered eating, or to focus on self-esteem or control issues that are often raised in individual therapeutic approaches.

In the first phase of weekly treatment, the parents are charged with re-nourishing their child, and take responsibility for planning, preparing, and plating all meals and snacks. Parents may consult with a dietitian to ensure that they are addressing all nutritional needs, especially since caloric requirements may be higher than parents expect in the initial phases of refeeding. However, this therapeutic approach assumes that parents know how to feed themselves, and know how to adequately feed a child; most have raised other healthy children, and, until illness struck, they were adequately nourishing the child currently struggling with an eating disorder. Externalizing the illness is an important step in helping family members understand that AN is not a choice; rather, it is an illness, and the patient needs empathetic, caring, yet firm and consistent structure and support to recover fully. Siblings are tasked with supporting their brother or sister by engaging them in fun and familiar activities, and are encouraged to express care and concern for them. They may act as a sounding-board for the patient to complain about parents, or to vent about treatment, or they may try to cheer their sibling through good-natured teasing and joking. That being said, they are not to take on the role of the "food police" and are not to monitor meals and snacks. Weight is measured at the start of each encounter and sets the tone for the ensuing session. If the patient is gaining weight as expected and required, the family is asked to describe things that are working well and to comment on strategies that have not been effective. If the patient has lost weight or is not making adequate progress, parents are encouraged to use their instincts and previous experience parenting this child to develop an approach for the coming week. Therapists act as eating disorder expert consultants to parents, who are viewed as the ultimate experts in their child and own families.

The transition to phase two of FBT occurs when the patient is weight-restored (or at least very close), and is eating meals and snacks with limited resistance. This phase focuses on supporting the patient as he or she slowly and gradually takes on more responsibility for planning and plating meals and snacks. Sessions tend to space out to biweekly frequency to allow families an opportunity to practice between sessions. The vast majority of adolescents do not like having their parents take responsibility for their nutrition, so the increased independence is often viewed as a reward for hard work and good decision-making. Parents need to monitor closely, as allowing the patient to serve his or her lunch or plan a snack should not rapidly lead to complete independence around meal planning. Instead, the parents should be willing to decrease oversight and supervision of eating as long as vital signs remain stable and weight continues to increase appropriately. If weight loss or plateau occurs, parents are encouraged to find ways to increase supervision and oversight of meal planning, preparation, and consumption.

Phase three of FBT stresses a return to age-appropriate independence around eating and a discussion of normal adolescent life issues and how these will be addressed within the family. During this time, the frequency may stretch out to monthly therapy visits. It is very common for parents in phase three of treatment to have concerns about chores, dating, curfews, and driving, while realizing that having time to focus on these issues demonstrates a significant improvement in eating-related concerns (Lock & Le Grange, 2013).

Research indicates that FBT is a level one, "well-established" treatment for adolescents with AN (Lock, 2015a), and superior to individual (Lock, 2010) interventions. It is considered a level three, "possibly efficacious" intervention for BN (LeGrange, 2007). When compared to systemic family therapy, it demonstrates faster weight restoration, fewer days in the hospital, and lower overall treatment costs (Agras, 2014). Adding an individual eating disorder therapist during FBT does not generally confer additional benefit. That being said, individual therapy may be indicated for comorbid conditions such as depression or anxiety beyond that associated with malnutrition or fear of weight gain.

Systemic Family Therapy

Systemic family therapy (SyFT) focuses on relationships and interactions among family members, exploring patterns of beliefs and behaviors, and using past experiences to try to solve the problem at hand. The therapist is neutral and non-directive and does not explicitly discuss food and eating concerns unless asked directly by the family. This therapy is manualized and delivered in 16 sessions over the course of nine months. When compared directly to FBT, there was no statistically significant difference in remission rates, suggesting that SyFT is an effective treatment for AN, especially in those with severe obsessive-compulsive symptoms (weight gain was greater in SyFT in this subgroup). The rate of weight gain is significantly faster in FBT, which is important in that costly medical hospitalization due to low weight and unstable vital signs is much more common early in treatment (Agras, 2014). As such, SyFT can be described as a level two, "probably efficacious" treatment for AN (Lock, 2015a). SyFT has not been studied in BN, BED, or ARFID.

Multi-Family Therapy

These group interventions bring together a number of families with one therapist with the intent to have families support each other and learn from each other, in addition to consultation with the eating disorder clinician. Parents report increased hope and self-efficacy, especially early in treatment. This approach is effective is promoting weight restoration, and highly acceptable to parents, with once study demonstrating greater than 90% completion of treatment (Blessit, 2015).

Cognitive Behavioral Therapy

Cognitive behavioral therapy (CBT) is a gold standard, problem-focused and action-oriented, manualized approach that was initially developed for the treatment of depression. The theory rests on the assumption that automatic thoughts and core beliefs influence the thoughts, feelings, and behaviors resulting from a situation or event. Errors in thinking, such as overgeneralizing, magnifying negatives, minimizing positives, and catastrophizing, are thought to lead to emotional distress and self-defeating behavior.

By examining the evidence for and against a particular set of beliefs in a given situation, the patient is able to challenge negative thoughts, which allows modification of the associated feelings and behaviors in a more adaptive manner. There are a number of CBT protocols that have been developed for the treatment of eating disorders; some incorporate cognitive restructuring and behavioral experiments, while others focus exclusively on behavioral interventions. Overall, CBT is an effective, evidence-based intervention for the treatment of both BN and BED in adults (Serpell, 2013), but it appears less effective in the treatment of AN. As with many of the other psychotherapeutic modalities, AN may not be as amenable to treatment with CBT owing to the ego-syntonic nature of the illness, which limits the patient's motivation for change and willingness to participate fully in the intervention.

CBT-E is a transdiagnostic protocol, which was developed for patients struggling with symptoms across the eating disorder spectrum. This is primarily a behavioral treatment, consisting of 20 sessions over 20 weeks (40 sessions over 40 weeks for very underweight patients) (Fairburn, 2008). The first stage allows the patient and therapist to gain a shared understanding of the eating issues in play by developing a very detailed and personalized formulation incorporating thoughts, feelings, and behaviors, and encouraging the patient to develop and maintain normal and regular eating patterns. Stage two provides an opportunity to review progress and plan for stage three, where the majority of the work occurs. Stage three targets the eating disorder maintaining mechanisms of poor body image and dietary restraint, while also encouraging the patient to address the effects of mood and life stress on eating behaviors. At the end of stage three, patient and therapist begin to discuss setbacks and relapse prevention; this extends into stage four, during which termination (including a "review" meeting several months after the last session) occurs (Fairburn, 2003).

The evidence base supporting CBT in children and adolescents is limited; CBT-E for AN is considered a level four, "experimental" intervention (Lock, 2015a; Grave, 2013), while CBT delivered in the guided self-help format is considered level three, "possibly efficacious" (Lock, 2015a; Schmidt, 2007). While CBT is considered a gold standard intervention in adults with BED, it has not been studied in children and teens.

Adolescent-Focused Therapy for Anorexia Nervosa

Otherwise known as ego-oriented individual therapy for AN, adolescent-focused therapy (AFT) is a manualized psychodynamic approach based in self-psychology (Fitzpatrick, 2010). The therapeutic relationship is used to promote improvement in the patient's ability to identify emotions and tolerate negative affective states that are typically avoided by symptoms of restrictive eating and excessive exercise. This, in turn, allows the adolescent to develop a healthier sense of self and the ego strength necessary to navigate separation and individuation from the family of origin. The therapist utilizes a nurturing and authoritative stance to illustrate the gravity of the situation and need for change, to educate the patient about the deleterious effects of malnutrition, and to firmly convey the expectation that the patient will maintain medical stability in order to stay out of the hospital. This is achieved by setting the expectation that the adolescent will abstain from exercise and increase nutritional intake to gain one-half to one pound (0.2–0.45 kg) per week. The therapist strives to externalize AN from the patient, demonstrating high regard for him or her, and genuine care and concern for his or her life.

Treatment consists of 32 individual sessions (although up to eight may be used for collateral sessions with parents, two are mandatory in the assessment phase) and four phases over the course of 12 months; visits occur weekly at the beginning of treatment and gradually taper over time. In the assessment phase, the therapist gathers a personal and developmental history including a discussion of the ways in which the patient manages stress, and exploration of school, social, and family function. Evaluating motivation for change is another important part of the initial sessions. In the early therapy phase, the clinician shifts focus to rapport building and begins to suggest interpretations of behaviors and emotional states. Affective displays are validated and encouraged, and the adolescent is empowered to work on increasing assertiveness. As they move into the middle therapy phase, the therapist is targeting the adolescent's resistance to change, reducing perfectionistic tendencies, and continuing to facilitate individuation. The final phase focuses on termination and processing issues related to ending treatment, such as generalizing therapeutic successes to other areas of one's life and internalizing relapse prevention skills.

Evidence for AFT suggests that it is "probably efficacious" for the treatment of adolescent AN. When compared to FBT, both interventions lead to significant clinical improvements. However, patients randomized to FBT had greater weight gain by BMI percentile and greater improvement in EDE at the end of treatment. Furthermore, fewer participants in the FBT arm required hospitalization than did those receiving individual AFT (Lock, 2010).

Dialectical Behavioral Therapy for Anorexia Nervosa, Bulimia Nervosa, and Binge Eating Disorder

Originally developed for the treatment of chronically suicidal adults with borderline personality disorders (BPD) (Linehan, 1993), dialectical behavioral therapy (DBT) is based on the theory that pervasive difficulties with regulating emotion can result in maladaptive coping strategies such as self-injury, disordered eating, compulsive exercise, and substance abuse. Current societal expectations of beauty and the thin ideal may contribute to the development of disordered eating, particularly in the setting of weight-related teasing or pressures to diet. The approach uses Zen-based acceptance and change strategies to mindfully and effectively navigate emotionally charged situations. Given that emotion dysregulation underlies a number of psychiatric conditions, DBT is now being used trans-diagnostically; it has been modified for use in adolescents (Miller, 2007), and is being actively studied in eating disorders, substance use disorders (SUD), and post-traumatic stress disorders (PTSD) (Linehan & Wilks, 2015).

A skills-based approach may allow patients to avoid binge eating or purging that is precipitated by stress or strong emotion, and DBT can be particularly helpful in the treatment of eating disorders in patients with comorbid conditions such as BPD or SUD, which are also amenable to DBT. Principles of mindful eating, "urge-surfing" (noticing and observing, but not acting on environmental triggers), and alternate rebellion (finding ways to express distress that are more in line with one's values and goals) have been used to modify the standard DBT skill set for the ED population (Safer, 2001). Radically open DBT targets those with disorders of over-control, such as AN; treatment focuses on reducing social isolation, cognitive rigidity, risk aversion, and inhibited emotional expression rather than on targeting emotional dysregulation (Lynch, 2015). Clinicians incorporate specific eating behaviors into the hierarchy of treatment targets, with life-threatening behaviors (continuing to purge despite dangerous electrolyte disturbance or intentionally restricting eating despite low weight) taking precedence over therapy interfering or quality of life interfering behaviors. Secondary treatment targets include achieving balance and resisting extreme behaviors (eg, no exercise versus excessive exercise, binge eating versus restrictive eating) (Wisniewski & Ben-Porath, 2015). Treatment generally consists of individual therapy meetings in concert with group skills-building sessions; adolescent-focused approaches have been shown to have some effectiveness (Salbach-Andrae, 2009), and may also use multi-family groups to incorporate family members into the treatment process. The combination of DBT and FBT in the treatment of adolescents with BN is actively being explored (Anderson et al., 2015; Murray et al., 2015).

Interpersonal Psychotherapy

Difficulty with interpersonal relationships is a key feature of many eating disorders, and may be present prior to the onset of disordered eating. Long-standing illness may also contribute, as resulting social isolation encouraged by ED pathology limits the development of healthy intimate relationships. Interpersonal difficulties often become evident in the adolescent and early adult years, when individuals begin to experience mature and close relationships; adolescence is also the time when eating disorders tend to present. Lack of satisfying relationships may affect mood, anxiety, and overall sense of self, and may become a maintaining mechanism for disordered eating. Interpersonal psychotherapy (IPT) was initially developed for the treatment of depression, but has been modified for use in treating eating disorders. It primarily addresses the patient's current interpersonal functioning, rather than directly focusing on eating symptoms and behaviors. By improving relationships, the hope is that the patient will develop more effective ways to manage stress, as well as more positive self-evaluation, which may decrease drive for thinness, dietary restraint, and other maladaptive eating behaviors (Murphy, 2012).

IPT is typically delivered in a three-phase format, over the course of approximately 20 sessions. Phase one (three to four sessions) focuses on educating the patient about the goals of treatment, engaging him or her in the treatment, and collaboratively identifying the interpersonal issues (taking an "interpersonal inventory") that are to be addressed in the remaining weeks of treatment. The therapist uses examples from the patient's own life to illustrate the ways in which problematic interpersonal experiences can influence symptoms. Discussion of specific eating disorder symptoms is limited to observing changes in frequency and intensity of eating behavior between sessions, and understanding the interpersonal context of these changes (Weissman, 2000).

Phase two may take up to 14 sessions, and is where the majority of the work of therapy occurs. Patient and therapist work together to address the problems previously identified, spending the majority of time on issues likely to have the most significant impact on functioning. The therapist employs a mostly non-directive stance, with the patient leading much of the discussion. However, the therapist does stress the importance of change in order for the patient to be more effective in relationships. Identified problems generally can be categorized into difficulties with interpersonal role disputes with prominent people in one's life (partner, employer, parent), role transitions (going to college, getting married, becoming a parent), and interpersonal deficits (scarcity of satisfying intimate relationships). Difficulty achieving life goals, and grieving the loss of a loved one may be an additional focus of treatment in some patients (Weissman, 2007).

Phase three focuses on solidifying and maintaining the changes achieved in phase two, while also developing a relapse prevention plan for the future. Sessions are scheduled at biweekly intervals, and typically take about three meetings to complete. Approximately 20 weeks after termination is complete, the therapist and patient meet a final time to review progress and to address any lapses or setbacks that may have occurred (Murphy, 2012).

Despite some initial anxiety that the eating disorder symptoms will not be adequately addressed without direct attention to them, patients tend to find IPT quite acceptable. Data for using IPT is generally limited to adults, and the evidence base for using IPT in AN is quite meager (McIntosh, 2005). However, empirical support in BED and BN is much more robust. Direct comparisons to CBT demonstrate that CBT is more effective at symptom reduction at the end of treatment, but that differences dissipate within eight months, suggesting that patients in the IPT group tend to continue to improve even after terminating therapy (Agras, 2000; Fairburn, 1993).

Acceptance and Commitment Therapy

Acceptance and commitment therapy (ACT) is an evidence-based therapy with roots in CBT that focuses exclusively on changing behaviors rather than targeting cognitions. It posits that one reason for the disappointing lack of efficacy seen in CBT may be the fact that AN is ego-syntonic, and, as such, many patients lack the motivation to change (Jurascio, 2010). Humans innately try to avoid experiences that cause uncomfortable thoughts and feelings; however, avoiding discomfort ultimately causes psychological distress by preventing the individual from taking the steps necessary to achieve life goals in line with his or her values. ACT aims to change one's reactions to uncomfortable thoughts and feelings by teaching mindfulness and distress tolerance techniques rather than focusing on trying to change the thoughts and feelings themselves, which is viewed as futile and likely to cause more distress. Instead, patients are encouraged to give up the quest for cognitive control and adopt an attitude of acceptance in order to move toward valued behaviors and goals. In effect, patients are asked to be more willing to tolerate negative affective states in order to lead a value-driven life (Juarascio et al., 2013).

ACT can be delivered individually (Jurascio, 2010), and is also thought to be effective in a group setting. A recent open trial suggests that a combination of ACT and separated family treatment with elements of FBT (parental mediated re-nourishment of the adolescent and exposure to feared foods) may reduce ED symptomatology (Timko, 2015).

Cognitive Remediation Therapy

Although inconsistent in children and adolescents, there is some data to suggest that individuals with AN may demonstrate cognitive inflexibility (poor set shifting) and weak central coherence which may predispose them to excessive focus on detail and an inability to "see the forest for the trees" (Garrett, 2014). These deficits are independent of IQ, and do not appear to resolve with weight restoration and correction of malnutrition. Unaffected sisters and parents of youth with AN have been shown to demonstrate a similar neuropsychological profile, which suggests a genetic component. Given that AN is such a difficult illness to treat, there is a rationale for the view that an inflexible thinking style may interfere with current psychological treatments. Cognitive rigidity may also negatively impact recruitment into therapeutic interventions and may lead to increased attrition, particularly in the early months of treatment (typically 1–2 month) (Lock & Le Grange, 2013).

Cognitive remediation therapy (CRT) was initially developed for use in brain injury and has been used to successfully treat cognitive processing difficulties associated with schizophrenia, autism, and OCD (Tchanturia, 2014). It is unique in that it does not focus on eating disorder symptoms. Rather, CRT uses fun cognitive puzzles and games to encourage and practice more flexible thinking, which has been very helpful in reducing attrition and engaging patients who may otherwise resist traditional therapies. A positive experience may facilitate engagement in more traditional interventions in the future, which is important as CRT may need to be paired with established treatments for optimal effectiveness. The process includes identifying the patient's cognitive strengths and weaknesses in a lighthearted manner, generalizing these to everyday life, and developing strategies to overcome difficulties (Lock & Le Grange, 2013). As it can be delivered in individual, group, family-based, (Lask, 2015) and self-help and/or career-driven (Lang, 2014) formats, it may provide a very accessible and cost-effective addition to the ED treatment arsenal.

Inpatient, Residential, Partial Hospitalization, and Intensive Outpatient Programs

Assuming that the patient is stable to be safely treated outside of the medical hospital, providers need to determine the most appropriate setting for ongoing care. Inpatient psychiatry units provide behavioral structure and support in a containing setting, and are generally not necessary unless the individual is actively suicidal or requires continuous supervision to prevent bingeing, purging, compulsive exercising, or acute food refusal.

Residential treatment centers provide structure and 24-hour support, but are not locked, and afford the opportunity for patients to have intensive therapy experiences, including in vivo exposure and response prevention food challenges. In the United States, they are selectively covered by insurance companies, while other countries having various methods for reimbursement, and patients may require 30-, 60-, or 90-day stays. Partial hospital programs (PHPs) allow for increased structure and support during the day, but also allow the individual to have some practice living at home a few hours each evening, and sleeping in their own beds. The structure of each day tends to be quite similar to the schedule of therapeutic groups, supported meals, and individual sessions available in residential treatment centers. Intensive outpatient programs (IOPs) provide evening support to individuals who are ready for re-entry to work or school but may benefit from additional support during vulnerable hours of the day. These programs tend to provide a supervised dinner as well as group and individual therapy activities.

It is common for hospitals to "step down" patients from inpatient medical or psychiatric units to residential treatment centers, and then on to PHP to IOP prior to a full return home. There is emerging evidence suggesting that day-programs (partial hospitalization) are not less effective than psychiatric admission (Herpertz-Dahlmann et al., 2014), although with generally few outcome studies (Brewerton & Costin, 2011a, 2011b), it is difficult to know the true efficacy of these interventions. Many patients can successfully restore weight in a highly structured setting, but tend to fall back into default patterns of restricting intake and exercising obsessively when they return to their home setting. As such, some programs are advocating keeping young patients at home as much as possible (assuming that it is medically safe), so that change can be undertaken as a family, and factors affecting recovery are addressed from the very start of treatment.

Psychotropic Medications

Food is the best medicine when treating eating disorders. Re-nourishment is the only intervention proven to be effective in treating AN, and effective psychotherapies focus on achieving this goal. There have been no studies to date with evidence supporting the use of psychotropic medications in children and adolescents to treat eating disorders (Golden, 2011). Fluoxetine at 60 mg has an indication from the Food and Drug Administration for the treatment of BN in adults (Goldstein, 1995), and lisdexamfetamine has recently been approved by the FDA for BED in adults (McElroy et al., 2015). The reasons for this are complicated. Medication studies in children and adolescents are notoriously difficult given concerns about safety in the developing brain. In addition, the ego-syntonic nature of the illness may interfere with recruitment in medication studies, as it leads many patients with eating disorders resist taking any medication that may cause an increase in appetite or weight gain (Halmi, 2008). Individuals at low weight tend to be more sensitive to medication side effects, and medications may not work as well in malnourished individuals given that they lack the building blocks necessary to manufacture neurotransmitters

(Barbarich, 2004) that may be necessary for clinical improvement. Finally, there is some speculation among researchers that eating disorders may require poly-pharmacy rather than mono-therapy, or that we just have not yet found the right target receptor or neurotransmitter necessary to treat eating disorders pharmacologically.

That being said, about 50% of patients seen in adolescent medicine eating disorders clinics report taking psychotropic medications (Golden, 2011). It can be useful to target comorbid conditions that may interfere with recovery from AN, so, as previously stated, taking a meticulous history of mood, anxiety, and inattention symptoms is imperative to determine whether symptoms are related to malnutrition, or if they are indicative of a separate, underlying comorbid condition.

Clinicians may be tempted to use psychotropic medications such as selective serotonin reuptake inhibitors (SSRIs) or benzodiazepines to target food-related anxiety and obsessive-compulsive rituals. Anecdotally, there have been some patients who are so fearful and anxious about eating that a rescue medication such as lorazepam or clonazepam has been necessary to get them started. However, in general, patients do better with learning coping strategies such as distraction, diaphragmatic breathing, progressive muscle relaxation, and guided imagery to deal with anxiety and to see that it dissipates over time as they are able to resist the urge to avoid eating. The SSRIs do not appear to have any benefit in treating adolescent eating disorders (Holtkamp, Konrad, et al., 2005), and despite an earlier study suggesting otherwise (Kaye, 2001), fluoxetine is not protective in preventing relapse (Walsh, 2006). The FDA has given fluoxetine 60 mg an indication for the treatment of BN in adults over 18, but similar studies have not been pursued in children and adolescents. Tricyclic antidepressants (Biederman et al., 1985), monoamine oxidase inhibitors (Walsh, Stewart, Roose, Gladis, & Glassman, 1984), and non-antidepressant medications such as topiramate (Nickel, 2005) and ondansetron (Faris, 2000) have also been studied in adults but have shown to have fairly limited efficacy and adverse side effects that significantly limit use. It is also important to note that bupropion (particularly at high doses) is relatively contraindicated in eating disorder patients due to lowered seizure threshold, which may be exacerbated by electrolyte shifts associated with purging (Horne, 1988).

Atypical antipsychotics have also been investigated by a number of groups, (McKnight, 2010), specifically targeting the extreme distortions around weight or shape and cognitive rigidity that, at times, seem quite similar to psychosis. There was also hope that increases in appetite, decreases in resting metabolic rate, and overall increases in weight demonstrated by patients using these medications for mood stabilization or treatment of psychosis would be replicated in the eating disorder population. However, studies have not demonstrated effectiveness, and many patients balk at taking a medication that lists increased appetite and weight gain as known side effects. Other patients have reported extremely distressing new onset binge eating and purging associated with starting these medications. In general, it is best to avoid using medications to stimulate appetite. "Anorexia" is really a misnomer in this population, as the vast majority of individuals report that they enjoy food, but are fearful of losing control of eating, and therefore choose not to eat instead. Long-standing restrictive behaviors can decrease hunger and satiety cues in the long run, but increasing appetite does not appear to have any beneficial effect in improving outcomes.

SERVICE AND POLICY IMPLICATIONS

Despite the fact that clinicians and researchers have developed and investigated a number of interventions aimed at treating eating disorders, there is much work yet to be done. Other than FBT in adolescent AN, none of the interventions available has compelling evidence to support use exclusively over the others. Furthermore, the majority of psychotherapies have been studied in adults, but have not been adequately investigated in children and adolescents. Obviously, this is important because eating disorders often arise in the adolescent years, and are now increasingly being seen in pre-pubertal children as well.

Given that eating disorders can be very chronic illnesses with a high mortality rate and significant impact on function in all domains, it is important that we continue to develop and investigate novel treatment interventions that are acceptable and sustainable. This is particularly germane from a cost-effectiveness standpoint; residential, partial hospital, and intensive outpatient programs provide a lot of structure and support, but they are also very expensive and can isolate patients from their families and other more developmentally normative activities. Family-based and group interventions can preserve valuable clinical resources, while utilizing parents and guardians in the treatment process, and allowing the family to work through dynamics that may be impeding recovery.

Clinicians who work with patients recovering from eating disorders also need to stay abreast of important developments in assessment and treatment. Medical providers across primary care and all subspecialties will come in contact with eating disorders, as patients may often present with vague complaints of fatigue, amenorrhea, gastrointestinal discomfort, or weight loss. Having eating disorders in the list of differential diagnoses may prevent costly and unnecessary subspecialty referrals and medical testing. Mental health providers must also stay current with evidence-based treatment approaches in order to avoid giving mixed messages or inappropriate treatment recommendations that may be based in older conceptualizations of eating disorders. As clinicians get more experience diagnosing and treating ARFID, work needs to be focused on developing evidence-based treatment approaches; although behavioral and family interventions seem useful, there are currently no empirical studies available to guide treatment.

Finally, we need to continue to work on disseminating evidence-based treatments beyond urban centers with major medical centers. Families in remote areas often struggle to find help, and many travel long distances for eating disorder treatment. Advances in tele-psychiatry, online trainings, and sophisticated guided self-help interventions may improve access to quality care, even in more remote settings without highly trained eating specialists available.

CONCLUSIONS

Eating disorders are common and have serious mental and physical health implications for children, adolescents, and young adults. While studies in this patient population are lacking, expert consensus dictates that the standard of care involves a multidisciplinary treatment team. From a psychotherapy perspective, evidence to date strongly favors FBT for the treatment of adolescent AN. The field will benefit from ongoing work to determine whether the evidence base for psychotherapies and psychotropic medications in the adult population can be extrapolated to children and adolescents.

References

Agras, W. W. (2000). A multicenter comparison of cognitive-behavioral therapy and interpersonal psychotherapy for bulimia nervosa. *Archives of General Psychiatry*, 459–466.

Agras, W. L. (2014). Comparison of 2 family therapies for adolescent anorexia nervosa: a randomized parallel trial. *JAMA Psychiatry*, 1279–1286.

American Psychiatric Association. (2013). *Diagnostic and statistical manual of mental disorders* (5th ed.). Washington, DC: American Psychiatric Publishing.

Anderluh, M., Tchanturia, K., Rabe-Hesketh, S., & Treasure, J. (2003). Childhood obsessive-compulsive personality traits in adult women with eating disorders: defining a broader eating disorder phenotype. *American Journal of Psychiatry*, 242–247.

Anderson, L. K., Murray, S. B., Ramirez, A. L., Rockwell, R., Le Grange, D., & Kaye, W. H. (2015). The integration of family-based treatment and dialectical behavior therapy for adolescent bulimia nervosa: philosophical and practical considerations. *Eating Disorders*, 325–335.

Bahia, A. M. (2012). PseudoBartter syndrome in eating disorders. *International Journal of Eating Disorders*, 150–153.

Bailey, D. M. (2000). Calcium accretion in girls and boys during puberty: a longitudinal analysis. *Journal of Bone and Mineral Research*, 2245–2250.

Barbarich, N. M. (2004). Use of nutritional supplements to increase the efficacy of fluoxetine in the treatment of anorexia nervosa. *International Journal of Eating Disorders*, 10–15.

Becker, D. G. (2015). Comorbidity of mood and substance use disorders in patients with binge-eating disorder: associations with personality disorder and eating disorder pathology. *Journal of Psychosomatic Research*, 159–164.

Biederman, J., Herzog, D. B., Rivinus, T. M., Harper, G. P., Ferber, R. A., Rosenbaum, J. F., … Schildkraut, J. J. (1985). Amitriptyline in the treatment of anorexia nervosa: a double-blind, placebo-controlled study. *Journal of Clinical Psychopharmacology*, 10–16.

Birmingham, C. S. (2005). The mortality rate from anorexia nervosa. *International Journal of Eating Disorders*, 143–146.

Blessit, E. V. (2015). Family therapy for adolescent anorexia nervosa. *Current Opinion in Psychiatry*, 455–460.

Brewerton, T., & Costin, C. (2011a). Long-term outcome of residential treatment for anorexia nervosa and bulimia nervosa. *Eating Disorders*, 132–144.

Brewerton, T., & Costin, C. (2011b). Treatment results of anorexia nervosa and bulimia nervosa in a residential treatment program. *Eating Disorders*, 117–131.

Fairburn, C. (2008). *Cognitive behavior therapy and eating disorders*. New York: The Guilford Press.

Fairburn, C. G. (2003). Cognitive behaviour therapy for eating disorders: a "transdiagnostic" theory and treatment. *Behavior Research and Therapy*, 509–528.

Fairburn, C. J. (1993). Psychotherapy and bulimia nervosa: the longer-term effects of interpersonal psychotherapy, behaviour therapy, and cognitive behaviour therapy. *Archives of General Psychiatry*, 419–428.

Faris, P. K. (2000). Effect of decreasing afferent vagal activity with ondansetron on symptoms of bulimia nervosa: a randomised, double-blind trial. *Lancet*, 792–797.

Fitzpatrick, K. M. (2010). Adolescent focused therapy for adolescent anorexia nervosa. *Journal of Contemporary Psychotherapy*, 31–39.

Forsberg, S., & Lock, J. (2015). Family-based treatment of child and adolescent eating disorders. *Child and Adolescent Psychiatric Clinics of North America*, 617–629.

Freeman, R. W. (2011). Consensus statement on the definition of orthostatic hypotension, neurally mediated syncope, and the postural tachycardia syndrome. *Autonomic Neuroscience*, 46–48.

Friborg, O. M., & Kaiser, S. Ø. (2014). Personality disorders in eating disorder not otherwise specified and binge eating disorder: a meta-analysis of comorbidity studies. *Journal of Nervous and Mental Disorders*, 119–125.

Garrett, A. L. (2014). Predicting clinical outcome using brain activation associated with set shifting and central coherence skills in anorexia nervosa. *Journal of Psychiatric Research*, 26–33.

Golden, N. (2011). Psychopharmacology of eating disorders in children and adolescents. *Pediatric Clinics of North America*, 121–138.

Golden, N., Keane-Miller, C., Sainani, K. L., & Kapphahn, C. (2013). Higher caloric intake in hospitalized adolescents with anorexia nervosa is associated with reduced length of stay and no increased rate of refeeding syndrome. *Journal of Adolescent Health*, 573–578.

Golden, N. K. (2015). Update on the medical management of eating disorders in adolescents. *Journal of Adolescent Health*, 1–6.

Golden, N. S. (1993). Amenorrhea in anorexia nervosa: neuroendocrine control of hypothalamic dysfunction. *International Journal of Eating Disorders*, 53–60.

Goldstein, D. W. (1995). Long-term fluoxetine treatment of bulimia nervosa. Fluoxetine Bulimia Nervosa Research Group. *British Journal of Psychiatry*, 660–666.

Grave, R. C. (2013). Enhanced cognitive behaviour therapy for adolescents with anorexia nervosa: an alternative to family therapy? *Behaviour Research and Therapy*, R9–R12.

Halmi, K. (2008). The perplexities of conducting randomized, double-blind, placebo-controlled treatment trials in anorexia nervosa patients. *American Journal of Psychiatry*, 1227–1228.

Hatchman, G. (2005). Boys with eating disorders. *The Journal of School Nursing*, 329–332.

Herpertz-Dahlmann, B., Schwarte, R., Krei, M., Egberts, K., Warnke, A., Wewetzer, C., ... Dempfle, A. (2014). Day-patient treatment after short inpatient care versus continued inpatient treatment in adolescents with anorexia nervosa (ANDI): a multicentre, randomised, open-label, non-inferiority trial. *Lancet*, 1222–1229.

Holtkamp, K. K., Konrad, K., Kaiser, N., Ploenes, Y., Heussen, N., Grzella, I., & Herpertz-Dahlmann, B. (2005). A retrospective study of SSRI treatment in adolescent anorexia nervosa: insufficient evidence for efficacy. *Journal of Psychiatric Research*, 303–310.

Holtkamp, K., Muller, B., Heussen, N., Remschmidt, H., & Herpertz-Dahlmann, B. (2005). Depression, anxiety, and obsessionality in long-term recovered patients with adolescent-onset anorexia nervosa. *European Child & Adolescent Psychiatry*, 106–110.

Horne, R. F. (1988). Treatment of bulimia with bupropion: a multicenter controlled trial. *Journal of Clinical Psychiatry*, 262–266.

Hudson, J. H. (2007). The prevalence and correlates of eating disorders in the national comorbidity survey replication. *Biological Psychiatry*, 348–358.

Jauregui-Garrido, B., & Jaurequi-Lobera, I. (2012). Sudden death in eating disorders. *Vascular Health and Risk Management*, 91–98.

Jones, D. V. (2004). Body image and the appearance culture among adolescent girls and boys: an examination of friend conversations, peer criticism, appearance magazines, and the internalization of appearance ideals. *Journal of Adolescent Research*, 323–339.

Juarascio, A., Shaw, J., Forman, E., Timko, C., Herbert, J., Butryn, M., ... Lowe, M. (2013). Acceptance and commitment therapy as a novel treatment for eating disorders: an initial test of efficacy and mediation. *Behavior Modification*, 459–489.

Jurascio, A. F. (2010). Acceptance and commitment therapy versus cognitive therapy for the treatment of comorbid eating pathology. *Behavior Modification*, 175–190.

Kamal, N., Chami, T., Andersen, A., Rosell, F. A., Schuster, M. M., & Whitehead, W. E. (1991). Delayed gastrointestinal transit times in anorexia nervosa and bulimia. *Gastroenterology*, 1320–1324.

Kaye, W. N. (2001). Double-blind, placebo-controlled administration of fluoxetine in restricting and restricting-purging-type anorexia nervosa. *Biological Psychiatry*, 644–652.

Keys, A. B. (1950). *The biology of human starvation*. Minneapolis: University of Minnesota Press.

Lang, K. T. (2014). Acceptability and feasibility of self-help cognitive remediation therapy for anorexia nervosa delivered in collaboration with carers: a qualitative preliminary evaluation study. *Psychiatry Research*, 387–394.

Lask, B. (2015). Family cognitive remediation therapy for anorexia nervosa. *Clinical Child Psychology and Psychiatry*, 207–217.

LeGrange, D. C. (2007). A randomized controlled comparison of family-based treatment and supportive psychotherapy for adolescent bulimia nervosa. *Archives of General Psychiatry*, 1049–1056.

Linehan, M. (1993). *Cognitive-behavioral treatment of borderline personality disorder*. New York: The Guilford Press.

Linehan, M., & Wilks, C. (2015). The course and evolution of DBT. *American Journal of Psychotherapy*.

Lock, J. (2008). Fitting square pegs in round holes: males with eating disorders. *Journal of Adolescent Health*, 99–100.

Lock, J. (2010). Randomized clinical trial comparing family-based treatment with adolescent-focused individual therapy for adolescents with anorexia nervosa. *Archives of General Psychiatry*, 1025–1032.

Lock, J. (2015a). An update on evidence-based psychosocial treatments for eating disorders in children and adolescents. *Journal of Clinical Child and Adolescent Psychology*, 1–15.

Lock, J. (2015b). Practice parameter for the assessment and treatment of children and adolescents with eating disorders. *Journal of the American Academy of Child and Adolescent Psychiatry*, 412–425.

III. INTERVENTIONS AND TREATMENTS

Lock, J. (2013). Is outpatient cognitive remediation therapy feasible to use in randomized clinical trials for anorexia nervosa? *International Journal of Eating Disorders*, 567–575.

Lock, J., Couturier, J., & Agras S. (2006). Comparison of long term outcomes in adolescents with anorexia nervosa treated with family therapy. *Journal of the American Academy of Child and Adolescent Psychiatry*, 666–672.

Lock, J., & Le Grange, D. (2013). *Treatment manual for anorexia nervosa: a family-based approach.* New York: The Guilford Press.

Lynch, T. H. (2015). Radically open dialectical behavior therapy for disorders of overcontrol: remembering our tribal nature. *American Journal of Psychotherapy.*

McElroy, S., Hudson, J. I., Mitchell, J. E., Willfley, D., Ferreira-Cornwell, M. C., … Gasior, M. (2015). Efficacy and safety of lisdexamfetamine for treatment of adults with moderate to severe binge-eating disorder: a randomized clinical trial. *JAMA Psychiatry*, 235–246.

McIntosh, V. J. (2005). Three psychotherapies for anorexia nervosa: a randomized, controlled trial. *The American Journal of Psychiatry*, 741–747.

McKnight, R. P. (2010). Atypical antipsychotics and anorexia nervosa: a review. *European Eating Disorder Review*, 10–21.

Mehler, P. B. (2015). Anorexia nervosa-medical complications. *Journal of Eating Disorders*, 1–8.

Miller, A. R. (2007). *Dialectical behavior therapy with suicidal adolescents.* New York: The Guilford Press.

Murphy, R. S. (2012). Interpersonal psychotherapy for eating disorders. *Clinical Psychology & Psychotherapy*, 150–158.

Murray, S. B., Anderson, L. K., Cusack, A., Nakamura, T., Rockwell, R., Griffiths, S., & Kaye, W. H. (2015). Integrating family-based treatment and dialectical behavior therapy for adolescent bulimia nervosa: preliminary outcomes of an open pilot trial. *Eating Disorders*, 336–344.

Nickel, C. T. (2005). Topiramate treatment in bulimia nervosa patients: a randomized, double-blind, placebo-controlled trial. *International Journal of Eating Disorders*, 195–300.

Safer, D. T. (2001). Dialectical behavior therapy for bulimia nervosa. *American Journal of Psychiatry*, 632–634.

Salbach-Andrae, H. B. (2009). Dialectical behavior therapy (DBT) and cognitive behavioral therapy (CBT) for adolescents with anorexia nervosa and bulimia nervosa in comparison. *Childhood and Development*, 180–190.

Schmidt, U. L. (2007). A randomized controlled trial of family therapy and cognitive behavior therapy guided self-care for adolescents with bulimia nervosa and related disorders. *American Journal of Psychiatry*, 591–598.

Seitz, J., Kahraman-Lanzerath, B., Legenbauer, T., Sarrar, L., Herpertz, S., Salbach-Andrae, H., … Herpertz-Dahlmann, B. (2013). The role of impulsivity, inattention and comorbid ADHD in patients with bulimia nervosa. *PLoS ONE*, e63891.

Serpell, L. S. (2013). Empirically-supported and non-empirically supported therapies for bulimia nervosa: retrospective patient ratings. *Journal of Eating Disorders*, 1, 41.

Skipper, A. (2012). Refeeding syndrome or refeeding hypophosphatemia: a systematic review of cases. *Nutrition in Clinical Practice*, 34–40.

Smink, F. R., van Hoeken, D., Oldehinkel, A. J., & Hoek, H. W. (2014). Prevalence and severity of DSM 5 eating disorders in a community cohort of adolescents. *International Journal of Eating Disorders*, 610–619.

Strober, M. F. (2007). The assoication of anxiety disorders and obsessive compulsive personality disorder with anorexia nervosa: evidence from a family study with discussion of nosological and neurodevelopmental implications. *International Journal of Eating Disorders*, S46–S51.

Strumia, R. (2013). Eating disorders and the skin. *Clinics in Dermatology*, 80–85.

Swanson, S. C. (2011). Prevalence and correlates of eating disorders in adolescents: results from the national comorbidity survey replication adolescent supplement. *Archives of General Psychiatry*, 714–723.

Takehiro, M. N. (2012). Gastric rupture with necrosis following acute gastric dilatation: report of a case. *Surgery Today*, 997–1000.

Tchanturia, K. L. (2014). Cognitive remediation in anorexia nervosa and related conditions: a systematic review. *European Eating Disorders Review*, 454–462.

Timko, C. Z. (2015). An open trial of acceptance-based separated family treatment (ASFT) for adolescents with anorexia nervosa. *Behavior Research and Therapy*, 63–74.

Wald, A. (2003). Is chronic use of stimulant laxatives harmful to the colon? *Journal of Clinical Gastroenterology*, 386–389.

Walsh, B. K. (2006). Fluoxetine after weight restoration in anorexia nervosa: a randomized controlled trial. *JAMA: The Journal of the American Medical Association*, 2605–2612.

Walsh, B. S., Stewart, J. W., Roose, S. P., Gladis, M., & Glassman, A. H. (1984). Treatment of bulimia with phenelzine: a double-blind, placebo-controlled study. *Archives of General Psychiatry*, 1105–1109.

Weissman, M. M. (2000). *Comprehensive guide for interpersonal psychotherapy*. New York: Basic Books.

Weissman, M. M. (2007). *Clinician's quick guide to interpersonal psychotherapy*. New York: Oxford University Press.

Wisniewski, L., & Ben-Porath, D. D. (2015). Dialectical behavior therapy and eating disorders; the use of contingency management procedures to manage dialectical dilemmas. *American Journal of Psychotherapy*.

III. INTERVENTIONS AND TREATMENTS

Seclusion in the Management of Highly Disturbed Children and Adolescents

M. Yurtbasi[1], G.A. Melvin[1], M.S. Gordon[1,2]

[1]Monash University, Notting Hill, VIC, Australia; [2]Monash Health,
Monash Medical Centre, Clayton, VIC, Australia

Amy[1] is a 15-year-old girl with a long history of borderline personality traits. She has a history of a number of sexual assaults perpetrated when she was a child by several adult males from outside her family. Amy has been admitted to an adolescent inpatient ward following escalating suicidal thoughts and several overdoses. Soon after arriving at the ward, Amy becomes agitated at not being allowed to leave and attempts to abscond with a plan to jump from a train platform into the path of an express train. She manages to leave the unlocked ward but is quickly brought back by six large male nursing staff who have to physically restrain her. In restraining her, the nurses are bitten and kicked by Amy. While Amy is given intra-muscular medication to calm her, she continues to bite and kick the staff for an additional 10 min. Several male staff are injured in the process. Two other very vulnerable patients on the ward witness Amy being restrained are very frightened. As a management strategy, the nursing staff feels that she is at too high a risk to be left on the open ward. The nursing staff decides as a management decision to place her in seclusion until the medication can work. This entails the six male staff members forcefully carrying her into a small room with one door and then locking her inside. After two hours Amy settles down and is then deemed to be safe to be let out onto the open ward.

Cases such as Amy's illustrate the position of seclusion on an inpatient ward, in which seclusion was used to manage a highly distressed adolescent who was considered, at the time, to be a risk to staff and other patients. The forceful nature of this incident may be counter to the therapeutic relationship. This chapter seeks to define and review the practice of seclusion as it relates to children and adolescents, identifies risk factors

[1] Pseudonym used and case de-identified to protect privacy.

Positive Mental Health, Fighting Stigma and Promoting Resiliency for Children and Adolescents
http://dx.doi.org/10.1016/B978-0-12-804394-3.00013-9

for seclusion, and offer a discussion on the interventions to reduce the practice. Although seclusion occurs in multiple settings, our emphasis here will be on psychiatric care provided in hospitals, with an additional discussion on the use of seclusion in schools.

The reduction in seclusion of children and adolescents admitted to emergency departments, medical, or psychiatric wards is a clinical and operational imperative for hospitals and health departments around the world. International policies and guidelines surrounding the use of seclusion typically specify that seclusion is only to be used as a response to dangerous behaviors and after other means have been exhausted (Department of Health, 2011; Department of Health and Human Services, 2006; Mental Health Commission of Canada, 2012; Ministry of Health: Canada, 2012; Royal College of Nursing, 2005). When a highly disturbed child or adolescent is admitted, they may display potentially dangerous, agitated, aggressive, or acting-out behavior that puts themselves, other patients, and the ward staff at very serious risk of harm. In the ward, staff have the option to respond to this potential threat by resorting to coercive measures including restraint, shackling, and seclusion. While seclusion is intended to be therapeutic, the use of seclusion itself may lead to additional psychiatric and physical morbidity (Bonner, Lowe, Rawcliffe, & Wellman, 2002; Hottinen et al., 2012). The use of seclusion has been criticized as being used extensively, inappropriately, and before other less restrictive measures (eg, debriefing, medication, time-out, sensory distraction) have been tried (Laiho et al., 2013). Seclusion has been inappropriately used as punishment for very vulnerable people who have been placed in the care of the hospital (Laiho et al., 2013; Livingstone, 2007).

The literature on restrictive interventions in hospitals for the management of disturbed children and adolescents is very limited. The scope and indications for these practices has not been well studied or reported. There are no randomized controlled trials evaluating the efficacy of seclusion. It has been noted in some studies that over a quarter of the young people admitted to a child and adolescent psychiatric inpatient facility may have experienced at least one restrictive intervention over the course of their admission (Duke, Scott, & Dean, 2014).

DEFINING SECLUSION

Broadly defined, seclusion is the sole confinement of an individual in a room they are unable to freely exit (Janssen et al., 2011; Van Der Merwe, Muir-Cochrane, Jones, Tziggili, & Bowers, 2013). Variations to this definition include specifying the need for locked doors and windows, forcing individuals to stay in a room while the door is open, limiting an individual to an area, also referred to as *open-area seclusion* (Bowers et al., 2007;

Janssen et al., 2011). Definitions vary between countries as well as between different states and wards, depending on the guidelines or regulations of the particular institution (see Table 13.1 for various international definitions of seclusion).

Although not a comprehensive list, Table 13.1 provides example definitions of seclusion and demonstrates the differences between definitions. These countries are among many that have identified the reduction and, where possible, the elimination of seclusion as a health priority (Department of Health, Victorian Government, 2009; Mental Health Commission of Canada, 2012; Royal College of Nursing, 2005). There are also variations in policy and guidelines within countries surrounding the use of seclusion. This may include limits on duration of seclusion, only secluding those with involuntary inpatient-status, defining the legitimate and illegitimate (eg, to discipline a patient) reasons for seclusion, and the requirement to exhaust all other alternative measures (Department of Health, 2011; Huckshorn, 2006; Kelly, 2011). Given these differences, it is challenging to compare seclusion practices and to establish a clear picture between different institutions, regions, and countries.

TABLE 13.1   International Definitions of Seclusion; Quoted From Source Material

Source	Location	Definition
State Government of Victoria (1986)	Australia	The sole confinement of a person at any hour of the day or night in a room of which the doors and windows are locked from the outside.
Department of Health and Human Services (2006)	USA	The involuntary confinement of a person in a room or an area where the person is physically prevented from leaving.
Royal College of Nursing (2005)	UK	The supervised confinement of a patient in a room, which may be locked to protect others from significant harm.
Janssen et al. (2008)	Netherlands	Locking a patient up alone in a specially designed seclusion room, clothed in (uncomfortable) safety robes either with or without his/her consent.
Mental Health Commission of Canada (2012); Ministry of Health: Canada (2012)	Canada	A physical intervention that involves containing a patient who is perceived to be in psychiatric crisis in a room that is either locked or "from which free exit is denied."
Steinert et al. (2007)	Germany	The patient is brought into a locked, isolated room and is not allowed to leave the room. Definition is also fulfilled if staff is located at an open door in order to prevent the patient from leaving the room.

PREVALENCE OF SECLUSION

There may be a lack of awareness in the broader community and among healthcare professionals regarding the prevalence of seclusion within psychiatric institutions. The use of seclusion varies widely with between 8.4–61% of inpatients to child and adolescent wards experiencing the practice (De Hert, Dirix, Demunter, & Correll, 2011; Swadi & Bobier, 2012) and 0.2–15.6% of inpatients or admissions to adult wards (De Hert et al., 2011; Swadi & Bobier, 2012; Steinert et al., 2010). While there are some wards that do not use seclusion, there are often other restrictive measures in place, such as pro-re-nata (PRN) medications, mechanical restraints, or physical holding (Bowers et al., 2007). Other institutions, such as schools that cater to intellectually disabled or developmentally delayed individuals, may be exempt from reporting seclusions and laws vary between countries and states on this matter, therefore it is not possible to judge the prevalence of seclusion in these places (Miller, 2011; Victorian Equal Opportunity and Human Rights Commission, 2012). While seclusion use has been found to be declining, in order to further reduce the incidence of restrictive practices, preventative action is needed. Through a deeper understanding of the risk factors for seclusion, clinicians can begin to address the issues and reduce seclusion use.

REASONS FOR SECLUSION

Seclusion is a treatment option available to ward staff when less restrictive attempts to contain the child or adolescent have been unsuccessful or are inappropriate (eg, sudden escalation in aggression leading to the serious injury of a co-patient or staff where diversionary tactics cannot be employed). A frequent trigger cited as a prelude to seclusion is that the patient is aggressive or out of control (Pogge, Pappalardo, Buccolo, & Harvey, 2013). However, while aggression is often cited as the reason for seclusion, aggression is usually undefined or broadly defined, leaving it open to interpretation and therefore leaving the use of seclusion open to abuse.

In the absence of a large body of research on the use of seclusion in child and adolescent populations, adult studies provide some insight into the use of seclusion. Keski-Valkama et al. (2010) found that in adults, seclusion and restraint were used more often due to agitation and disorientation rather than violent behavior. Kaltiala-Heino, Tuohimaki, Korkeila, and Lehtinen (2003) found that adult patients were secluded for a number of reasons including violence, threatening violence, breaking property, threatening to break property, agitation/disorientation, and unclassifiable reasons (such as "others were afraid of the patient"). However, Allen, De Nesnera, Moreau, and Barnett (2014) reported age differences in reasons for seclusion between children, adolescents, and adults. The majority of children and adolescents were secluded for behavioral issues, such as outbursts at meal times, while adults were mostly secluded due to escalating psychiatric symptoms, such as paranoia and hallucinations that resulted in aggression. These studies used retrospective hospital records to obtain the reasons for seclusion and often used generalized terms when documenting seclusion incident reports, making it difficult to ascertain the precise reasons for seclusion. It may be speculated that general reporting of seclusion is an outcome of vague guidelines given to staff around documentation, potential misuse, lack of emphasis on seclusion, or time pressures.

IDENTIFYING FACTORS ASSOCIATED WITH SECLUSION

Seclusion is a multi-factorial phenomenon, therefore factors associated with seclusion are complex. Particular groups of patients are more likely to be secluded than others. Children and adolescents who are secluded share a number of common characteristics. Awareness of the variables associated with seclusion can inform the identification of patients at high-risk of seclusion who can then have tailored management plans put into place to reduce and ideally prevent the use of the practice. Broadly speaking, the two main sources of variance for seclusion are (1) patient factors and (2) ward factors.

Patient Factors

Gender, Age, and Ethnicity

When other variables are adjusted for, males are secluded as often as females (Bridgett, Valentino, & Hayden, 2012; Gullick, McDermott, Stone, & Gibbon, 2005; Stellwagen & Kerig, 2009; Stewart, Baiden, & Theall-Honey, 2013). This finding runs counter to the commonly held belief that males who are potentially more aggressive are secluded more often. Children are more frequently secluded compared with adolescents, while secluded adolescent patients remain in seclusion for longer periods of time than younger patients (Donovan, Plant, Peller, Siegel, & Martin, 2003; Fryer, Beech, & Byrne, 2004; Pogge et al., 2013). There are several reasons for possible differences in seclusion practices across the different ages. Ward nursing staff may accept seclusion as an age-appropriate response for younger children, which results in higher rates of seclusion of younger patients (Pogge et al., 2013; Saks, 2010). Children, when very anxious, have marked mood dysregulation which requires shorter time to settle than adolescents who may suffer with other more severe psychiatric conditions such as mania and psychosis. Younger children may be secluded for less dangerous behaviors than adolescents and require less time in seclusion, whereas adolescents may be secluded for behaviors that are deemed more problematic and as a result they remain in seclusion for extended periods of time (Allen et al., 2014).

Belonging to a particular ethnic group has not been associated with seclusion. Studies in Finland and the United States have found no significant association between ethnicity and seclusion (Sourander, Ellila, Valimaki, & Piha, 2002; Stellwagen & Kerig, 2009), however they may lack power due to the relatively smaller numbers of non-Caucasian inpatients in their facilities (Sourander et al., 2002; Stellwagen & Kerig, 2009).

Involuntary Admission

Involuntary or emergency admissions are frequently associated with higher rates of seclusion for children and adolescents as well as adults (Donovan et al., 2003; Georgieva, Vesselinov, & Mulder, 2012; Korkeila, Tuohimaki, Kaltiala-Heino, Lehtinen, & Joukamaa, 2002; Swadi & Bobier, 2012). Two reasons for this are that voluntary patients cannot be secluded without consent, and if voluntary patients require seclusion, they would rapidly become involuntary (Department of Health, 2011; Ulla, Maritta, & Riittakerttu, 2012). In addition, the very nature of involuntary admission denotes greater agitation or vulnerability of the inpatient from the start of the admission than patients who have the capacity to voluntarily consent to admission.

Longer Length of Stay

Longer length of stay is also associated with seclusion (Pogge et al., 2013; Stewart et al., 2013; Swadi & Bobier, 2012). Children and adolescents who are secluded have significantly longer admissions than those who are not secluded, while patients who stay longer have a greater opportunity for seclusion. These seclusions predominantly occur in the first weeks of admission. It may be that seclusion is seen by clinical staff as a marker of the need for longer treatment (Pogge et al., 2013).

Aggression

Histories of aggression and aggressive behavior are associated with higher rates of seclusion (Fryer et al., 2004; Melvin, Pacewicz, & Gordon, 2014; Sourander et al., 2002). Aggression is cited as a reason for seclusion, resulting in higher rates of seclusion among those displaying aggressive behavior (Baeza et al., 2013; Pogge et al., 2013; Swadi & Bobier, 2012). The relationship between aggression and seclusion is not linear. If ward staff are aware of that a patient has a history of aggression, they may respond with restrictive measures sooner than for a patient who does not have a history of aggression (Vruwink et al., 2012). Therefore, it is noteworthy but not surprising that aggression has been strongly associated with higher rates of seclusion.

Diagnosis

The relationship between psychiatric diagnosis and seclusion in child and adolescent inpatient groups is inconsistent across studies. This mixed finding may be indicative of methodological discrepancies across the literature. Studies in which diagnosis has not been significantly associated with seclusion tend to have unique exclusionary criteria and examine particular diagnoses, rather than investigating the significance of any diagnosis, or they exclude those with psychosis, or combine seclusion and restraint into a single variable (Donovan et al., 2003; Pogge et al., 2013; Stellwagen & Kerig, 2009). Some studies report the rate of diagnosis for those who have been secluded but do not perform inferential statistics, in such studies it is unclear whether patients with certain diagnoses are significantly more likely to be secluded (Bridgett et al., 2012; Ulla et al., 2012). Psychosis or other psychotic disorders have been associated with higher rates of seclusion in child and adolescent inpatient populations (Melvin et al., 2014; Sourander et al., 2002; Swadi & Bobier, 2012) as well as adult inpatient populations (Janssen et al., 2013; Raboch et al., 2010; Tunde-Ayinmode & Little, 2004). While it appears that psychosis may increase the chances of being secluded, this is not always the case (Pogge et al., 2013). Patients will have different levels of severity of symptoms for the same disorder, which may explain some of the variance in outcomes. Responding to psychiatric symptoms (eg, hallucinations and delusions) is at times recorded as the reason for seclusion, less so in child and adolescent inpatient populations compared to adult inpatients (Allen et al., 2014). In addition, Fryer et al. (2004) found that children and adolescents with attention deficit or disruptive behavior disorders were more likely to be secluded, however this finding has not been replicated. Given that diagnosis has not been a consistent finding in relation to seclusion, other authors have looked at levels of functioning and psychopathology symptoms.

Psychopathology and Functioning

Measures of global functioning and psychopathology have consistently been associated with seclusion. Those with lower levels of functioning and more severe psychopathology are more likely to be secluded than their counterparts (De Hert et al., 2011). For example, inpatients with higher Total Problem Behavior scores on the Child Behavior Checklist, Youth Self-Report, and higher Callous-Unemotional traits in the Antisocial Process Screening Device were more likely to experience seclusion (Gullick et al., 2005; Stellwagen & Kerig, 2009). In addition, patients with lower scores on adaptive functioning scales (General Health Questionnaire—Functioning Scale, Child and Adolescent Functioning Assessment Scale, Sociale Redzaamheidsschaal—Z (Social Reliance Scale—Z), and the Children's Global Assessment Scale) had higher rates of seclusion (Gullick et al., 2005; Melvin et al., 2014; Scheirs, Blok, Tolhoek, Aouat, & Glimmerveen, 2012; Sourander et al., 2002; Stewart et al., 2013). These findings complement the results of Gullick et al. (2005), who found that children with higher externalizing and internalizing scores were more likely to be secluded. Measures of functioning and psychopathology may be more accurate in predicting seclusion than diagnosis, as they are tailored to the individual and account for a variety of reasons rather than diagnostic categories.

Temperament

Bridgett et al. (2012) found that dimensions of temperament, effortful control (inhibiting impulsive responses and planning) and fearfulness (fearfulness of real/perceived danger), were associated with increased rates of seclusion. In a sample of children and adolescents, they found that poor effortful control, and higher temperamental fear uniquely predicted seclusion. The research indicates that assessment of temperament shows promise in detecting those children and adolescents who may be at increased risk of challenging behaviors that will require early intervention and clear management plans at point of admission to prevent an escalation to seclusion.

Medication

There is limited information regarding the impact and associations between a child or adolescent patient's use of PRN medication or regular medication, and seclusion incidence. Studies tend to investigate the use of PRNs separately as a form of chemical restraint and do not associate them with seclusion. For example, Donovan et al. (2003) noted that as seclusion episodes decreased, PRN use increased, whereas Gullick et al. (2005) reported that of concurrent use of seclusion with PRNs, only 4.5% of secluded inpatients had received PRNs prior to seclusion. Neither study used inferential statistics to test the significance of these findings. Conversely, Swadi and Bobier (2012) found that PRN medications were the most frequent intervention used prior to seclusion. Adult research has found that secluded inpatients receive significantly more PRN and regular medications than non-secluded inpatients (Repo-Tiihonen, Paavola, Halonen, & Tiihonen, 2002; Tunde-Ayinmode & Little, 2004). Such research needs to be replicated within child and adolescent populations to determine if the same effects are evident in younger inpatient groups. These findings could have implications for the appropriate use of both PRNs and seclusion, given that neither are evidence-based practices. The lack of such research in child and adolescent populations is a major gap in the literature. It would be important to know how successful diversion-ary tactics like medication PRNs are in preventing seclusion. It would be important to chart the use of PRNs during seclusion. It may be that seclusion is used in some instances as a first-line treatment and medication is used after the person has been secluded. Further, it may be that the use of PRNs *themselves* lead to seclusion where the patient develops adverse behavioral effects (for example, mental akathisia from antipsychotics, paradoxical reaction of benzodiazepines, anticholinergic confusion from benztropine).

History of Maltreatment and Family Factors

Amy's case at the start of the chapter highlights the association between past abuse and increased risk for seclusion. In a US study, Bridgett et al. (2012) coded the presence or absence of a history of maltreatment in child and adolescent inpatients, via patients' medical and child-protection records, using the Maltreatment Classification System. Their findings revealed that majority of the patients had a history of maltreatment. Child and adolescent patients with a history of any type of abuse or maltreatment tend to be secluded significantly more often than those without a history of maltreatment (Bridgett et al., 2012; Fryer et al., 2004). In these studies, type of abuse (physical, sexual, verbal, emotional, or psychological) did not make a significant difference, rather the presence of any type of abuse resulted in higher rates of seclusion (Fryer et al., 2004). However, Fryer et al. (2004) did note a trend in higher rates of seclusion for boys who had been physically abused compared with girls. Further, in Fryer's cohort, the witnessing of domestic violence was not associated with seclusion rates (Fryer et al., 2004).

Other factors such as poorer parental mental health, recent stressful life events, being a ward of the state, and poorer family function are also found to be risk factors for seclusion (Gullick et al., 2005; Sourander et al., 2002; Stewart et al., 2013). A possible explanation for this may be that children and adolescents who come from dysfunctional families have maladaptive behavioral and communication strategies, which leads to negative communication with nursing staff and then, in turn, leads to seclusion on the ward. Another possible explanation is that the patients may come from families with high levels of expressed emotion, in which verbal and physical aggression is common ways of expressing distress. Such theories require evaluation in determining the contribution toward seclusion. It has been reported that the 88.5% of children and adolescents within psychiatric care have experienced maltreatment (Bridgett et al., 2012). It is conceivable that those patients who are secluded represent those young people who have experienced higher levels of adversity in their childhood. It is difficult to know what is the cause and effect, as those young people who have a history of maltreatment are very likely to have experienced a matrix of other negative family factors (eg, parental mental illness, poverty, protective issues). Further research is needed to untangle the relationship between specific adverse family factors and seclusion.

Environmental Factors Associated with Seclusion

Other than patient factors, the most important source of variance in seclusion practice relates to ward environmental factors. Potential ward factors include staffing levels, staff sick leave, staff training, time of the day, day of the week, and the model of care of the unit. Seclusion can be seen as a marker of clinical care provided in the ward environment. While any one patient may be very challenging and necessitate seclusion when all less restrictive strategies are exhausted, the frequent and repeated use of particularly prolonged seclusion across a number of patients on the same ward may raise questions about ward environment factors that need to be identified and addressed.

Ward Culture

Ward culture is a broad concept, which includes the beliefs, attitudes, values, expectations, and atmosphere of a particular ward or institution (Laiho et al., 2014). The culture dictates how nursing staff responds to those under their care, including the use of restrictive practices (Laiho et al., 2014; Vatne & Fagermoen, 2007). While ward culture is sure to play an integral role to seclusion outcomes, it is a variable which is difficult to measure or quantify. Furthermore, ward cultures are also influenced by numerous other factors, such as staff experience and management of past patients with aggression, staff training in restraint, the layout and size of the ward, staff turnover and sick leave, patient turnover on the ward, the availability of diversionary strategies (such as a de-escalation, phone calls to family, use of sensory modalities), the nature and extent of prescribing of appropriate regular and PRN psychotropic medications by ward doctors, and staff compliance with ward policy and hospital guidelines. All of these practices and ward experiences may in combination contribute to higher or lower rates of seclusion practices on any given inpatient service, however clear evidence of their influence is currently lacking.

Staffing and Temporal Factors

The investigation of the relationship between environmental factors and seclusion within child and adolescent populations is lacking. The available evidence based on adult populations has found associations between seclusion and lower male to female staff ratio, less experienced staff and less variability in clinical experience (Happell & Gaskin, 2011). Most seclusions occur during the first week of admission, suggesting that patients may need more help adjusting to their situation than they currently receive (Fryer et al., 2004; Keski-Valkama et al., 2010) and the need to identify high-risk patients at point of admission. Additional ward variables are likely to vary from service to service. Additional research to understand why some wards have been able to reduce seclusion levels while other wards have not is needed.

Environmental Factors

Elements such as those investigated by van der Schaaf, Dusseldorp, Keuning, Janssen, and Noorthoorn (2013) show the impact of the physical environment on inpatient outcomes over a one-year period. In a sample of over 14,000 men and women aged between 10 and 100 years, they found that 14 design features significantly impacted on seclusion outcomes, including factors that resulted in higher and lower rates of seclusion. Protective factors included "total private space per patient," "level of comfort,"and "greater visibility on the ward," while risk factors included "presence of an outdoor space," "special safety measures" (eg, warning system), and "a large number of patients in the building." It would be valuable to replicate such a study specifically within child and adolescent groups, as hospitals could then make informed decisions when altering their ward design or building new hospitals.

There is a particular need for additional research on environmental and staffing variables associated with seclusion in child and adolescent groups, in addition to research based on child and adolescent experiences and perceptions of seclusion. These areas are currently lacking in research particularly among this population, and given the differences between age groups in seclusion outcomes and reasons for seclusion, it is crucial to investigate children and adolescents separately from adults.

Seclusion in Schools

Seclusion is used within schools that cater for children with developmental disabilities (eg, autism spectrum disorder, intellectual disabilities), conditions that are often associated with challenging behaviors and aggression (Emerson et al., 2001). There is very little research on seclusion in schools (Villani, Parsons, Church, & Beetar, 2012). Schools require specific research as their settings are different from hospitals, for example schools do not administer PRN medication (Villani et al., 2012). Furthermore, unlike hospitals or residential settings, approval and regulation from medical staff is not required for restraint and seclusion (Villani et al., 2012). Within some jurisdictions (Victoria, Australia, and USA) teachers are not mandated to report the use of seclusion and many schools do not have policies regarding the use of seclusion (Victorian Equal Opportunity and Human Rights Commission, 2012; Villani et al., 2012) leading to potential inappropriate management strategies such as locking of children in rooms, a strategy which is equivalent to seclusion. Furthermore, the differences between time-out and seclusion within schools are unclear, making it difficult to evaluate these different practices separately.

Occasionally in the media, anecdotal evidence highlights the inappropriate use of seclusion. In April 2015, it was reported in the mainstream newspapers in Australia that a 10-year-old boy with autism had a 2-meter by 2-meter cage built by his school in Canberra to manage his challenging behaviors (Doran, 2015). Numerous allegations about the use of restrictive practices in schools have been made following the death of students during restraint procedures (Villani et al., 2012). As a consequence, some special education schools in the United States implemented practice parameters for the use of seclusion and restraint, and there are proposed changes to the federal Individuals with Disabilities Education Act (Miller, 2011; Villani et al., 2012). It is also acknowledged that time-out (defined as restricting or removing an individual from their environment) is a one of the most utilized interventions for those with behavioral issues, particularly for boys with emotional or behavioral disorders (Everett, 2010). Time-out and seclusion follow the same principles, however time-out does not use locked, empty seclusion rooms to restrict children and adolescents. Teachers have reported they feel ill-equipped to use seclusion with students, and that the teachers have not received adequate training to do so (Victorian Equal Opportunity and Human Rights Commission, 2012).

Given the lack of formal research in this area, Villani et al. (2012) reviewed data from school compiled by advocacy groups. They collected six years of retrospective data (2002–07) on the use of seclusion and restraint from a private special education school. This school provides its staff with four-day behavioral management training, therefore the training would likely be considered better than many other schools. Villani et al. (2012) found younger students were restrained or secluded more often than older students, and older students were secluded for longer durations, although less frequently, consistent with research based on psychiatric wards. Furthermore, they found substantial variability in duration of seclusion, as a result of particular students that were outliers. As with hospital seclusion, Villani et al. (2012) also noted that strong leadership was key in reducing the use of restrictive measures. This leadership includes involvement and direction from those in leadership positions, vision, and goals for staff, and making executive decisions. The report concluded that was that there is close to no evidence base on the use of seclusion in schools, teachers' lack formal training to deal with these issues, and there is an overwhelming need for more research in this area.

There have been some interventions within special schools that aimed to reduce the use of restrictive practices. Cannella-Malone, Tullis, and Kazee (2011) suggested that implementing an exercise routine throughout the school day for difficult students could reduce the incidence of problem behaviors and thereby decrease the use of seclusion. This was a case-series based on three students. The exercise program almost eradicated their problem behaviors, which suggests this promising intervention warrants further investigation.

Another effective attempt was phased withdrawal to reduce "time-out," a practice similar to seclusion, in a residential program for adolescents and adults with developmental disabilities (Iwata, Rolider, & Dozier, 2009). The sample included 90 adolescents, most of whom had behavioral problems. Eleven students who had extreme aggressive behavior were not included in the study. Of the remaining individuals, 39 had been placed in time-out at the commencement of the study. Over the one-year study period, time-out was removed for these 39 students and was successfully eliminated for 36 of them; three students had to have time-out reinstated. This high success rate suggests that it is possible to eliminate restrictive practices for most adolescents with developmental disabilities through a gradual withdrawal of the restrictive practices with a replacement with other measures. For most individuals, time-out could be replaced with alternative measures such as "extinction or response cost" (token economy), while there was a 92% success rate, it was acknowledged that for a small group of adolescents time-out was still necessary. This indicates that it may not be feasible to eliminate restrictive practices, though for most, it can be largely eliminated.

ETHICAL ISSUES OF SECLUSION

There is a power imbalance between the authority who secludes and the individual who is secluded. Adult and child and adolescent patients have reported that they believe seclusion is a form of manipulation used to threaten them so they behave the way staff would like them to behave (Martinez, Grimm, & Adamson, 1999; Meehan, Bergen, & Fjeldsoe, 2004). Patients who have experienced seclusion report that it is the fear of seclusion that alters their behavior, suggesting seclusion is perceived as punishment (Martinez et al., 1999). While punishment may deter young people from misbehaving, it is often viewed as being inappropriate in the health care setting and contravenes a common seclusion guideline, which states that seclusion must be used as a last resort.

Many individuals who are secluded have traumatic histories (Petti, Somers, & Sims, 2003), as do many other individuals in psychiatric wards, residential care, intermediate facilities, and other settings that care for highly disturbed children and adolescents (Petti et al., 2003). A significant ethical argument against the use of seclusion is that seclusion can traumatize young people who have experienced physical, emotional, or sexual abuse in the past (Bonner et al., 2002; Sequeira & Halstead, 2002).

Seclusion has the added potential problem of traumatizing staff members who implement seclusion (Bonner et al., 2002).

There is limited research that examines the experiences of children and adolescents who have been secluded. There are several studies examining adult-lived experiences and perceptions of seclusion, which in the main provide robust criticisms of the practice (Faschingbauer, Peden-McAlpine, & Tempel, 2013; Mayers, Keet, Winkler, & Flisher, 2010; Soininen et al., 2013). Further, there is very little information on the perceptions of staff members that are responsible for secluding individuals. However, based on the available research it is evident that there is a discrepancy between the perspectives of those in authority and those who are secluded. While nurses tend to view seclusion as a helpful and even therapeutic technique, patients feel it is used inappropriately and is not beneficial for them, finding it violating, isolating, and dehumanizing (Meehan et al., 2004; Sambrano & Cox, 2013). Seclusion, as experienced by the patient, provides a strong impetus to justify or deny the therapeutic role for seclusion and significantly reduce the practice.

THE EFFICACY OF SECLUSION

The justification for any treatment provided to a patient is ideally based on evidence-based care. Seclusion currently lacks an evidence base for its therapeutic use. There are no randomized controlled trials evaluating the efficacy of the practice, nor evidence of the effects of seclusion on individuals (Gaskin, 2013; Sailas & Fenton, 2000). The reasons is that it is a significant clinical, ethical, and research challenge to devise a truly randomized trial which would allocate a potentially aggressive young person to either seclusion or another strategy. While the majority of research and clinical opinion wish to see seclusion reduced or eliminated, Prinsen and van Delden (2009) argue that the issue of seclusion is not straightforward. Furthermore, some argue it is unrealistic to abolish seclusion; that it is "lacking in clinical reality" (Liberman, 2006). For example, even with the best care and seclusion-reduction techniques, it has been argued that dangerous behaviors such as assault by patients toward other patients or staff cannot be completely eliminated, and therefore there is a need to have restrictive alternatives in place as a precautionary measure. While seclusion may be unwanted, arguments may be used both for and against its use. For example, Prinsen and van Delden (2009) show that the impact on autonomy may be used to both dissuade and support the use of seclusion. On the one hand, seclusion forces an individual against his/her will, thereby violating his/her autonomy, while on the other hand seclusion may be used to help an individual regain their autonomy when he/she is in a highly disturbed state (Prinsen & van Delden, 2009). However, such reasoning does not suffice if seclusion is misused, which is certainly the case with seclusion-as-punishment.

SPECIFIC AND GENERAL SECLUSION REDUCTION INTERVENTIONS

In addition to identifying patients and ward variables that increase the risk of seclusion, interventions that up-skill inpatient competency in handling situations that prevent seclusion are worth considering. Collaborative Problem Solving (CPS) is a manualized intervention based on cognitive-behavioral techniques, that was designed to reduce aggression in children and adolescents and thereby reduce restrictive practices (Greene, Ablon, & Martin, 2006). The model "conceptualizes the aggressive behavior of children as the by-product of lagging cognitive skills in the global domains of flexibility, frustration tolerance, and problem solving" and has effectively reduced the use of seclusion and restraint (Greene et al., 2006). In a study conducted by Greene et al. (2006), a multidisciplinary team of 34 staff members was trained to use the CPS model through two weekly-supervised sessions. Pre- and post-data showed that there was a significant decrease in the number of restraints and seclusion in the 15 months following training. Furthermore, the number of staff and patient injuries also significantly declined. Seclusion is touted as a safety measure that protects inpatients and staff from injury, however Greene et al. (2006) demonstrated that with appropriate training, it is not only possible to reduce the use of restrictive practices, but also to reduce danger to staff and patients. In a larger study, Martin, Krieg, Esposito, Stubbe, and Cardona (2008) compared the rates of restraint and seclusion on child and adolescent psychiatric ward for 3 years prior and 1.5 years after implementing CPS. Seclusion and restraint significantly declined, as did the duration of seclusion and restraint. While controlled evaluations of CPS pose ethical and practical challenges it appears that these uncontrolled studies show the program can be efficacious in reducing seclusion and improving practices on the ward.

In 1999 two mental health crisis centers began to implement an intervention to eliminate the use of seclusion and restraint in their centers. They successfully managed to reach zero seclusions per month in less than one year, and continued to show improvements (including decrease in staff injuries) in a 58-month follow-up (Ashcraft & Anthony, 2008). Subsequently the same crisis centers had reported zero seclusions and restraints over the two-year period (Ashcraft, Bloss, & Anthony, 2012). The intervention involved changes to a number of areas including policy, leadership, training, and both staff and consumer feedback. This demonstrates that with continued support and ongoing training significant long-term change is possible. Similarly, Azeem, Aujla, Rammerth, Binsfeld, and Jones (2011) implemented a successful strategy of trauma-informed/strength-based care for reducing seclusion in child and adolescent populations. The model focused on improving leadership, informed practice based on available evidence (eg, risk factors of seclusion), staff development, tools to reduce restrictive practices (eg, de-escalation techniques), involving patients and family in decision-making, and debriefing staff and patients after the use of restraint or seclusion. Seclusion declined by more than half as many episodes in the six months following the program as there were before its implementation.

Evidently, there are a number of interventions that appear to be successful, each different from the other. This begs the question, are there common underlying elements across these interventions? Some common elements of successful interventions that may be contributing to change include strong support from leaders and additional training for staff members in managing difficult behaviors (Gaskin, 2013). Furthermore, the use of assessment tools and feedback for staff are often incorporated into successful programs (Gaskin, 2013; Romijn & Fredericks, 2012). One of the most challenging aspects of seclusion interventions is the attempt to change ward culture. If a program successfully changes the way staff members perceive and respond to aggressive or threatening behavior, in addition to changing the way they think about seclusion, they have the potential to create a long-lasting change in the ward. Attempting to change the behavior of child and adolescent patients is also a component of seclusion reduction programs, and increasing patients' capacity to cope with strong emotions and aggressive impulses may contribute to reduced seclusion rates.

It is highly likely that there is a positive non-specific effect of the implementation of an intervention and awareness raising of seclusion in the ward, regardless of the components of the intervention; unfortunately no randomized controlled trials currently exist to show whether these successful interventions uniquely contribute to seclusion reduction, or which interventions are most efficacious.

THE USE OF LEGISLATION AND POLICY

Policies from many countries specify that seclusion is only to be used as a last resort (Department of Health, 2011; Department of Health and Human Services, 2006; Mental Health Commission of Canada, 2012; Ministry of Health: Canada, 2012; Royal College of Nursing, 2005). For example, Ashcraft et al. (2012) investigated the implementation of a "no force first" policy in a crisis center of the Recovery Innovations mental health agency; these programs operate in the United States and

New Zealand. Following a successful model of care that was introduced in 1999 that eliminated the use of seclusion and restraint, the "no force first" policy aimed to build on their previous work by eliminating any use of force, particularly the use of PRN medications (chemical restraint). Over a two-year period data revealed that only 0.45% of those in the crisis center received PRNs. The interest in implementing this policy was to ensure that the elimination of seclusion and restraint did not result in a substitution of other coercive measures (namely chemical restraint). The policy included a number of positive strategies such as redirecting the mission of Recovery Innovations to recovery rather than stabilizing individuals; also training and employing peers who have themselves experienced coercion through restrictive practices.

PROMOTING CHANGE

Research findings suggest that in order to change the culture within a ward, there needs to be multilevel support, strong leadership, with a vision and message from the senior management that the hospital is committed to reducing seclusion practices (Azeem et al., 2011). While zero seclusion may be aspirational for a number of inpatient units, the overall expectation is that seclusion is the last resort in the care pathway. Seclusion reduction can be addressed through engagement and input from hospitals: (1) the nursing staff, (2) the medical staff, (3) Quality and Safety unit, (4) the Mental Health Program management, and (5) patients and parent/carers.

The ethos of the ward at the level of the nursing staff, medical and administrative staff would be to aim for "zero" seclusion. Successful interventions shown to reduce seclusion include staff training, regular feedback, and addressing the preconceived ideas and attitudes of staff regarding seclusion, for example by helping staff to view seclusion as a non-therapeutic, last resort that is a "treatment failure" (Gaskin, 2013; Romijn & Fredericks, 2012).

The reduction of seclusion involves input from medical staff. Medical reporting via the registrar to the consultant in the use of seclusion at the time the patient is being secluded; review of the patient by the registrar over the time the patient is secluded; and review with debriefing on discharge from seclusion provides real-time checks and balances on this restrictive practice.

The discussion of seclusion at the hospital quality and safety meetings on a case-by-case basis provides a mechanism to identify ward factors which may contribute to seclusion. The hospital quality and safety unit provides an "arms-length" oversight of the use of seclusion in order to provide frank feedback to the ward staff on their success or otherwise of their interventions.

The use of seclusion needs to be a standing item for discussion on the mental health program meeting agenda. Data should be used to monitor seclusion rates that are then presented and then discussed at the mental health program level in order to provide higher level monitoring and oversight. While seclusion rates can vary significantly from month to month, overall trends will indicate if the levels are of concern.

CONCLUSIONS

Seclusion is an undesirable practice that negatively impacts children and adolescents who are subjected to it. It has been argued that it is not possible to completely dispense with seclusion altogether, as the clinical reality is that other strategies to deal with aggression will not be sufficient to cover all possible scenarios. The responsibility of ensuring the patient is safe toward his- or herself, toward co-patients, and staff may necessitate the availability of seclusion as a last resort whose use is very limited, well-monitored by senior management, and justified on a case-by-case basis. The limited research in this population necessitates further consideration of this topic in order to make informed decisions in the management of children and adolescents with difficult behaviors.

References

Allen, D., De Nesnera, A., Moreau, M. A., & Barnett, R. J. (2014). Seclusion and restraint use in children and adults: differences between age groups. *Journal of Psychosocial Nursing and Mental Health Services, 52*(3), 20–25.

Ashcraft, L., & Anthony, W. (2008). Eliminating seclusion and restraint in recovery-oriented crisis services. *Psychiatric Services, 59*(10), 1198–1202.

Ashcraft, L., Bloss, M., & Anthony, W. A. (2012). The development and implementation of "no force first" as a best practice. *Psychiatric Services, 63*(5), 415–417.

Azeem, M. W., Aujla, A., Rammerth, M., Binsfeld, G., & Jones, R. B. (2011). Effectiveness of six core strategies based on trauma informed care in reducing seclusions and restraints at a child and adolescent psychiatric hospital. *Journal of Child and Adolescent Psychiatric Nursing, 24*(1), 11–15. http://dx.doi.org/10.1111/j.1744-6171.2010.00262.x.

Baeza, I., Correll, C. U., Saito, E., Amanbekova, D., Ramani, M., Kapoor, S., … Carbon, M. (2013). Frequency, characteristics and management of adolescent inpatient aggression. *Journal of Child and Adolescent Psychopharmacology, 23*(4), 271–281. http://dx.doi.org/10.1089/cap.2012.0116.

Bonner, G., Lowe, T., Rawcliffe, D., & Wellman, N. (2002). Trauma for all: a pilot study of the subjective experience of physical restraint for mental health inpatients and staff in the UK. *Journal of Psychiatric and Mental Health Nursing, 9*, 465–473.

Bowers, L., van der Werf, B., Vokkolainen, A., Muir-Cochrane, E., Allan, T., & Alexander, J. (2007). International variation in containment measures for disturbed psychiatric inpatients: a comparative questionnaire survey. *International Journal of Nursing Studies, 44*(3), 357–364. http://dx.doi.org/10.1016/j.ijnurstu.2006.01.005.

Bridgett, D. J., Valentino, K., & Hayden, L. C. (2012). The contribution of children's temperamental fear and effortful control to restraint and seclusion during inpatient treatment in a psychiatric hospital. *Child Psychiatry and Human Development*, 43(6), 821–836. http://dx.doi.org/10.1007/s10578-012-0298-x.

Cannella-Malone, H. I., Tullis, C. A., & Kazee, A. R. (2011). Using antecedent exercise to decrease challenging behavior in boys with developmental disabilities and an emotional disorder. *Journal of Positive Behavior Interventions*, 13(4), 230–239. http://dx.doi.org/10.1177/1098300711406122.

De Hert, M., Dirix, N., Demunter, H., & Correll, C. U. (2011). Prevalence and correlates of seclusion and restraint use in children and adolescents: a systematic review. *European Child & Adolescent Psychiatry*, 20(5), 221–230. http://dx.doi.org/10.1007/s00787-011-0160-x.

Department of Health. (2011). *Seclusion in approved mental health services: Chief Psychiatrist's guideline*. Melbourne: Australia.

Department of Health, Victorian Government. (2009). *Creating safety: Addressing restraint and seclusion practices project report, December 2009, Victoria, Australia*. Retrieved from http://health.vic.gov.au/chiefpsychiatrist/creatingsafety/index.htm.

Department of Health and Human Services. (2006). *Medicare and Medicaid programs; Hospitals conditions on participation: Patients' rights* (42 CFR Part 482). USA.

Donovan, A., Plant, R., Peller, A., Siegel, L., & Martin, A. (2003). Two-year trends in the use of seclusion and restraint among psychiatrically hospitalized youths. *Psychiatric Services*, 54(7), 987–993.

Doran, M. (2015). *Use of cage for boy with autism at Canberra school prompts call for national education standard*. ABC News. Retrieved from http://www.abc.net.au/news/2015-04-03/experts-slam-need-to-cage-boy-wth-autism-at-canberra-school/6369470.

Duke, S. G., Scott, J., & Dean, A. J. (2014). Use of restrictive interventions in a child and adolescent inpatient unit- predictors of use and effect on patient outcomes. *Australasian Psychiatry*, 22(4), 360–365. http://dx.doi.org/10.1177/1039856214532298.

Emerson, E., Kiernan, C., Alborz, A., Reeves, D., Mason, H., Swarbrick, R., … Hatton, C. (2001). The prevalence of challenging behaviors: a total population study. *Research in Developmental Disabilities*, 22(1), 77–93. http://dx.doi.org/10.1016/S0891-4222(00)00061-5.

Everett, G. E. (2010). Time-out in special education settings: the parameters of previous implementation. *North American Journal of Psychology*, 12(1), 159–170.

Faschingbauer, K. M., Peden-McAlpine, C., & Tempel, W. (2013). Use of seclusion: finding the voice of the patient to influence practice. *Journal of Psychosocial Nursing and Mental Health Services*, 51(7), 33–38.

Fryer, M. A., Beech, M., & Byrne, G. J. A. (2004). Seclusion use with children and adolescents: an Australian experience. *Australian and New Zealand Journal of Psychiatry*, 38, 26–33.

Gaskin, C. J. (2013). *Reducing restrictive interventions: Literature review and document analysis*. Melbourne, Australia.

Georgieva, I., Vesselinov, R., & Mulder, C. L. (2012). Early detection of risk factors for seclusion and restraint: a prospective study. *Early Intervention in Psychiatry*, 6(4), 415–422. http://dx.doi.org/10.1111/j.1751-7893.2011.00330.x.

Greene, R. W., Ablon, J. S., & Martin, A. (2006). Use of collaborative problem solving to reduce seclusion and restraint in child and adolescent inpatient units. *Psychiatric Services*, 57(5), 610–612.

Gullick, K., McDermott, B., Stone, P., & Gibbon, P. (2005). Seclusion of children and adolescents: psychopathology and family factors. *International Journal of Mental Health Nursing*, 14, 37–43.

Happell, B., & Gaskin, C. J. (2011). Exploring patterns of seclusion use in Australian mental health services. *Archives of Psychiatric Nursing*, 25(5), e1–e8. http://dx.doi.org/10.1016/j.apnu.2011.04.001.

III. INTERVENTIONS AND TREATMENTS

Hottinen, A., Valimaki, M., Sailas, E., Putkonen, H., Joffe, G., Noda, T., & Lindberg, N. (2012). Underaged patients' opinions toward different containment measures: a questionnaire survey in Finnish adolescent psychiatry. *Journal of Child and Adolescent Psychiatric Nursing*, 25(4), 219–223. http://dx.doi.org/10.1111/jcap.12006.

Huckshorn, K. A. (2006). Re-designing state mental health policy to prevent the use of seclusion and restraint. *Administration and Policy in Mental Health*, 33(4), 482–491. http://dx.doi.org/10.1007/s10488-005-0011-5.

Iwata, B. A., Rolider, N. U., & Dozier, C. L. (2009). Evaluation of timeout programs through phased withdrawal. *Journal of Applied Research in Intellectual Disabilities*, 22, 203–209.

Janssen, W. A., Noorthoorn, E. O., de Vries, W. J., Hutschemeakers, G. J., Lendemeijer, H. H., & Widdershoven, G. A. (2008). The use of seclusion in the Netherlands compared to countries in and outside Europe. *International Journal of Law and Psychiatry*, 31(6), 463–470. http://dx.doi.org/10.1016/j.ijlp.2008.09.002.

Janssen, W. A., Noorthoorn, E. O., Nijman, H. L., Bowers, L., Hoogendoorn, A. W., Smit, A., & Widdershoven, G. A. (2013). Differences in seclusion rates between admission wards: does patient compilation explain? *The Psychiatric Quarterly*, 84(1), 39–52. http://dx.doi.org/10.1007/s11126-012-9225-3.

Janssen, W. A., van de Sande, R., Noorthoorn, E. O., Nijman, H. L., Bowers, L., Mulder, C. L., … Steinert, T. (2011). Methodological issues in monitoring the use of coercive measures. *International Journal of Law and Psychiatry*, 34(6), 429–438. http://dx.doi.org/10.1016/j.ijlp.2011.10.008.

Kaltiala-Heino, R., Tuohimaki, C., Korkeila, J., & Lehtinen, V. (2003). Reasons for using seclusion and restraint in psychiatric inpatient care. *International Journal of Law and Psychiatry*, 26, 139–149.

Kelly, B. D. (2011). Mental health legislation and human rights in England, Wales and the Republic of Ireland. *International Journal of Law and Psychiatry*, 34(6), 439–454. http://dx.doi.org/10.1016/j.ijlp.2011.10.009.

Keski-Valkama, A., Sailas, E., Eronen, M., Koivisto, A. M., Lonnqvist, J., & Kaltiala-Heino, R. (2010). The reasons for using restraint and seclusion in psychiatric inpatient care: a nationwide 15-year study. *Nordic Journal of Psychiatry*, 64(2), 136–144. http://dx.doi.org/10.3109/08039480903274449.

Korkeila, J., Tuohimaki, C., Kaltiala-Heino, R., Lehtinen, V., & Joukamaa, M. (2002). Predicting use of coercive measures in Finland. *Nordic Journal of Psychiatry*, 56(5), 339–345.

Laiho, T., Kattainen, E., Astedt-Kurki, P., Putkonen, H., Lindberg, N., & Kylma, J. (2013). Clinical decision making involved in secluding and restraining an adult psychiatric patient: an integrative literature review. *Journal of Psychiatric and Mental Health Nursing*, 20(9), 830–839. http://dx.doi.org/10.1111/jpm.12033.

Laiho, T., Lindberg, N., Joffe, G., Putkonen, H., Hottinen, A., Kontio, R., & Sailas, E. (2014). Psychiatric staff on the wards does not share attitudes on aggression. *International Journal of Mental Health Systems*, 8, 14. http://dx.doi.org/10.1186/1752-4458-8-14.

Liberman, R. P. (2006). Elimination of seclusion and restraint: a reasonable goal? *Psychiatric Services*, 57(4), 576.

Livingstone, A. (2007). *Creating safety: Addressing seclusion practices, a literature review, Victoria, Australia*. Retrieved from http://health.vic.gov.au/chiefpsychiatrist/creatingsafety/index.htm.

Martin, A., Krieg, H., Esposito, F., Stubbe, D., & Cardona, L. (2008). Reduction of restraint and seclusion through collaborative problem solving: a five-year prospective inpatient study. *Psychiatric Services*, 59(12), 1406–1412.

Martinez, R. J., Grimm, M., & Adamson, M. (1999). From the other side of the door: patient views on seclusion. *Journal of Psychosocial Nursing and Mental Health Services*, 37(3), 13–22.

Mayers, P., Keet, N., Winkler, G., & Flisher, A. J. (2010). Mental health service users' perceptions and experiences of sedation, seclusion and restraint. *The International Journal of Social Psychiatry*, 56(1), 60–73. http://dx.doi.org/10.1177/0020764008098293.

Meehan, T., Bergen, H., & Fjeldsoe, K. (2004). Staff and patient perceptions of seclusion: has anything changed? *Journal of Advanced Nursing, 47*(1), 33–38.

Melvin, G., Pacewicz, M., & Gordon, M. (2014). Which patients are secluded on an adolescent inpatient unit? A retrospective study. In *Paper presented at the International Association for Child and Adolescent Psychiatry and Allied Professions Durban, South Africa.*

Mental Health Commission of Canada. (2012). *Changing directions, changing lives: The mental health strategy for Canada.* Retrieved from http://strategy.mentalhealthcommission.ca/pdf/strategy-text-en.pdf.

Miller, J. P. (2011). Physical education: amending the individuals with Disabilities Education Act to restrict restraint and seclusion in public and private schools. *Family Court Review, 49*(2), 400–414.

Ministry of Health: Canada. (2012). *Secure rooms and seclusion standards and guidelines: A literature and evidence review.* Retrieved from http://www.health.gov.bc.ca/library/publications/year/2012/secure-rooms-seclusion-guidelines-lit-review.pdf.

Petti, T., Somers, J., & Sims, L. (2003). A chronicle of seclusion and restraint in an intermediate-term care facility. *Adolescent Psychiatry, 27*, 83–116.

Pogge, D. L., Pappalardo, S., Buccolo, M., & Harvey, P. D. (2013). Prevalence and precursors of the use of restraint and seclusion in a private psychiatric hospital: comparison of child and adolescent patients. *Administration and Policy in Mental Health, 40*(3), 224–231. http://dx.doi.org/10.1007/s10488-011-0396-2.

Prinsen, E. J., & van Delden, J. J. (2009). Can we justify eliminating coercive measures in psychiatry? *Journal of Medical Ethics, 35*(1), 69–73. http://dx.doi.org/10.1136/jme.2007.022780.

Raboch, J., Kalisova, L., Nawka, A., Kitzlerova, E., Onchev, G., Karastergiou, A., ... Kallert, T. W. (2010). Use of coercive measures during involuntary hospitalization: findings from ten European Countries. *Psychiatric Services, 61*(10), 1012–1017. http://dx.doi.org/10.1176/appi.ps.61.10.1012.

Repo-Tiihonen, E., Paavola, P., Halonen, P., & Tiihonen, J. (2002). Seclusion treatment measures and serum cholesterol levels among Finnish male forensic psychiatric patients. *The Journal of Forensic Psychiatry, 13*(1), 157–165. http://dx.doi.org/10.1080/09585180210123212.

Romijn, A., & Fredericks, J. M. (2012). Restriction on restraints in the care for people with intellectual disabilities in the Netherlands: lessons learned from Australia, UK, and United States. *Journal of Policy and Practice in Intellectual Disabilities, 9*(2), 127–133. http://dx.doi.org/10.1111/j.1741-1130.2012.00345.x.

Royal College of Nursing. (2005). *Violence: The short-term management of disturbed violent behaviour in in-patient psychiatric settings and emergency departments.* United Kingdom: National Institute for Health and Clinical Excellence.

Sailas, E., & Fenton, M. (2000). Seclusion and restraint for people with serious mental illnesses (review). *The Cochrane Database of Systematic Reviews*, CD001163.

Saks, E. R. (2010). *Refusing care: Forced treatment and the rights of the mentally ill.* University of Chicago Press.

Sambrano, R., & Cox, L. (2013). 'I sang Amazing Grace for about 3 hours that day': understanding Indigenous Australians' experience of seclusion. *International Journal of Mental Health Nursing, 22*(6), 522–531. http://dx.doi.org/10.1111/inm.12015.

van der Schaaf, P. S., Dusseldorp, E., Keuning, F. M., Janssen, W. A., & Noorthoorn, E. O. (2013). Impact of the physical environment of psychiatric wards on the use of seclusion. *The British Journal of Psychiatry: the Journal of Mental Science, 202*, 142–149. http://dx.doi.org/10.1192/bjp.bp.112.118422.

Scheirs, J. G., Blok, J. B., Tolhoek, M. A., Aouat, F. E., & Glimmerveen, J. C. (2012). Client factors as predictors of restraint and seclusion in people with intellectual disability. *Journal of Intellectual & Developmental Disability, 37*(2), 112–120. http://dx.doi.org/10.3109/13668250.2012.682357.

Sequeira, H., & Halstead, S. (2002). Control and restraint in the UK: service user perspectives. *The British Journal of Forensic Practice, 4*(1), 9–18.

III. INTERVENTIONS AND TREATMENTS

Soininen, P., Valimaki, M., Noda, T., Puukka, P., Korkeila, J., Joffe, G., & Putkonen, H. (2013). Secluded and restrained patients' perceptions of their treatment. *International Journal of Mental Health Nursing*, 22(1), 47–55. http://dx.doi.org/10.1111/j.1447-0349.2012.00838.x.

Sourander, A., Ellila, H., Valimaki, M., & Piha, J. (2002). Use of holding, restraints, seclusion and time-out in child and adolescent psychiatric in-patient treatment. *European Child & Adolescent Psychiatry*, 11(4), 162–167. http://dx.doi.org/10.1007/s00787-002-0274-2.

State Government of Victoria. (1986). *Mental health act 1986*. Victoria: Australia.

Steinert, T., Lepping, P., Bernhardsgrutter, R., Conca, A., Hatling, T., Janssen, W., … Whittington, R. (2010). Incidence of seclusion and restraint in psychiatric hospitals: a literature review and survey of international trends. *Social Psychiatry and Psychiatric Epidemiology*, 45(9), 889–897. http://dx.doi.org/10.1007/s00127-009-0132-3.

Steinert, T., Martin, V., Baur, M., Bohnet, U., Goebel, R., Hermelink, G., … Voigtlander, W. (2007). Diagnosis-related frequency of compulsory measures in 10 German psychiatric hospitals and correlates with hospital characteristics. *Social Psychiatry and Psychiatric Epidemiology*, 42(2), 140–145. http://dx.doi.org/10.1007/s00127-006-0137-0.

Stellwagen, K. K., & Kerig, P. K. (2009). Relating callous-unemotional traits to physically restrictive treatment measures among child psychiatric inpatients. *Journal of Child and Family Studies*, 19(5), 588–595. http://dx.doi.org/10.1007/s10826-009-9337-z.

Stewart, S. L., Baiden, P., & Theall-Honey, L. (2013). Factors associated with the use of intrusive measures at a tertiary care facility for children and youth with mental health and developmental disabilities. *International Journal of Mental Health Nursing*, 22(1), 56–68. http://dx.doi.org/10.1111/j.1447-0349.2012.00831.x.

Swadi, H., & Bobier, C. (2012). Lessons from an investigation of seclusion at an older adolescent inpatient unit. *Australasian Psychiatry: Bulletin of Royal Australian and New Zealand College of Psychiatrists*, 20(2), 98–101. http://dx.doi.org/10.1177/1039856212437431.

Tunde-Ayinmode, M., & Little, J. (2004). Use of seclusion in a psychiatric acute inpatient unit. *Australasian Psychiatry*, 12(4), 347–351.

Ulla, S., Maritta, V., & Riittakerttu, K. H. (2012). The use of coercive measures in adolescent psychiatric inpatient treatment: a nation-wide register study. *Social Psychiatry and Psychiatric Epidemiology*, 47(9), 1401–1408. http://dx.doi.org/10.1007/s00127-011-0456-7.

Van Der Merwe, M., Muir-Cochrane, E., Jones, J., Tziggili, M., & Bowers, L. (2013). Improving seclusion practice: implications of a review of staff and patient views. *Journal of Psychiatric and Mental Health Nursing*, 20(3), 203–215. http://dx.doi.org/10.1111/j.1365-2850.2012.01903.x.

Vatne, S., & Fagermoen, M. S. (2007). To correct and to acknowledge: two simultaneous and conflicting perspectives of limit-setting in mental health nursing. *Journal of Psychiatric and Mental Health Nursing*, 14, 41–48.

Victorian Equal Opportunity and Human Rights Commission. (2012). *Held back: The experiences of students with disabilities in Victorian schools*. Victoria: Australia.

Villani, V. S., Parsons, A. E., Church, R. P., & Beetar, J. T. (2012). A descriptive study of the use of restraint and seclusion in a special education school. *Child Youth Care Forum*, 41, 295–309.

Vruwink, F. J., Noorthoorn, E. O., Nijman, H. L., Vandernagel, J. E., Hox, J. J., & Mulder, C. L. (2012). Determinants of seclusion after aggression in psychiatric inpatients. *Archives of Psychiatric Nursing*, 26(4), 307–315. http://dx.doi.org/10.1016/j.apnu.2011.10.004.

Index

Edwards Brothers Malloy
Ann Arbor MI. USA
August 29, 2016